W9-CYC-298

Surgical Management of Nasal Obstruction: Rhinologic Perspective

Guest Editor

SAMUEL S. BECKER, MD

OTOLARYNGOLOGIC CLINICS OF NORTH AMERICA

www.oto.theclinics.com

April 2009 • Volume 42 • Number 2

SAUNDERS an imprint of ELSEVIER, Inc.

W.B. SAUNDERS COMPANY
A Division of Elsevier Inc.

1600 John F. Kennedy Boulevard • Suite 1800 • Philadelphia, Pennsylvania 19103-2899

http://www.theclinics.com

OTOLARYNGOLOGIC CLINICS OF NORTH AMERICA Volume 42, Number 2
April 2009 ISSN 0030-6665, ISBN-13: 978-1-4377-0596-6, ISBN-10: 1-4377-0596-0

Editor: Joanne Husovski

Otolaryngologic Clinics of North America (ISSN 0030-6665) is published bimonthly by Elsevier, Inc., 360 Park Avenue South, New York, NY 10010-1710. Months of issue are February, April, June, August, October, and December. Business and Editorial Offices: 1600 John F. Kennedy Blvd., Suite 1800, Philadelphia, PA 19103-2899. Customer Service Office: 6277 Sea Harbor Drive, Orlando, FL 32887-4800. Periodicals postage paid at New York, NY and additional mailing offices. Subscription prices is $264.00 per year (US individuals), $488.00 per year (US institutions), $129.00 per year (US student/resident), $347.00 per year (Canadian individuals), $613.00 per year (Canadian institutions), $390.00 per year (international individuals), $613.00 per year (international institutions), $199.00 per year (international & Canadian student/resident). Foreign air speed delivery is included in all *Clinics'* subscription prices. All prices are subject to change without notice. **POSTMASTER:** Send address changes to *Otolaryngologic Clinics of North America*, Elsevier Periodicals Customer Service, 11830 Westline Industrial Drive, St. Louis, MO 63146. **Customer Service: 1-800-654-2452 (US). From outside the United States, call 1-314-453-7041. Fax: 1-314-453-5170. E-mail: journalscustomerservice-usa@ elsevier.com (for print support) or journalsonlinesupport-usa@elsevier.com (for online support).**

Reprints. For copies of 100 or more of articles in this publication, please contact the Commercial Reprints Department, Elsevier Inc., 360 Park Avenue South, New York, NY 10010-1710. Tel.: 212-633-3812; Fax: 212-462-1935; E-mail: reprints@ elsevier.com.

Otolaryngologic Clinics of North America is also published in Spanish by McGraw-Hill Interamericana Editores S.A., P.O. Box 5-237, 06500 Mexico D.F., Mexico.

Otolaryngologic Clinics of North America is covered in *MEDLINE/PubMed (Index Medicus), Current Contents/Clinical Medicine, Excerpta Medica, BIOSIS, Science Citation Index,* and *ISI/BIOMED.*

Printed in the United States of America.

Contributors

GUEST EDITOR

SAMUEL S. BECKER, MD
Director of Rhinology, Becker Nose and Sinus Center, Voorhees, New Jersey

AUTHORS

ADAM M. BECKER, MD
Department of Otolaryngology–Head and Neck Surgery, Medical College of Georgia, Augusta, Georgia

SAMUEL S. BECKER, MD
Director of Rhinology, Becker Nose and Sinus Center, Voorhees, New Jersey

PAOLO CAMPISI, MSc, MD, FRCSC, FAAP
Assistant Professor, Department of Otolaryngology–Head and Neck Surgery, Hospital for Sick Children, University of Toronto, Toronto, Ontario, Canada

ROY R. CASIANO, MD
Professor of Otolaryngology and Director, Center for Sinus and Voice Disorders, Department of Otolaryngology–Head and Neck Surgery, University of Miami-Leonard Miller School of Medicine, Miami, Florida

RAKESH KUMAR CHANDRA, MD
Assistant Professor, Department of Otolaryngology, Northwestern University's Feinberg School of Medicine, Chicago, Illinois

NIPUN CHHABRA, MD
Department of Otolaryngology–Head and Neck Surgery, Case Western Reserve University & University Hospitals Case Medical Center, Cleveland, Ohio

J. JARED CHRISTOPHEL, MD
Chief Resident, Department of Otolaryngology–Head and Neck Surgery, University of Virginia Health System, Charlottesville, Virginia

ARTEMUS T. COX III, MD, FACS
Assistant Professor of Surgery, Facial Plastic and Reconstructive Surgery, The University of Alabama-Birmingham, Birmingham, Alabama

MARIKA R. DUBIN, MD
Resident, Department of Otolaryngology–Head and Neck Surgery, University of California, San Francisco, California

JAMES A. DUNCAVAGE, MD
Department of Otolaryngology, Vanderbilt University Medical Center, Nashville, Tennessee

JEAN ANDERSON ELOY, MD
Assistant Professor of Surgery and Director of Rhinology and Sinus Surgery, Department of Surgery; and Division of Otolaryngology–Head and Neck Surgery, University of Medicine and Dentistry of New Jersey, New Jersey Medical School, Newark, New Jersey

NICHOLAS FETTMAN, MD
Department of Otolaryngology–Head and Neck Surgery, St. Louis University, St. Louis, Missouri

VITO FORTE, MD, FRCSC
Otolaryngologist-in-Chief, Hospital for Sick Children; Professor, Department of Otolaryngology–Head and Neck Surgery, Hospital for Sick Children, University of Toronto, Toronto, Ontario, Canada

CHARLES W. GROSS, MD, FACS
Professor of Otolaryngology–Head and Neck Surgery and Pediatrics, Division of Rhinology, Department of Otolaryngology–Head and Neck Surgery, University of Virginia Health System, Charlottesville, Virginia

RICHARD J. HARVEY, MD
Rhinology and Skull Base Surgery, Department of Otolaryngology/Skull Base Surgery, St. Vincent's Hospital, Darlinghurst, Sydney, New South Wales, Australia

STEVEN M. HOUSER, MD, FACS, FAAOA, FARS
Assistant Professor, Department of Otolaryngology–Head and Neck Surgery, Case Western Reserve University & University Hospitals Case Medical Center; Department of Otolaryngology–Head and Neck Surgery, MetroHealth Medical Center, Cleveland, Ohio

LARRY H. KALISH, MS, MMed, FRACS
Department of Otorhinolaryngology, Concord Hospital, Sydney, NSW, Australia

STILIANOS E. KOUNTAKIS, MD, PhD, FACS
Professor and Vice Chairman, Department of Otolaryngology–Head and Neck Surgery, Medical College of Georgia, Augusta, Georgia

BRIAN KULBERSH, MD
Resident, Department of Otolaryngology–Head and Neck Surgery, The University of Alabama-Birmingham, Birmingham, Alabama

ANDREW P. LANE, MD
Associate Professor, Department of Otolaryngology–Head and Neck Surgery, Division of Rhinology and Sinus Surgery, Johns Hopkins University School of Medicine, Baltimore, Maryland

DAVID NESKEY, MD
Otolaryngology Resident, Department of Otolaryngology–Head and Neck Surgery, University of Miami-Leonard Miller School of Medicine, Miami, Florida

JOAO F. NOGUEIRA, MD
Department of Otorhinolaryngology, Professor Edmundo Vasconcelos Hospital, Sao Paulo ENT Center, Rua Afonso Braz São Paulo, Brazil

LESLIE A. NURSE, MD
Department of Otolaryngology, Vanderbilt University Medical Center, Nashville, Tennessee

MONICA OBEROI PATADIA, MD
Chief Resident, Department of Otolaryngology, Northwestern University's Feinberg School of Medicine, Chicago, Illinois

SPENCER C. PAYNE, MD
Assistant Professor, Division of Rhinology & Sinus Surgery, Department of Otolaryngology–Head and Neck Surgery, Charlottesville, Virginia

STEVEN D. PLETCHER, MD
Assistant Professor, Department of Otolaryngology–Head and Neck Surgery, University of California, San Francisco, California

JAMES D. RAMSDEN, PhD, BM, BCh, FRCS
Honorary Senior Clinical Lecturer, ENT Department, University of Oxford, John Radcliffe Hospital, Oxford, United Kingdom

JOEY RAVIV, MD
Assistant Professor, Department of Otolaryngology, Northwestern University's Feinberg School of Medicine, Chicago, Illinois

THOMAS SANFORD, MD
Department of Otolaryngology–Head and Neck Surgery, St. Louis University, St. Louis, Missouri

NATHAN B. SAUTTER, MD
Assistant Professor, Oregon Sinus Center Division of Rhinology & Sinus Surgery, Department of Otolaryngology–Head and Neck Surgery, Oregon Health & Science University, Portland, Oregon

RODNEY J. SCHLOSSER, MD
Director and Professor of Rhinology and Skull Base Surgery, Department of Otolaryngology–Head and Neck Surgery, Medical University of South Carolina, Charleston, South Carolina

KRISTIN A. SEIBERLING, MD
Department of Surgery, Otolaryngology–Head and Neck Surgery, The Queen Elizabeth Hospital, South Australia, Australia

PATRICK O. SHEAHAN, MD
Research Fellow, Rhinology and Skull Base Surgery, Department of Otolaryngology–Head and Neck Surgery, Medical University of South Carolina, Charleston, South Carolina

MICHAEL J. SILLERS, MD, FACS
Alabama Nasal and Sinus Center, Birmingham, Alabama

RAJ SINDWANI, MD
Department of Otolaryngology–Head and Neck Surgery, St. Louis University, St. Louis, Missouri

TIMOTHY L. SMITH, MD, MPH
Professor, Oregon Sinus Center Division of Rhinology & Sinus Surgery, Department of Otolaryngology–Head and Neck Surgery, Oregon Health & Science University, Portland, Oregon

ALDO C. STAMM, MD, PhD
Department of Otorhinolaryngology, Professor Edmundo Vasconcelos Hospital, Sao Paulo ENT Center, Rua Afonso Braz São Paulo SP, Brazil

BRUCE K. TAN, MD
Chief Resident, Department of Otolaryngology–Head and Neck Surgery, Johns Hopkins University School of Medicine, Baltimore, Maryland

PETER-JOHN WORMALD, MD, FRACS, FCS (SA)
Department of Surgery, Otolaryngology–Head and Neck Surgery, The Queen Elizabeth Hospital, University of Adelaide, South Australia, Australia

Contents

This article provides a review of contemporary techniques in nasal septal surgery. Relevant anatomy and physiology of the nose and nasal septum are discussed. The essentials of a complete diagnostic evaluation are outlined. The evolution of surgical approaches to the correction of a deviated septum, including classic submucosal resection, traditional septoplasty, and open techniques, is covered. Complications of septoplasty are reviewed, with an emphasis on prevention and treatment. The recently popularized endoscopic septoplasty, a significant advance in septal surgery, is addressed elsewhere in this issue.

Endoscopic septoplasty has gained popularity since Lanza and colleagues and Stammberger first described the technique. This technique has several advantages over the traditional "headlight" septoplasty. These advantages include superior visualization, accommodation of limited and minimally invasive septoplasty, and usefulness as an effective teaching tool. This article reviews and illustrates the endoscopic septoplasty technique and discusses its limitations and advantages.

This article addresses the challenge of persistent nasal airway obstruction following septoplasty, specifically as it relates to revision septoplasty. Emphasis is on the importance of and the steps to be taken in making a complete and correct diagnosis of the problem before any surgery is performed. The authors present two categories of revision surgery: surgery involving the cartilaginous septum and surgery involving the bony septum, because they believe the evaluation and management of these areas are distinct. This article presents a discussion of airflow dynamics, options to objectively assess nasal volume and patency, examination of the septum, and surgical approaches and techniques.

The use of nasal packing following septoplasty has been proposed to serve multiple purposes. One of the most common reasons for use of packing is to prevent postoperative complications such as bleeding and formation of either synechiae or a septal hematoma. Stabilization of the remaining cartilage to prevent postoperative deviation is another reason that packing may be used. Although it appears intuitive that packing may prevent or decrease the incidence of these complications, evidence supporting this assertion is limited at best. Furthermore, certain types of nasal packing have been demonstrated to increase postoperative pain and have been implicated as a causative factor of catastrophic complications, such as toxic shock. With limited evidence to suggest a beneficial effect and a potential for deleterious side-effects, the routine use of postoperative packing following septoplasty should be questioned.

literature, that not everyone undergoing a turbinectomy procedure suffers from the debilitating symptoms of either atrophic rhinitis or empty nose syndrome. Thus, it behooves us to evaluate this latter entity with a more critical eye, so that we can avoid creating future sufferers and provide relief to those who have already been afflicted.

THE CLINICS ARE NOW AVAILABLE ONLINE!

Access your subscription at:
www.theclinics.com

Preface

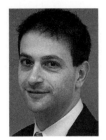

Samuel S. Becker, MD
Guest Editor

Nasal airway obstruction—the inability to obtain free passage of air through the nose—afflicts millions of patients worldwide. Severity ranges from mild blockage, such as that caused by slight septal deviation, to life-threatening nasal blockage from choanal atresia. Treatment options are equally wide ranging.

Many aspects of nasal airway obstruction may be mitigated by medical management alone. For instance, swelling from allergic rhinitis typically responds well to allergy treatment. In a number of cases, however, medical intervention is insufficient. When medical management fails, and anatomic abnormalities contribute significantly to nasal obstruction, surgical intervention may be indicated. Septal deviation, turbinate hypertrophy, internal and external nasal valve collapse, sinusitis, polyps, encephaloceles, and tumors are just a few of the varied sources of nasal obstruction. Equally diverse are the surgical means available to the contemporary otolaryngologist to address these anatomic abnormalities.

In this two-part issue of the *Otolaryngologic Clinics of North America*, experts in the surgical management of the nasal airway address the range of anatomic abnormalities that contribute to nasal obstruction, and describe in detail the surgical methods available for treatment of these problems. In Part 1, expert rhinologists address sinonasal aspects of surgery for nasal obstruction. In Part 2, experts in rhinoplasty describe surgical interventions for nasal obstruction from a facial plastic surgery perspective. Together, these two issues should increase the otolaryngologist's armamentarium for the comprehensive surgical management of nasal airway obstruction.

Samuel S. Becker, MD

E-mail address:
sam.s.becker@gmail.com (S.S. Becker)

Otolaryngol Clin N Am 42 (2009) xiii
doi:10.1016/j.otc.2009.02.003

Nasal, Septal, and Turbinate Anatomy and Embryology

David Neskey, MD[a], Jean Anderson Eloy, MD[b],*, Roy R. Casiano, MD[a,c]

KEYWORDS

- Nasal anatomy • Septal anatomy
- Nasoseptal anatomy • Turbinate anatomy
- Nasoseptal embryology • Nasal obstruction

This article describes the development and anatomy of the nasal septum and structures of the lateral nasal wall. A clear understanding of the development and anatomic variations of the nasal septum and structures of the lateral nasal wall is vital for successful treatment of nasal obstruction. With knowledge of the specific location and anatomic reason for a patient's nasal obstruction, clinicians can better identify the specific structure responsible for the obstruction and thus implement a more targeted approach to treatment.

NASOSEPTAL EMBRYOLOGY

The tissue that gives rise to the face and nasal structures derives from three different embryonic sources: the ectoderm, the neural crest, and the mesoderm. The ectoderm provides an overlying cover and, through its interactions with mesenchymal layers, a pattern for developing structures.[1,2] Neural crest cells provide the majority of facial mesenchymal tissue.[1,2] The paraxial and prechordal mesoderm provides precursors for myoblasts that differentiate into voluntary craniofacial muscles.[2]

At 4 weeks' gestation, five identifiable primordial structures surround the stomodeum, a depression below the developing brain and the first sign of a future face. These five structures are the frontonasal prominence, the right and left maxillary prominances, and the right and left mandibular prominences. The maxillary and mandibular

[a] Department of Otolaryngology – Head and Neck Surgery, University of Miami-Leonard Miller School of Medicine, Miami, FL 33136, USA
[b] Rhinology and Sinus Surgery, Department of Surgery; Division of Otolaryngology – Head and Neck Surgery, University of Medicine and Dentistry of New Jersey, New Jersey Medical School, 140 Bergen Street, Suite E1620, PO Box 1709, Newark, NJ 07101, USA
[c] Center for Sinus and Voice Disorders, Department of Otolaryngology – Head and Neck Surgery, University of Miami-Leonard Miller School of Medicine, Miami, FL 33136, USA
* Corresponding author. Rhinology and Sinus Surgery, Division of Otolaryngology-Head and Neck Surgery, University of Medicine and Dentistry of New Jersey – New Jersey Medical School, 90 Bergen Street, Suite 8100, PO Box 1709, Newark, NJ 07101.
E-mail address: jean.anderson.eloy@gmail.com (J.A. Eloy).

Otolaryngol Clin N Am 42 (2009) 193–205
doi:10.1016/j.otc.2009.01.008
0030-6665/09/$ – see front matter © 2009 Elsevier Inc. All rights reserved.

prominences lie superolaterally and inferolaterally bilaterally respectively. By the end of the fourth week of gestation, paired thickenings of ectoderm appear on the fronto-nasal prominence superior and lateral to the stomodeum.[2] These oval placodes develop into the nose and nasal cavities (**Fig. 1**).

During the fifth week, mesenchymes on the periphery of the nasal placodes prolif-erate to form horseshoe elevations. The lateral and medial limbs are termed nasolat-eral and nasomedial processes respectively. Mesenchymal tissue surrounding the nasal placodes continues to proliferate and thicken, resulting in a perceived depres-sion of the placodes. These depressions are subsequently called the nasal pits and are the primordia of anterior nares and nasal cavities (see **Fig. 1**).[2]

From 5 weeks' gestation, the nasal pits continue to deepen toward the oral cavity. By 6 and one-half weeks, only a thin oronasal membrane separates the oral cavity from the nasal cavities.[1] This oronasal membrane subsequently disintegrates, leading to a communication to the nasal cavities posterior to the primary palate. These regions

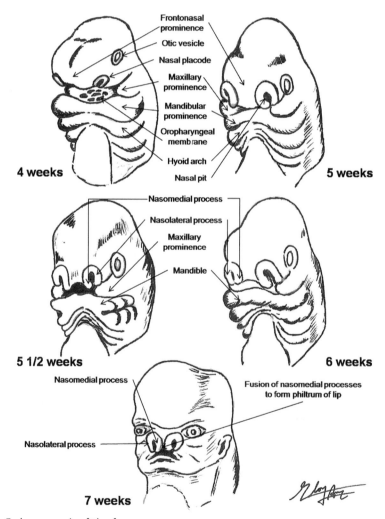

Fig. 1. Embryogenesis of the face.

of continuity are the primordial choanae. As the palatal shelves fuse and the secondary palate develops, the nasal cavity lengthens, resulting in the junction of the nasal cavity and the pharynx.[1,2]

Beginning from the fourth to sixth week of gestation, the paired maxillary processes grow medially toward each other and toward the paired nasomedial processes.[1] By the end of the sixth week, the nasolateral processes begin to fuse with the maxillary processes to form the ala nasi and the lateral border of the nostril bilaterally (see **Fig. 1**). Along the junctions of the nasolateral and maxillary processes lie the nasola-crimal grooves. Ectoderm within these grooves thickens to form epithelial cords, which then detach and canalize to form nasolacrimal ducts and lacrimal sacs. By late fetal period, nasolacrimal ducts extend the medial corners of the eyes to the inferior meatuses in the lateral wall of the nasal cavity.[2]

The nasomedial prominences continue to expand but remain unfused until the seventh or eighth week of gestation, when they merge with superficial components of the maxillary processes. The fusion lines between these processes are the nasal fins. As mesenchymes penetrate this articulation, a continuous union is formed, completing most of the upper lip and upper jaw bilaterally (see **Fig. 1**). The nasomedial processes then merge with each other, forming the intermaxillary segment and subsequently displacing the frontonasal prominence posteriorly. The intermaxillary segment formed from the nasomedial processes is the precursor to several structures, including the primary palate, the tip and crest of nose, and a portion of the nasal septum.[1]

The nasal septum grows inferiorly from the nasofrontal prominence to the level of the palatal shelves following fusion to form the secondary palate (**Fig. 2**). Anteriorly, the septum is contiguous with the primary palate originating from the nasomedial processes. The initial site of palatal fusion occurs posterior to the incisive foramen and extends both anteriorly and posteriorly. The fusion point between the primary and secondary palate is the incisive foramen (see **Fig. 2**).[3]

At the end of its development, the nasal septum divides the nasal cavity into two separate chambers. The nasal septum's components are the quadrangular cartilage, the perpendicular plate of the ethmoid, the vomer, the maxillary crest, the palatal crest, and the membranous septum (**Fig. 3**).

The tubular vomeronasal organ first appears as bilateral epithelial thickening on the nasal septum. By the fortieth day of gestation, this primordial structure has invaginated along the septum. The structure thus end in a blind pouch and subsequently separates from the septal epithelium. In other species, the vomeronasal organ is lined with chemoreceptors similar to those in the olfactory epithelium. This epithelium projects into the accessory olfactory bulb, which connects to the amygdala and other limbic centers.[4]

LATERAL NASAL WALL EMBRYOLOGY

At 8 weeks' gestation, a cartilaginous nasal capsule surrounds the nasal cavity and is continuous with the cartilage of the nasal septum. Three soft tissue elevations or preturbinates can be identified within the nasal cavity. Even at this early stage, the preturbinates are oriented in size and position comparable with the adult inferior, middle, and superior turbinates (see **Fig. 2**).[5]

By 9 to 10 weeks, the cartilage capsule develops into two cartilaginous flanges that penetrate the soft tissue elevations of the inferior and middle turbinate. A small elevation of cartilage located at the entrance to the middle meatus ultimately forms the uncinate process. This cartilage originates from the medial wall of the lateral cartilage capsule. As the uncinate begins to develop, a ridge of bone originating from the

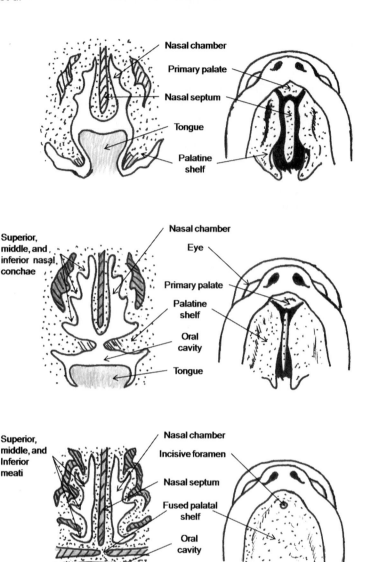

Fig. 2. Embryogenesis of the nasal cavity and palate.

hard palate advances posteriorly to replace the lateral cartilaginous capsule and becomes the posterolateral wall of the nose.[5]

Around 11 to 12 weeks' gestation, the primordial ethmoidal infundubulum develops as a space lateral to the uncinate process in the middle meatus. From this space, a short tract running inferolaterally toward the maxillary bone precursor is the initial development of the maxillary sinus. As the primordial maxillary sinus grows, a vertical plate of bone extending from the primitive maxilla lengthens posteriorly to separate the lower part of the orbit from the lateral cartilaginous capsule. Additionally a second vertical bony plate extends cephalad from the hard palate and forms the posteroinferior lateral wall of the nasal cavity.[5]

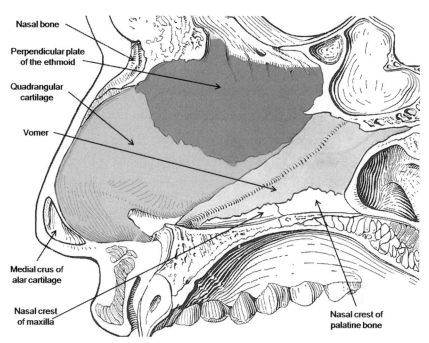

Nasal bone

Perpendicular plate
of the ethmoid

Quadrangular
cartilage

Vomer

Medial crus of
alar cartilage

Nasal crest
of maxilla

Nasal crest of
palatine bone

Fig. 3. Schematic depiction of a sagittal view of the nasal septum and surrounding structures.

By 15 to 16 weeks' gestation, the inferior, middle, and superior turbinates are well formed. Additionally the primordial maxillary sinus is surrounded by a sleeve of cartilage and has grown from the space lateral to the uncinate, the ethmoid infundibulum, toward the apex of maxilla inferiorly. Posterior protrusions from the ethmoid infundibulum continue to enlarge and will become the posterior ethmoid cells.[5]

At 17 to 18 weeks' gestation, the thick cartilage cap of the primitive maxillary sinus leads the continuing extension of the sinus anteriorly, laterally, and inferiorly. This channel runs medial to the nasolacrimal duct near its origin at the orbit. Initial ossification of the cartilaginous precursor of the inferior turbinate also occurs at the angle where the inferior turbinate budded from the lateral cartilaginous capsule. Protrusions posteriorly into the sphenoid bone are visualized.[5] Over the next 3 to 4 weeks, ossification progresses to involve the superior aspect of nasolacrimal duct near the orbit and the middle turbinate. As with its inferior counterpart, ossification of the middle turbinate commences at its site of origin from the lateral cartilaginous capsule.

By 24 weeks' gestation, the primordial maxillary sinus has invaginated into the woven bone of the maxilla. Laterally, a bony plate separates the channel from the orbit and medially a plate of bone separates the inferior turbinate from the lateral cartilaginous capsule. In addition, the nasolacrimal duct is firmly encased in a tube of bone superiorly near the eye.[5]

The development of the lateral nasal wall is close to complete by 24 weeks' gestation. By this time, the superior and middle turbinates have developed and ossified from the ethmoid bone, while the inferior turbinate has emerged from two origins, the maxilla and the lateral cartilaginous capsule. Based on the initial mucosal thickening, turbinate development appears to be a primary process, and meatal ingrowth occurs secondarily.[5]

VARIATIONS LEADING TO NASAL OBSTRUCTION
Deviated Nasal Septum

A few large studies have investigated the prevalence of nasal septal deviation and have concluded that a nondeviated septum is present in only 7.5% to 23% of patients, while septal deformities are far more common.[6,7] Because septal deflection has a high prevalence and multiple patterns of deformity, clinicians needed a classification system to help them sort and describe cases. Mladina[7] developed such a system (**Table 1**). This system divides septal deformities into seven types. Types 1 and 2 represent a spectrum of septal deformities involving a unilateral vertical ridge in the valve region. A type 2 deformity is severe enough to disturb the function of the valve. In a type 3 deformity, a unilateral vertical ridge is at the level of the head of the middle turbinate. A type 4 deformity has characteristics that combine those of a type 3 deformity with those of either types 1 or 2. A type 4 deformity is often described as an S-shaped deformity. Types 5 and 6 deformities are horizontally based deformities. A type 5 deformity has a horizontal crest that is frequently in contact with the lateral nasal wall (**Fig. 4**). A type 6 deformity has a prominent maxillary crest contralateral to the deviation and an obvious septal crest on the deviated side. A type 7 deformity combines the characteristics of any of the other six types.[8] Although this classification system thoroughly describes anatomic variations of septal deviations, it does not identify sources for these differences.

Another system, which divides septal deformities into anterior cartilaginous deviation and combined (cartilaginous and bony) septal deformity, correlates a cause for nasal septal deflections.[6] Anterior cartilage deviation is typically localized to the anterior quadrilateral cartilage and is frequently associated with asymmetry of the external bony pyramid and dislocation of cartilage off the anterior nasal spine. This deformity is more common in newborns delivered vaginally, particularly those delivered from persistent occipitoposterior positions, than from newborns delivered via cesarean. The deformity can also occur, though rarely, in newborns delivered via cesarean secondary to the pressure on the head during internal rotation. The internal rotation stage of delivery forces the face and shoulder against the pelvic wall, which can lead to deformity of the nasal cartilage and distortion of the bony pyramid.[9] Combined septal deformity involves all septal components, including the vomer bone, the perpendicular plate of the ethmoid, and the quadrilateral cartilage. Deformities can include a spur at the vomer ethmoid junction or a C- or S-shaped bending of cartilage and a compensatory hypertrophy of turbinate opposite the side of the deviation. There are typically associated deformities of the cheek, external nares, palate, and malocclusion of the teeth. Therefore, a combined septal deformity is part of a greater generalized facial deformity.

Table 1	
Mladina classification for nasal septal deviation	
Septal Deformity	**Description**
Type 1	Unilateral vertical ridge in the valve region
Type 2	Similar to type 1 but more severe obstruction and disturbance of nasal valve
Type 3	Unilateral vertical ridge at the level of the head of the middle turbinate
Type 4	Combination of type 3 with either type 1 or 2
Type 5	Horizontal septal crest in contact with the lateral nasal wall
Type 6	Prominent maxillary crest contralateral to the deviation with a septal crest on the deviated side
Type 7	Combination of previously described septal deformity types

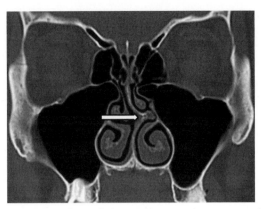

Fig. 4. Coronal CT in a patient with nasal obstruction secondary to a type 5 leftward deviated nasal septum (*arrow*).

The maxillary molding theory, in giving possible explanations for septal deformities, considers anterior septal deviation and combined septal deformity to be variations in a single spectrum of deformities stemming from stresses and strains on the skull of the fetus.[6,10] During pregnancy, the fetus is subjected to various torsions and pressures and the skull bones are malleable to these forces. Skull bones are not elastic. Once they are displaced, these bones will continue to grow in their altered alignment. Depending on the severity, direction, and location of the pressure, local deformities may develop, including anterior septal deviation. If the force is great enough, the septum can be compressed against the solid skull base, resulting in a splaying of the cartilage at the vomer ethmoid junction and creating a C- or S-shaped deformity.[6]

Torsional strains can cause unequal parietal bone molding. This unilateral pressure can cause medial displacement of the maxilla and subsequent malocclusion of the teeth and elevation of the palate on the side of the pressure. Palatal elevation causes a tilting of the vomer away from the compressing forces, leading to septal deviation.[6] Although forces during parturition are probably responsible for most septal deformities, a genetic component may be involved in posterior deformities.

The maxilla has solid articulations posteriorly with the skull. Therefore, when external forces are applied, the resulting deformities are typically located anteriorly. Given this anatomic arrangement, it appears that posterior deformities have a genetic component or a normal component to maxillary complex development, whereas anterior deformities are more often related to extrinsic forces.[11]

Inferior Turbinate Hypertrophy

Inferior turbinate hypertrophy is a common cause of surgically correctable nasal obstruction. No clear developmental reasons have been given for this condition. Three different variations are often encountered and include bony, soft tissue, and mixed hypertrophy. Bony turbinate hypertrophy is usually caused by a prominent (broad) inferolateral turn of the turbinate. Very large but normally shaped obstructing inferior turbinates are also described. However, these are not as prevalent as the prominent inferolateral turn. Soft tissue hypertrophy is very common and represents the majority of cases of inferior turbinate hypertrophy. The common underlying pathophysiology in soft tissue hypertrophy is chronic rhinitis and other conditions that cause chronic mucosal inflammation (**Fig. 5**). Mixed inferior turbinate hypertrophy involves anatomic bony hypertrophy in the setting of chronic rhinitis (**Fig. 6**). Although very uncommon,

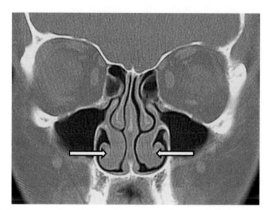

Fig. 5. Coronal CT demonstrating bilateral hypertrophy of the soft tissue component of the inferior turbinate. Note the prominent overlying soft tissue component (*arrows*) from chronic rhinitis.

pneumatization of the inferior turbinate (**Fig. 7**) may cause inferior turbinate hypertrophy and leads to nasal obstruction.

Paradoxical Middle Turbinate

Paradoxical middle turbinate refers to an inferomedially curved middle turbinate edge with its concave surface adjacent to the septum (**Fig. 8**). This anatomic variant alone is not pathologic, but can lead to significant narrowing of the middle meatus and cause ostiomeatal complex obstruction with resultant rhinosinusitis. Although not frequently seen, when associated with a bulbous middle turbinate, paradoxical middle turbinate can potentially lead to nasal obstruction. This finding usually occurs bilaterally.

Concha Bullosa

A concha bullosa represents pneumatization of the middle turbinate. This anatomic variant is usually found bilaterally with variable asymmetry (**Fig. 9**A). However, unilateral conchae bullosa are not uncommon (**Fig. 9**B). Although a concha bullosa is not a pathologic entity, it can lead to nasal obstruction when overly pneumatized.

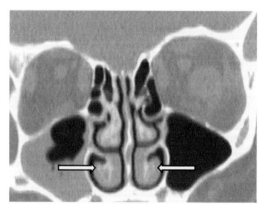

Fig. 6. Coronal CT demonstrating mixed inferior turbinate hypertrophy with prominent inferolateral turns as well as marked overlying soft tissue component (*arrows*).

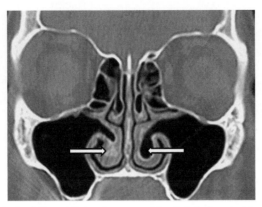

Fig. 7. Coronal CT depicting bilateral pneumatized inferior turbinates (*arrows*). An uncommon finding, this entity can potentially lead to unilateral or bilateral nasal obstruction.

Unilateral concha bullosa is often associated with a deflection of the nasal septum away from the side of the concha. The degree of septal deflection usually parallels the size of the concha bullosa. Since the middle turbinate is part of the ethmoid complex, concha bullosa is typically seen in patients with highly pneumatized ethmoid sinuses.

Choanal Atresia

Choanal atresia is a congenital obstruction of the posterior nasal apertures. This abnormality can occur unilaterally or bilaterally (**Fig. 10**) with a female-to-male ratio nearing 2:1.[12] The incidence of choanal atresia is estimated to be 1 in 5000 to 7000 live births with the unilateral anomaly occurring more frequently.[13] When the unilateral atresia is present, the right side is affected twice as often with a corresponding septal deviation on the affected side.[13] Traditionally, choanal atresia has been described as bony, membranous, or mixed membranous-bony with the bony entity being the most common, accounting for approximately 90% of cases.[14] Recently, the mixed

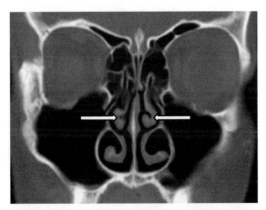

Fig. 8. Coronal CT showing bilateral paradoxically curved middle turbinates (*arrows*). Although not a usual cause of nasal obstruction, when associated with septal deflection or inferior turbinate hypertrophy, this variation can significantly worsen nasal obstruction.

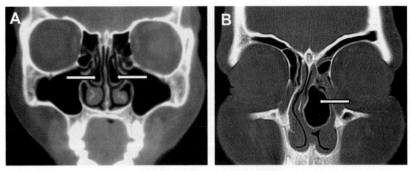

Fig. 9. (*A*) Coronal CT showing bilateral conchae bullosa (*arrows*). (*B*) Coronal CT demonstrating markedly enlarged unilateral concha bullosa (*arrow*) with contralateral septal deflection.

membranous–bony atresias have been found to be the most common defect, occurring in 70% of cases.[15] Choanal atresia can be an isolated finding but is associated with other anomalies in 50% of cases. The most commonly described association is with CHARGE syndrome (CHARGE stands for cluster of characteristics that include *coloboma* of the eye, *heart* defects, *atresia* of the choanae, *retardation* of growth or development, *genital* or urinary abnormalities, and *ear* abnormalities and deafness). Association with Crouzon syndrome and other syndromes have also been described.[15–17]

Since the initial description of choanal atresia by Roederer in 1755, several theories have been developed to explain the etiology of the atresia plate.[14] The four basic principles that have come to be accepted are:

Persistence of the buccopharyngeal membrane from the foregut[14]
Abnormal persistence or location of mesoderm-forming adhesions in the nasochoanal region[18]
Abnormal persistence of the nasobuccal membrane of Hochstetter[14]
Misdirection of neural crest migration with subsequent mesodermal flow[18]

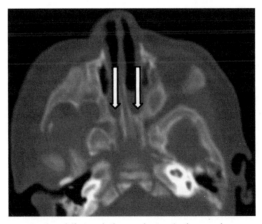

Fig. 10. Axial CT demonstrating bilateral choanal atresia (*arrows*).

Other theories that have been proposed but not commonly accepted include:

Resorption of the floor of the secondary nasal fossa
Incomplete dorsal extension of the nasal cavity

Most believe that the latter two hypotheses are likely to result in nasal stenosis as opposed to choanal atresia.

The development of choanal atresia can only be understood with a fundamental knowledge of embryologic development. The first 12 weeks of gestation are critical for facial development. The neural crest cells migrate to preordained locations in the branchial arch mesenchyme at the end of fourth week of gestation. In the next 2 weeks, cellular proliferation and migration within the various facial processes occur, leading to the development of identifiable structures, including the columella, philtrum, and upper lip. Additionally, the nasal processes proliferate around the nasal pits, while the nasal pits are furrowing deeper within the mesenchyme. As the nasal pits migrate posteriorly, they ultimately meet the frontal portion of the stomodeum with only a sheet of tissue separating them. This thin sheet of tissue is termed the *nasobuccal membrane* and typically ruptures to create a nasal cavity with the primary choanae. As development continues, the primary of primitive choanae undergoes further alterations as fusion of septal elements and palate moves the choana more posteriorly to form the secondary choana.[19]

Pyriform Aperture Stenosis

Congenital pyriform aperture stenosis (CPAS) was first described by Brown and colleagues[20] in 1989. Although its exact cause is unknown, this very rare disorder is thought to be secondary to overgrowth of the nasal process of the maxilla during the fourth to eighth week of gestation.[20,21] CPAS is usually bilateral, although unilateral presentation can occur.[20] The pyriform aperture represents the narrowest most anterior bony part of the nasal airway and small changes in the diameter at this site can significantly affect nasal airway resistance and cause nasal obstruction (**Fig. 11**). It is deemed stenotic if the maximum transverse diameter of each aperture is less

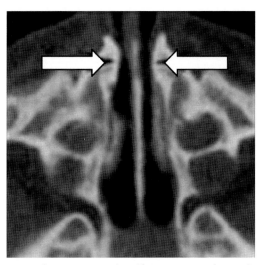

Fig. 11. Axial CT demonstrating a narrowed pyriform aperture (*arrows*).

than or equal to 3 mm or when the combined aperture width is less than 8 mm.[20] CPAS is associated with a central maxillary incisor in about 63% of cases.[22] There may also be a relationship between CPAS and holoprosencephaly since a central maxillary incisor is also commonly found in the latter, and a case report of monozygotic twins reported that one twin presented with holoprosencephaly and the other with CPAS.[23,24]

REFERENCES

1. Carlson BM. Development of head and neck. In: Human embryology and developmental biology. St Louis: Mosby; 1994. p. 283–6.
2. Moore KL, Persaud TVN. The developing human. Clinically oriented embryology. 6th edition. Philadelphia: WB Saunders; 1998.
3. Markus AF, Delaire J, Smith WP. Facial balance in cleft lip and palate. I. Normal development and cleft palate. Br J Oral Maxillofac Surg 1992;30(5):287–95.
4. Bhatnagar KP, Smith TD, Winstead W. The human vomeronasal organ: Part IV. Incidence, topography, endoscopy, and ultrastructure of the nasopalatine recess, nasopalatine fossa, and vomeronasal organ. Am J Rhinol 2002;16(6):343–50.
5. Bingham B, Wang RG, Hawke M, et al. The embryonic development of the lateral nasal wall from 8 to 24 weeks. Laryngoscope 1991;101(9):992–7.
6. Gray LP. Deviated nasal septum. Incidence and etiology. Ann Otol Rhinol Laryngol 1978;87(3 Pt 3 Suppl 50):3–20.
7. Mladina R, Čujić E, Šubarić M, et al. Nasal septal deformities in ear, nose, and throat patients: an international study. Am J Otol 2008;29(2):75–82.
8. Mladina R, Subaric M. Are some septal deformities inherited? Type 6 revisited. Int J Pediatr Otorhinolaryngol 2003;67(12):1291–4.
9. Jeppesen F, Windfeld I. Dislocation of the nasal septal cartilage in the newborn. aetiology, spontaneous course and treatment. Acta Obstet Gynecol Scand 1972; 51(1):5–15.
10. Gray LP. Septal and associated cranial birth deformities: Types, incidence and treatment. Med J Aust 1974;1(15):557–63.
11. Grymer LF, Pallisgaard C, Melsen B. The nasal septum in relation to the development of the nasomaxillary complex: a study in identical twins. Laryngoscope 1991;101(8):863–8.
12. Josephson GD, Vickery CL, Giles WC, et al. Transnasal endoscopic repair of congenital choanal atresia: long-term results. Arch Otolaryngol Head Neck Surg 1998;124(5):537–40.
13. Deutsch E, Kaufman M, Eilon A. Transnasal endoscopic management of choanal atresia. Int J Pediatr Otorhinolaryngol 1997;40(1):19–26.
14. Flake CG, Ferguson CF. Congenital choanal atresia in infants and children. Ann Otol Rhinol Laryngol 1964;73:458–73.
15. Stankiewicz JA. The endoscopic repair of choanal atresia. Otolaryngol Head Neck Surg 1990;103(6):931–7.
16. Arnaud-Lopez L, Fragoso R, Mantilla-Capacho J, et al. Crouzon with acanthosis nigricans. Further delineation of the syndrome. Clin Genet 2007;72(5): 405–10.
17. Inan UU, Yilmaz MD, Demir Y, et al. Characteristics of lacrimo-auriculo-dento-digital (LADD) syndrome: case report of a family and literature review. Int J Pediatr Otorhinolaryngol 2006;70(7):1307–14.
18. Hengerer AS, Strome M. Choanal atresia: a new embryologic theory and its influence on surgical management. Laryngoscope 1982;92(8 Pt 1):913–21.

19. Hengerer AS, Brickman TM, Jeyakumar A. Choanal atresia: embryologic analysis and evolution of treatment, a 30-year experience. Laryngoscope 2008;118(5):862–6.
20. Brown OE, Myer CM III, Manning SC. Congenital nasal pyriform aperture stenosis. Laryngoscope 1989;99(1):86–91.
21. Osovsky M, Aizer-Danon A, Horev G, et al. Congenital pyriform aperture stenosis. Pediatr Radiol 2007;37(1):97–9.
22. Lo FS, Lee YJ, Lin SP, et al. Solitary maxillary central incisor and congenital nasal pyriform aperture stenosis. Eur J Pediatr 1998;157(1):39–44.
23. Tavin E, Stecker E, Marion R. Nasal pyriform aperture stenosis and the holoprosencephaly spectrum. Int J Pediatr Otorhinolaryngol 1994;28(2–3):199–204.
24. Krol BJ, Hulka GF, Drake A. Congenital nasal pyriform aperture stenosis in the monozygotic twin of a child with holoprosencephaly. Otolaryngol Head Neck Surg 1998;118(5):679–81.

Diagnosis of Nasal Airway Obstruction

Rakesh Kumar Chandra, MD*, Monica Oberoi Patadia, MD,
Joey Raviv, MD

KEYWORDS

- Nasal obstruction • Deviated septum • Nasal valve
- Cottle maneuver • Nasal endoscopy • Acoustic rhinometry
- Rhinomanometry • Nasal airflow • Inferior turbinate
- Chronic sinusitis • Nasal polyps

Nasal obstruction is an important symptom of many underlying disorders and is a common cause of otolaryngology visits. Kimmelman[1] has estimated that approximately 5 billion dollars are spent annually to relieve nasal airway obstruction, and an estimated 60 million dollars are spent on surgical procedures intended to relieve nasal airway obstruction. Patients will often use the term congestion, which may either refer to mucus secretions or obstructive nasal pathology. This article describes diagnosis of the latter.

DIFFERENTIAL DIAGNOSIS

Nasal obstruction is a symptom and not a diagnosis. The evaluation of nasal obstruction has both objective and subjective measures. Nasal patency can be quantified objectively based on the anatomy of the nasal cavity or the physiology of nasal airflow. The subjective feeling of nasal obstruction depends on additional factors such as pressure receptors, thermal receptors, pain receptors, secretions, and others.[2] Ultimately, the etiology of nasal obstruction is polyfactorial. For this reason, the differential diagnosis of nasal obstruction (**Fig. 1**) is broad, including physiologic and anatomic pathology. It is important to remember that patients may have a combination of these factors contributing to the symptom of nasal obstruction.

Anatomic Causes

The nasal valve is described as the narrowest portion of the human airway.[3] Anatomically, it is broken down into an internal and external nasal valve. The endonasal anatomic region of the internal nasal valve was first described by Mink in 1903. The anatomic boundaries of this internal nasal valve include the dorsal nasal septum

Department of Otolaryngology, Northwestern University, Feinberg School of Medicine, Chicago, IL 60611, USA
* Corresponding author.
E-mail address: rickchandra@hotmail.com (R.K. Chandra).

Otolaryngol Clin N Am 42 (2009) 207–225
doi:10.1016/j.otc.2009.01.004
0030-6665/09/$ – see front matter © 2009 Elsevier Inc. All rights reserved.

Neoplasms	Inflammatory
Benign Juvenile nasopharyngeal angiofibroma (JNA) Hemangioma Dermoid Papilloma Neurofibroma Nasal osteoma Benign salivary gland tumor Rhinophyma **Malignant** Esthesioneuroblastoma Malignant salivary gland neoplasm Nasopharyngeal carcinoma Basal cell carcinoma Adenocarcinoma Lymphoma Mucosal melanoma Squamous cell carcinoma Sarcoma Verrucous carcinoma Metastatic lesion	Rhinosinusitis Nasal polyposis Samter's Triad/Aspirin Sensitivity Triad Inferior turbinate hypertrophy Rhinitis Allergic rhinitis (seasonal or perennial) Non-allergic rhinitis (NAR) Non-allergic rhinitis with eosinophilia (NARES) Infectious rhinitis (bacterial, viral, fungal) Vasomotor rhinitis Atrophic rhinitis Rhinitis medicamentosa **Infectious** Syphilis Human Immune Deficiency Virus Nasal vestibulitis
Congenital/Anatomic	**Trauma**
Choanal atresia Adenoid hypertrophy Naso-septal deviation Nasal tip ptosis Internal/external nasal valve incompetence Septal perforation Concha bullosa Cystic Fibrosis Ciliary Dysmotility	Synechiae Facial nerve paralysis Overaggressive osteotomies Post rhinoplasty nasal valve narrowing Empty nose syndrome (complete turbinate resection) Cocaine abuse Septal perforations
Medication	**Systemic**

Anti-thyroid medications
Birth control pills
Estrogen replacements
Hypertensive medications
  Calcium channel blockers
  Beta blockers
	Wegener's granulomatosis
	Sarcoidosis
	Midline lethal granuloma
	Rhinoscleroma
	Histiocytosis X
	Tuberculosis

Neurogenic	**Other**
Encephalocele Glioma CSF leak	Nasal foreign body Hypothyroidism Pregnancy Obesity

Fig. 1. Differential diagnosis for nasal airway obstruction.

medially, the internal caudal edge of the upper lateral cartilage laterally, and the anterior head of the inferior turbinate as the posterior boundary. Normally the angle between the nasal septum and upper lateral cartilage is 10 to 15 degrees in the leptorrhine nose, and is usually a little wider in the platyrrhine nose. This internal nasal valve, the narrowest segment of the nasal airway, has a cross-sectional area of approximately 40 to 60 mm^2. It accounts for approximately two thirds of total nasal airway resistance, and hence, collapse or stenosis of this area is thought to be one of the most common causes of nasal obstruction (**Fig. 2A–C**).[4]

The boundaries of the external nasal valve, also known as the nasal vestibule, includes the caudal edge of the lateral crus of the lower lateral cartilages, the alar fibro-fatty tissue, and the membranous septum.[5] The nasal vestibule is the first component of the nasal resistor. Studies have shown 30 L/min as the limiting flow during inspiration at which nasal airway collapse occurs in this area.[6] It is important to differentiate between the nasal valve proper and the nasal valve area. The nasal valve area, as described by Kasperbauer and Kern,[7] is the area extending posteriorly from the actual nasal valve to the bony pyriform aperture and extending inferiorly to the nasal floor.

On inspiration, the high velocity of air passing through the nasal valve will cause a decrease in intraluminal pressure. These Bernoulli's forces create a vacuum effect on the upper lateral cartilages, ultimately causing collapse of the upper lateral cartilage.[4] The resiliency of the upper and lower lateral cartilages counteract Bernoulli forces during deep inspiration and prevent internal and external nasal valve collapse. Airway collapse of the external nasal valve is prevented by activation of the dilator naris muscles during inspiration, whereas positive pressure is the driving force for nasal vestibule dilation during expiration.

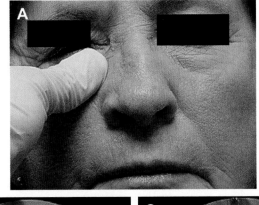

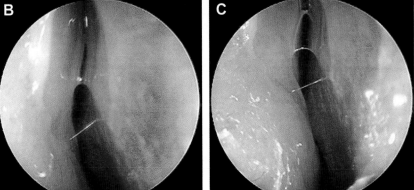

Fig. 2. (*A*) Performance of the Cottle maneuver. View of the right nasal valve before (*B*) and during (*C*) the Cottle maneuver.

Previous trauma, especially previous rhinoplasty, is the most common cause of a weakened nasal valve. The already narrowed nasal valve can further be limited as a result of a deviated nasal septum. As stated by Poiseuille's law, airflow through the nose is proportional to the radius of the airway raised to the fourth power. As air is inhaled through the nasal cavity, airflow accelerates as it enters the nasal valve. It follows that any small deflection of the nasal septum can lead to exponential effects on nasal airflow, and hence, influences nasal obstruction.

Septal deviation has also been associated with significantly longer mucociliary clearance times than normal controls. Notably, normalization of mucociliary clearance has been observed after septoplasty.[8,9] It is important to remember, however, that not every abnormality of the septum requires correction, as anterior deviations in the nasal valve region are more likely than posterior deviations to cause symptoms of obstruction.

Pneumatization of the middle turbinate, or concha bullosa, is a common anatomic variant found in approximately 25% of the population.[10] A study reviewing 202 consecutive CT scans found pneumatization of the vertical lamella of the middle turbinate in 46.2%, of the inferior or bulbous segment in 31.2%, and the lamella and bulbous portion in 15.7% of cases.[11] Most concha bullosae are small and asymptomatic. However, a large concha bullosa or massive bilateral concha bullosa is thought to contribute to nasal obstructive symptoms.[12] Concha bullosa is thought to be a significant etiology of nasal middle meatal obstructive syndrome, the symptoms of which include headaches, impaired nasal breathing and anosmia.[10] Septal deviation and middle turbinate concha bullosa often occur concurrently.[13] Nearly 80% of patients with a dominant concha bullosa have a concurrent deviated septum. There is also a strong association between unilateral concha bullosa and contralateral septal deviation. Naturally, the influence of septal deviation and concha bullosa on the symptom of nasal obstruction will depend on several factors, including the degree of anatomic compromise and inflammatory comorbidities.

Patients with fixed anatomic obstructions may experience intermittent symptoms secondary to the nasal cycle and other autonomic phenomena. The phenomenon of the nasal cycle was studied by Lang and colleagues[14] who measured fluctuations in nasal cross-sectional area during the nasal cycle using acoustic rhinometry. They were able to show changes in unilateral nasal cross-sectional area during the nasal cycle; however, little variation was noticed at the nasal valve itself. This may explain why the nasal cycle is often unnoticed unless other pathology exists, such as septal deviation, allergic rhinitis, and so forth. Nasal resistance is also affected by physical exertion. Physical exertion is thought to decrease nasal resistance either by sympathetic stimulation or by a simple redistribution of blood to the heart, lungs and peripheral muscles.[15] In accordance with Ohm's Law, a decrease in nasal airway resistance requires less work to produce the same amount of flow, which is beneficial during times of physical exertion. This may also account for episodic symptomatic improvement in patients with fixed obstructive pathologies.

Many anatomic causes of nasal obstruction can be understood in the context of measures used to correct or compensate for the abnormal anatomy. The site of anatomic compromise can also be gleaned from the effect of nonsurgical maneuvers. For example, Portugal and colleagues[15] demonstrated a reduction in nasal airway resistance with external nasal dilators (also referred to as the Breathe-Right device), with better results in the Caucasian nose. The study was limited to only 20 subjects, 10 Caucasian and 10 African American, whose airway resistance and minimal cross-sectional areas were analyzed using anterior rhinomanometry and acoustic rhinometry at rest and 15 minutes after exercise. The Breathe-Right device was found to exert its main effect in the upper lateral cartilage region of the nasal valve, with an overall airway improvement of 21%.

Precise anatomic assessment is also important to predict which patients may benefit from improvement of nasal obstruction through rhinoplasty, and what maneuvers will be necessary.[4] Boccieri and colleagues[16] reported the use of spreader grafts in a series of 60 subjects undergoing primary rhinoplasty. All subjects fell into one of three groups who are prone to internal nasal valve collapse after primary rhinoplasty: those with narrow nose syndrome, with a narrow nasal vault and bulbous tip, and those with a crooked nose. Preoperative and postoperative rhinometric analysis indicated significant improvement in nasal valve obstruction, particularly in subjects with narrow nose syndrome or narrow nasal vault and bulbous tip. Subjects with a crooked nose had a less significant improvement. Boccieri and colleagues concluded that preoperative evaluation can identify patients who may be prone to nasal valve collapse after primary rhinoplasty, and that primary use of spreader grafts can support the internal nasal valve and alleviate need for a second surgery in the future.

Given the dynamic nature of the nasal valve, neuromuscular anatomic causes of nasal obstruction must also be considered. This may be a significant factor in patients with loss of facial musculature tone due to aging or facial paralysis. Facial paralysis results in a nonfunctional dilator naris muscle and aging can weaken the fibroareolar tissues of the nasal sidewalls, each leading to collapse of the nasal valve during inspiration.[4] The impact of facial musculature tone upon nasal obstruction is well illustrated by Vaiman and colleagues[17] who published two studies reporting on the treatment of nasal valve collapse with transcutaneous and intranasal electrical stimulation of the nasal musculature. The first was a prospective trial with electrotherapy versus placebo. Electrotherapy consisted of three 15-minute sessions per week for 10 weeks, with 10 to 12 months of follow-up. Sixty percent of subjects in the study group had a subjective improvement and 40% had objective improvement. Comparatively, 35% of the placebo group noted subjective improvement and 5% had objective improvement. Follow-up showed rapid decline in benefits and they concluded that electrotherapy alone was not a beneficial treatment of the nasal valve collapse. The second study built upon the first but focused more on muscle-building therapies. The report included three cohorts of subjects with clinical nasal valve collapse. Group one received transcutaneous and intranasal electrical stimulation of the nasal muscles only. For group two, treatment included biofeedback training and a home exercise program for specific nasal movements. Treatment for group three included the home exercises, electrical stimulation, and surface and intranasal electromyographic biofeedback-assisted specific strategies for nasal muscle education. Group two and three had 80% and 75% objective improvement, respectively. Group one had poorer results. They concluded that for select patients wanting to avoid surgery, relief of nasal valve collapse can be achieved with nonsurgical means.[18] This data exemplifies the significant contributions of nasal and facial neuromusculature toward patency of the nasal valve.

Sinonasal Inflammatory Disease

Allergic rhinitis is the most common allergic condition in the world, and nasal congestion is notable for one of its most prominent and troublesome symptoms.[19] Rhinitis patients appear to be more sensitive to decreases in cross-sectional nasal area. For example, nasal obstruction when lying down is a frequent complaint by patients. Nasal resistance is highest when the patient is in the supine position, and decreases as the head is elevated. This is most likely attributed to a nasal mucosal reaction to venous changes that alter local blood flow, secondary to compression of the neck veins or hydrostatic pressures.[20] When the patient is in the lateral decubitus position, the dependent inferior turbinate is engorged and the turbinate in the superior position is constricted. Two other studies attributed the increase in nasal obstruction while in the supine position to the activities of the central autonomic nervous system or the autonomic shoulder and axillary sensory information linked to nasal reflexes.[21] The perception of positional nasal obstruction is noted to be significantly higher in patients with rhinitis symptoms when compared with normals.[20]

A study by Ciprandi and colleagues[22] in June 2008 evaluated 100 subjects: 50 with short-term and 50 with long-term persistent allergic rhinitis. This study is the first to conclude that duration of persistent allergic rhinitis may lead to progressive worsening of nasal airflow, as determined by rhinomanometry (discussed later). It is important to recognize that asthma and allergic rhinitis are important comorbid factors, such that allergic rhinitis should be managed empirically in any patient with asthma and nasal obstructive symptoms while any additional workup is pending. The incidence of allergic rhinitis in patients with asthma may be as high as 80%.[23] Although a complete discussion of rhinosinusitis is beyond the scope of this issue, it should be noted that nasal obstruction is a major symptom in all forms, acute and chronic.[24]

Medical and Hormonal Causes

Because those with allergic rhinitis and chronic rhinosinusitis often self-medicate before specialty evaluation, patients must be queried regarding chronic intranasal decongestant use, including sympathomimetic amines (ephedrine/phenylephrine) and imidazoline derivatives (oxymetazoline and xylometazoline). These medications risk development of the syndrome of rhinitis medicamentosa with rebound nasal congestion, which typically occurs 5 to 7 days after use of the intranasal medication. Knipping and colleagues[25] note that a loss and destruction of ciliated epithelial cells results in the disruption of mucociliary clearance and an increase in vascular permeability resulting in interstitial edema.

Systemic medical therapies may result in increased nasal obstructive symptoms. The most common of these include antihypertensive medications such as reserpine, hydralazine, guanethidine, methyldopa, and prazosin. Beta-blockers, such as propranolol and nadolol, and antidepressants and antipsychotics, including thioridazine, chlordiazepoxide amitriptyline and perphenazine, can also cause congestion. Hypothyroidism may result in nasal obstruction. Chavanne[26] noticed an increase in nasal congestion and secretions in subjects who had undergone total thyroidectomy. The exact etiology of hypothyroid rhinitis is uncertain and is estimated to occur in approximately 40% to 60% of patients in a hypothyroid state.[27] One proposed mechanism of effect is secondary to vascular dilation of the nasal mucosa. Antithyroid medications can mimic these symptoms, which should resolve upon withdrawal of the offending substance.[28]

Rhinitis of pregnancy, also called rhinopathia gravidarum, has been frequently discussed in the literature; yet, the exact etiology of this is unknown. It is thought to occur in 5% to 32% of pregnant women, and is most prevalent during the first trimester. Isolated pregnancy rhinitis should resolve after the gestational period, such that ongoing symptoms should prompt additional workup. The assumed etiology is a combination of generalized increases in interstitial fluid volume, compounded by the direct effect of estrogen on the nasal mucosa, which causes increased vascularity and mucosal edema.[29] Electron micrographic and histochemical studies performed by Toppozada and colleagues[30] on the respiratory epithelium of pregnant women have suggested that an over activity of the parasympathetic system leading to increased glandular secretion and vascular congestion is responsible for the state of nasal congestion.

This over activity of the parasympathetic system may be an allergic response to placental proteins, fetal proteins, or a woman's own sex hormones. Bowser and Rie-derer[31] noted a possible direct influence of progesterone on fibroblasts, and therefore, on the consistency of the nasal extracellular matrix. Additionally, this group proposed that estrogen and progesterone might cause rhinopathic symptoms indirectly by changing the concentration of neurotransmitters (eg, substance P, nitric oxide) and their receptors. Wolstenholme and colleagues[32] recently studied 11 women on day 1 and 14 pre- and postcombined oral contraceptive therapy. These women had anterior rhinoscopy, peak inspiratory flow rate, acoustic rhinometry, anterior rhinomanometry, mucociliary clearance time, and rhinitis quality-of-life questionnaire scores recorded. The study concluded that modern day combined oral contraceptive pills have no effect on nasal physiology.

Traumatic Causes

Accidental trauma and sinonasal surgery may result in complications such as septal perforations, adhesions, nasal stenosis and empty nose syndrome. These conditions may precipitate obstructive symptoms through three mechanisms: (1) physical blockage of airflow, (2) induction of sinusitis, and (3) impaired sensation of airflow.

A detailed discussion of nasal trauma is beyond the scope of this issue, but it deserves mention that over resection of the inferior (or even middle) turbinates may result in empty nose syndrome,[33] which, paradoxically, presents with nasal dryness or a sensation of nasal congestion. Causes for the symptom of nasal obstruction in these patients include disruption of normal airflow patterns, lack of surface area responsible for sensation of airflow, and ozena. These observations underscore the need for turbinate preservation during rhinoplasty and sinus surgery.

Neoplastic Causes

The entire spectrum of sinonasal neoplasms may present with nasal obstruction, which is the most common presenting complaint. This symptom, which may be associated with other nonspecific symptoms such as unilateral epistaxis or anosmia, often triggers otolaryngology referral for endoscopy or imaging. It is also noteworthy that the diagnosis of malignancy is often delayed as the most common symptoms, including facial pain/numbness, nasal obstruction, and epistaxis, are vague from the patient's perspective.[34] Squamous cell carcinoma is the most common malignant tumor of the sinonasal tract. The most common benign tumors include osteomas, which are rarely the primary cause of nasal obstruction, and inverting papillomas, which may transition to squamous cell carcinoma in 5% to 15% of cases.[35,36] Two other entities deserve mention: juvenile nasopharyngeal angiofibroma and pyogenic granuloma. Juvenile nasopharyngeal angiofibroma must be considered in young patients with epistaxis. Nasal obstruction is still the most common symptom, seen in 80% to 90% of these cases. The finding of a large obstructing lesion along the anterior nasal septum, especially in a pregnant patient, likely represents a pyogenic granuloma,[37] which is a reparative vascular lesion rather than a true neoplasm.

Atypical and Idiopathic Lesions

Atypical inflammatory disorders including Wegener's granulomatosis, tuberculosis, sarcoidosis, rhinoscleroma, and rhinosporidiosis may present with nasal lesions, friable mucosa, or crusting, and hence, symptoms of obstruction. Cocaine abuse must be ruled out in patients with such findings. An important diagnosis to consider in the differential is extranodal NK/T-cell lymphoma, which may initially manifest as an intranasal purple granulomatous mass with bleeding. This rapidly progresses to widespread local tissue destruction involving the midface. A finding of nasopharyngeal lymphoid hypertrophy in an adult should be further investigated and an HIV test should be recommended. The prevalence of nasopharyngeal lymphoid hypertrophy in patients with early stages of HIV infection is anywhere from 56% to 88%. This hypertrophy and nasal obstruction may improve as the patient's immunocompromised state declines.[38]

HISTORY AND PHYSICAL EXAMINATION

A complete history and head and neck examination are critical to accurately diagnosing the underlying etiology of a patient's nasal obstructive symptoms. It is important to query patients about over the counter medication use, possible allergic triggers (eg, pets) and previous surgery, as some will deny prior aesthetic procedures. Observations that may be present on physical examination include midface deformities that may result from chronic mouth breathing. Patients with allergic rhinitis may exhibit the classic allergic shiners or allergic salute. Facial nerve function should be assessed, as paralysis of the splinting muscles of the nasal ala may result in a functional nasal airway obstruction. Middle ear effusions may be a manifestation of chronic nasopharyngeal inflammation, adenoid hypertrophy, or an obstructing mass near the eustachian tube. Purulent discharge or facial tenderness suggests sinusitis.

The nose should be examined with consideration of airflow dynamics and the sites of increased resistance. A suggested method is to focus on external support structures, followed by an assessment of internal support structures, and lastly evaluate internal soft- tissue structures. If the patient has a prior history of rhinoplasty, note if the patient's nasal bridge has been overly narrowed by osteotomies. Severe tip ptosis can also contribute to nasal airway obstruction because it may redirect airflow superiorly, which can be perceived as nasal airway obstruction. If nasal tip ptosis is indeed contributing to symptoms, tilting the tip superiorly will considerably improve the patient's symptoms. The patient should be observed during quiet and deep inspiration and the physician should assess upper and lower lateral cartilage competency. Early collapse during inspiration would suggest valve incompetence.

The first area of interest endonasally is the internal nasal valve which is the smallest cross-sectional area in the nasal cavity. Care must be taken not to distort the valve with the nasal speculum, and often the valve can be adequately examined by simply lifting the nasal tip superiorly.[39] The Cottle maneuver, a test of nasal valve integrity, can be performed by retracting the cheek laterally, pulling the upper lateral cartilage away from the septum and widening the internal nasal valve angle (see **Fig. 2**A–C). If the patient's symptoms are relieved with this maneuver, this suggests the cause of the nasal airway obstruction is related to the nasal valve area (eg, dorsal septal deviation, lack of upper lateral cartilage integrity). False negatives can be seen with synechiae in the nasal valve which prevents the valve from opening during the maneuver.[39] Aggressive lateral osteotomies can result in over medialization of the ascending process of the maxilla resulting in a decrease in the cross-sectional area of the posterior lateral nasal valve area, also resulting in a false negative finding during the Cottle maneuver. Another simple technique involves using a cotton swab or nasal speculum to lateralize the upper lateral cartilage from inside the nose, and the patient is again asked if their symptoms are improved. This technique enables direct observation of the nasal valve area as it widened.

Complete examination of the septum, turbinates, meati, and internal valve is best accomplished with diagnostic nasal endoscopy. This should be performed before and after decongestion (**Fig. 3**A, B) to assess the decongestant response and to

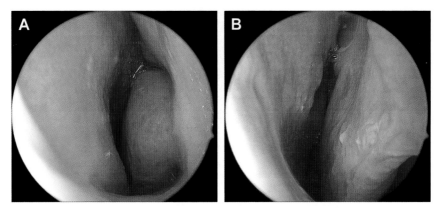

Fig. 3. The inferior turbinate before (*A*) and after (*B*) decongestion with oxymetazoline.

rule out posterior septal deviations, middle turbinate resection or scarring to the lateral nasal wall, inflammatory disease, polyps, foreign bodies, and neoplasms. If the nasal airway obstruction improves with decongestion alone, this suggests a mucosal inflammatory disorder of the inferior turbinates.[40] No response suggests the etiology of the obstruction is of a rigid, structural nature such as nasal valve obstruction, septal deviation, or bony hypertrophy of the inferior turbinate. It should be noted that some mucosal inflammatory disorders may also exhibit lack of decongestive response, including rhinitis medicamentosa or diffuse nasal polyposis. Recently, Lanfranchi and colleagues[41] published a report on the importance of nasal endoscopy in the preoperative examination of patients with nasal obstruction who present for rhinoplasty. This series of 96 subjects undergoing rhinoplasty revealed that preoperative endoscopy allowed the diagnosis of pathology requiring additional surgery in 28 subjects (30%). The pathologies included concha bullosa, posterior septal deviations, adenoid hypertrophy, choanal stenosis, and one intranasal tumor. During endoscopy, the surgeon must maintain vigilance to rule out neoplasia (**Fig. 4**) and to recognize subtle signs of atypical inflammatory disease such as mucosal nodularity, crusting, friable mucosa, or synechiae. An algorithm is presented (**Fig. 5**).

Radiologic Evaluation

Because the source of obstruction is not always evident by patient history and physical, radiography may be required to assist with diagnosis. CT can be used to evaluate structural/bony abnormalities such as a deviated septum, nasal bone fractures, choanal atresia, and sinus disease. CT may also reveal unexpected anatomic findings such as concha bullosa of the inferior turbinate or foreign body. MRI, because of its soft tissue detail, is better suited for evaluating the integrity of the dura and for further assessment of certain nasal masses (such as encephalocele or glioma).

Objective Evaluation and Diagnostic Studies

Although subjective evaluation of nasal obstruction can be accomplished using a nasal obstruction visual analog scale (NO-VAS),[2] it is often preferable to obtain quantitative objective assessment. Hygrometry was one of the first objective measures of the nasal airway. This technique was described by Zwaardemaker in 1894 and involved having the patient breathe onto a mirror. The diameter of the fog produced by each nostril was compared.[42] In 1902, Spiess described the "hum-test," a technique where he

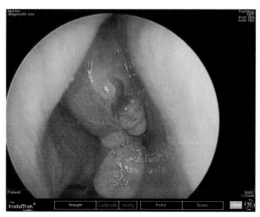

Fig. 4. Diagnostic nasal endoscopy in a subject whose only complaint was nasal obstruction. Findings revealed inverting papilloma.

used the change in the timbre of sound produced during humming while externally occluding the decongested nasal side to assess nasal airway patency.[43]

Today, methods for objective assessment of nasal airway include:

- Peak nasal inspiratory flow (PNIF)
- Acoustic rhinometry (AR)
- Rhinomanometry (RM)

Software-based analysis of acoustic signals is also in evolution. These objective measures have uses in both research, and less frequently, in clinical settings. For

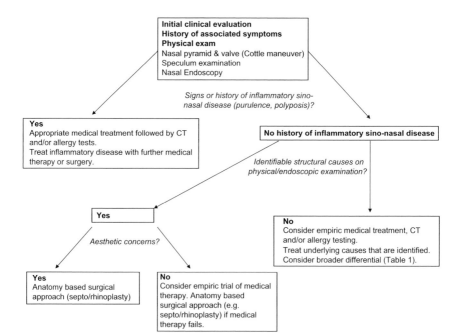

Fig. 5. Algorithm for differential diagnosis of nasal airway obstruction.

example, these studies can be used pre- and postdecongestion in an attempt to predict the efficacy of certain medical and surgical therapies. Lund stresses the importance of objective testing because of the high patient dissatisfaction rate (30%) after surgery to resolve nasal airway obstruction.[44] Acoustic rhinometry and rhinomanometry can also be used for nasal provocational studies in patients with suspected allergic rhinitis and recently has been used for assisting in the diagnosis of obstructive sleep apnea and sleep disordered breathing. These studies are commonly used in the research setting, but clinical use is not widespread in the United States due to expense, availability of equipment, variability of operator, and inconsistencies with consensus data correlating subjective measures with objective measures.[2,45]

Peak Nasal Inspiratory Flow

PNIF is a noninvasive, easy to perform method commonly used to assess nasal patency. It is a physiologic measure indicating the peak nasal airflow in liters per minute achieved during maximal forced nasal inspiration.[46] Given that the transnasal pressure differences are not recorded, PNIF is thought to be susceptible to high variability based on effort and cooperation from the subject and correct instructions from the investigator.[2,46] This use of maximum effort also increases the incidence of turbulent airflow. Another concern with PNIFs is the lack of this measurement representing true physiologic conditions, as normal breathing starts at a significantly lower tidal volume.[46] Ultimately, the method is suggested to be reliable for assessment of nasal patency as it has proved to be reproducible and in concordance with other objective tests. Furthermore, respiratory comorbidity could potentially affect the PNIF measurements by limiting the inspiratory effort.

Acoustic Rhinometry

In 1989, Hilberg and colleagues[43] were the first to use AR to measure the cross-sectional area in the nasal airway. AR is a simple, noninvasive, and relatively cheap way to measure nasal airway cross-sectional area as a function of longitudinal distance along the nasal passageway following the path of an acoustic impulse. It is the most common method used for measurements of nasal cavity geometry.[47] Nasal passage volumes can be calculated from contiguous cross-sectional values.[43] The method is appropriate for anatomic assessment and structure of the nasal airway, drug actions and surgical changes in the nasal cavity including change in the mucovascular components of the nasal valve area, and changes based on certain pathology such as nasal polyposis or septal deviation.[2,47,48]

The technology of AR was originally devised for oil investigation, however, it wasn't until the 1970s that it was first used in the field of medicine to perform measurements in the distal airway.[49] The acoustic rhinometer consists of a sound source, wave tube, microphone, filter, amplifier, digital convertor, and a computer. A sound wave is transmitted into the nasal cavity which is then reflected back from the nasal passages and converted into digital impulses, which are then constructed on a rhinogram.[50] This rhinogram provides a two-dimensional anatomic assessment of the nasal airway. The cross-sectional area of the nose differs at different points from the nasal rim, and these variances are detected by changes in acoustic impedance. Each notch on the rhinogram represents a different anatomic constriction in the nasal cavity (**Fig. 6**).[50] The first notch represents the nasal valve and is usually the minimal cross-sectional area (MCV) in the normal nose. The second notch represents anterior portions of the inferior turbinate or middle turbinate, while the third notch is estimated to be in the area of the middle/posterior end of the middle turbinate.[51] Each notch identifies a site of limitation of nasal airflow and can be used to locate the site of obstruction in the nose (see **Fig. 6**).

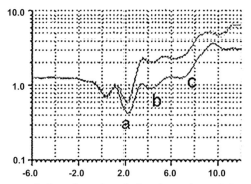

Fig. 6. Acoustic rhinogram before (*lower*) and after (*upper*) nasal decongestion. The x-axis reflects the distance from the nostril and the y-axis is the cross-sectional area of the nasal airway. Note the increase in cross-sectional area after decongestion, most pronounced at notch (b) and (c). Notch (a) represents the MCA at the nasal valve. Notch (b) represents cross-sectional area at the anterior portions of the inferior turbinate and middle turbinate. Notch (c) reflects the area of the middle/posterior end of the middle turbinate.

AR has been independently validated against other anatomic measures and standardized values have been established by several authors.[47,52] A high correlation of cross-sectional area has been found when comparing acoustic rhinometry to MRI after nasal decongestion[47,53] and CT for accuracy of cross-sectional area measurements in the nose based on cadaver studies.[47] With technological advancements, CT volumetry (CTV) has been noted to be among the best imaging modalities available for evaluating the nasal cavity and paranasal sinus geometry with a phantom test revealing less than 1% error in segmented compared with actual volumes.[47] For this reason, Dastidar and colleagues[47,54] conducted a study in 1999 to compare 48 nasal cavities with nasal stuffiness via measurements with acoustic rhinometry versus high-resolution CTV. MCAs and volumes were measured and compared by way of each method. Measurements of volume were found to have a strong correlation that was statistically significant ($P<.05$) in the anterior and mid-nasal cavities, but became less accurate posteriorly. Others have also suggested that measurements from the posterior nasal cavity are unreliable due to a loss of acoustic energy resulting in underestimation.[55] In the study comparing AR and CTV, measurements of MCAs were surprisingly poorly correlated between each of the methods.[47]

At present, close to two decades after its introduction, AR is a popular method used to evaluate nasal patency in the research setting. It has several clinical applications, especially in determining objective improvement after surgery or nasal steroid therapy. Difficulties in using AR in the clinical setting include continued adjustments of technique and validation, and inconsistency in user operation.[55]

Rhinomanometry

RM is a functional assessment of airflow and involves measurement of transnasal pressure and airflow. From these measurements one can assess the mean pressure, volume, work (pressure×flow) and resistance (pressure/flow) associated with each breath. Resistance from each side of the nose can be compared with each other and with total nasal resistance, enabling the physician to identify how each nasal passage is contributing to the patient's complaint. The resulting plot, with the x-axis representing the pressure differential and the y-axis representing flow, produces an

S-shaped curve. The most common method of reporting results is with inspiratory airflow. The machine consists of a pressure transducer for measuring posterior nasal pressure, a pneumotachometer for measurement of flow, a mask for measurement of anterior nasal pressure and flow, and a computer for converting these measurements into digital signals.

In RM, posterior nasal pressure is measured in one of three ways. Anterior RM, introduced by Coutade[44] in 1902, involves placement of a transducer in the nostril not being tested. Because there is no flow in this nostril, the pressure at the anterior end of this nostril is equal to the pressure in the posterior end of this nostril. Transnasal pressure differences and nasal airflow are recorded at the same time for each side and the dynamic changes of airway resistance are assessed.[46] This is the most common method used because it is usually well tolerated and it is easier for the patient to cooperate. A limitation of anterior rhinomanometry includes the inability of accurate measurements with septal perforations. Another disadvantage is that a direct measurement of total nasal resistance cannot be made because each nostril is measured separately. Estimations of total nasal resistance can be obtained by calculations; however, these results are not as accurate as direct measurement.

Another method of measuring the nasal pressure differential is with posterior (peroral) RM, introduced by Spiess[44] in 1899. With this method, the pressure detector is in the posterior oropharynx by way of tubing passed through the mouth. It is only method which can accurately assess the contribution of adenoid hypertrophy to nasal airway obstruction, however it is not tolerated as well as anterior RM. The third method of measuring transnasal pressure is postnasal RM. This involves placement of a posterior nasopharyngeal tube by way of the test or non-test nostril. Postnasal RM is also not commonly used secondary to difficulties with patient tolerance.

During RM, airflow can be generated by active or passive means. Active rhinomanometry, the most common technique used today, involves using the patient's own respiratory efforts as the source of airflow. Passive RM involves pumping air through the nose at a known rate. This method does not imitate true nasal physiology and has been found to reflexively increase mucosal thickness, which could affect the accuracy of its measurements.[49]

The measurement of airflow during RM can be accomplished by direct or indirect means. With direct methods, airflow is measured at the nasal outlet by way of a nozzle or mask. Masks are most commonly used today because the nozzle can alter the relationship of the nasal ala with airflow.[49] Indirect methods of airflow measurement are slightly more complicated, using body plethysmography to measure changes in intrathoracic volume to extrapolate air flow.

Odiosoft Rhino

Odiosoft rhino (OR) is a new objective technique that converts the frequency of sound generated by nasal airflow into cross-sectional area measurements. The theory behind the technology is that nasal airflow generates a higher frequency sound as turbulence increases.[56] This noninvasive technique, developed by Seren,[57] involves a microphone, nasal probe, sound card, and a computer. The nasal probe is connected to a microphone situated 1 cm from the nostril, and the subject is asked to close the other nostril, avoiding any distortion of the test nostril. The sound created during breathing is directly measured with the odiosoft rhino technique, unlike acoustic rhinometry which measures reflected sounds to calculate nasal cross-sectional area. A recent study published in 2006 shows this method provides a sensitive and specific assessment of nasal airway patency with better correlation to patient symptom scores when compared with AR.[58] Although these findings are encouraging, the search continues for an ideal modality of objective testing.

Variability with Objective Testing

There are several factors which have the ability to cause inconsistencies with objective testing. Hasegawa and Kern[59] noted that the nasal cycle could cause variations in unilateral readings; therefore, most authorities in objective nasal airway testing recommend nasal decongestion before testing to reduce this variability. Several studies have shown a reduction of nasal resistance with exercise[59,60] and an increase in resistance with supine position,[61] aspirin use,[62] and smoking.[63] Ethnicity can also be a source of variability in the nasal airway. Ohki and colleagues[64] found the greatest nasal resistance in Caucasians, intermediate resistance in Asians, and the lowest nasal resistance in African Americans. Morgan and colleagues[65] were able to show similar ethnic trends with nasal cross-sectional area using AR.

In 1981, to minimize the variability of RM, the International Committee on Standardization of Rhinomanometry came out with a set of guidelines.[66] Active, anterior RM was labeled as the preferred method of testing. Testing should be performed during the same time of day, after the patient has been resting for at least 30 minutes, and in an environmentally controlled room without any external sunlight. The pressure transducer should be sealed to the nostril with tape without any deformation of the nostril and a transparent face mask should be used to ensure no kinking in tubing. Recommendations for standardization of data reporting suggested pressure should be reported in units Pascal (Pa), flow reported in units cm^3/second, and resistance reported in units Pa/cm^3/sec. The committee also recommended that resistance results be reported at a standard pressure of 150 Pa or "Radius 2" (the intersecting point on the rhinometry graph between 200 cm^3/sec and 200 Pa).

In 2005, the most recent consensus statement for both AR and RM suggested additional guidelines in an attempt to further standardize objective nasal airway testing.[67] The committee recommended using trained technicians, citing a 3- to 8-fold increase in accuracy. They also made recommendations for standardized decongestion, using two applications that were 5 minutes apart. For those patients who could not generate pressures of 150 Pa, the committee agreed with reporting resistance at 75,100 and 150 Pa, as long as the specific pressure was reported. The committee also recommended a standard reference resistance device for RM. The European Rhinologic Society has also suggested a similar standard nose calibration device for AR.[21]

COMPARISON OF ASSESSMENT TOOLS

Schumacher[21] suggests that since RM is a functional test of nasal airway, it may be a better screening tool for nasal airway obstruction. A complimentary role for AR has been suggested as it is better suited for the identification of the site of obstruction.[68] Scadding found comparable results between the two modalities when used for screening, however AR had better patient tolerance and was easier to perform.[69] Passali and colleagues[70] found that RM was more sensitive and specific for patients with functional nasal obstruction (such as rhinitis). In contrast, AR was found to be more sensitive and specific when evaluating nasal airway obstruction secondary to structural abnormalities. In Passali's study, the results of both objective tests had no correlation with either mucociliary transport time or subject symptom scores.

There are several advantages and disadvantages to each method of nasal airway testing. Acoustic rhinometry is rapid (usually takes 10 seconds for each nostril), minimally invasive, and can identify the exact site of obstruction in the nose.

Disadvantages include expense and availability, although the cost of acoustic rhinometry is declining and is currently less expensive than rhinomanometry.[71] Acoustic rhinometry is also unable to accurately measure beyond narrow apertures (ie, the nasal valve) and is less accurate in the posterior aspect of the nasal cavity.[67]

Advantages to rhinomanometry are that it is a more functional test, and in certain circumstances, can be done on both nostrils simultaneously. Disadvantages include time (usually takes 20–30 minutes), and an inability to identify the site of obstruction.[71] Rhinomanometry also cannot be used in cases of total or near-total nasal obstruction because of the patient's inability to generate sufficient nasal airway pressure and flow.

There are some inherent flaws in both rhinomanometry and acoustic rhinometry. Both tests fail to take tip ptosis or alar collapse into account, as measurements are taken distal to this site. Both testing methodologies also have problems with variability, which is largely operator dependent. Another concerning flaw of both methods is their poor correlation with patient complaint scores. Tomkinson and Eccles[72] found poor correlation between subjective patient complaints and acoustic rhinometry, despite significant correlation of acoustic rhinometry with CT, MRI and rhinoscopy. Gordon and colleagues[73] found that 22% of subjects undergoing septoplasty had persistent subjective obstruction postoperatively despite showing improved rhinomanometric scores. Because of these inconsistencies, objective testing cannot reliably be used to predict successful outcomes after medical or surgical therapy. Although these tests do not provide absolute values to correlate with symptoms, some argue that those patients with high end resistance/cross-sectional obstruction values are more likely to have subjective improvement after intervention.

Several recent studies have attempted to further elucidate the correlation between objective and subjective testing of nasal obstruction. Kjaergard and colleagues[2] sought to determine the correlation between NO-VAS and AR and PNIF. This cross-sectional study included 2523 consecutive subjects referred to the Ear, Nose, and Throat Department in Sørlandet Hospital, Kristiansand, Norway, for evaluation of chronic nasal or sleep related complaints. Three AR curves from both nasal cavities were averaged to get a mean curve for each side, to account for variations in the nasal cycle. Recordings were obtained from the anterior segment (0–3 cm) which represented the nasal vestibule and nasal cavities, and the middle segment (35.2 cm) which represented the turbinate region where the mucosa has a large congestive capacity. MCA (cm^2) between 0 and 3 cm (MCA1), 3 to 5.2 cm (MCA2), and 0 to 5.2 cm (MCA3) behind the nostril and nasal cavity volumes (NCV; cm^3) between 0 and 3 cm (NCV1) and 3 to 5.2 cm (NCV2) behind the nostril were also obtained. For PNIF, three satisfactory maximal inspirations were obtained with the subject in an upright position. Subjects were symptomatically stratified in three categories of increasing severity based on NO-VAS. NO-VAS category significantly correlated with five of six objective measures of nasal obstruction: MCA2 ($P<.001$), MCA3 ($P<.001$), NCV1 ($P<.001$), NCV2 ($P = .002$) and PNIF ($P<.001$). The lack of association between MCA1 and NO-VAS was explained by the authors due to the functional valve area being located in the middle segment of the nasal cavity in a large number of subjects in this study. The study ultimately demonstrated a highly significant association between the subjective sensation of nasal obstruction and the corresponding measures for area, space, and airflow. Despite the statistically significant associations between the objective and subjective measures of nasal obstruction, the correlation coefficients remained relatively low ($r^2 = 0.13$–0.35) in this study. Limitations from this study also include possible selection bias, as the sample included a preponderance of men who were being evaluated for sleep related disorders or chronic nasal complaints. Smokers were also overrepresented.

Tahamiler and colleagues[56] compared OR with RM in 79 normal subjects. NO-VAS data was also collected. The authors observed a statistically significant correlation ($P<.05$) in bilateral nares between OR findings and expiration RM at 2000 to 4000 Hz and 4000 to 6000 Hz. NO-VAS of nasal obstruction and OR expiratory results were significantly correlated bilaterally only at the 2000 to 4000 Hz frequency interval. There were no correlations noted between NO-VAS, OR, and anterior RM at any inspiratory levels.[56]

In summary, the current literature provides provocative data suggesting that objective measurement of nasal obstruction is indeed possible. Further research is necessary, however, to establish an objective method that is rapid, cost effective, well tolerated by patients, and anatomically precise. In the meantime, clinical assessment, including nasal endoscopy, remains the cornerstone of diagnosis.

REFERENCES

1. Kimmelman CP. The problem of nasal obstruction. Otolaryngol Clin North Am 1989;22(2):253–64.
2. Kjaergaard T, Cvancarova M, Steinsvag SK. Does nasal obstruction mean that the nose is obstructed? Laryngoscope 2008;118(8):1476–81.
3. Bridger GP. Physiology of the nasal valve. Arch Otolaryngol 1970;92:543–53.
4. Wittkopf M, Wittkopf J, Ries RW. The diagnosis and treatment of nasal valve collapse. Curr Opin Otolaryngol Head Neck Surg 2008;16(1):10–3.
5. Howard BK, Rohrich RJ. Understanding the nasal airway: principles and practice. Plast Reconstr Surg 2002;109(3):1128–46.
6. Kerr A. Rhinology. In: Kerr AG, editor. Scott-Brown's otolaryngology. 6th edition. Oxford (UK): Butterworth-Heinemann; 1997.
7. Kasperbauer JL, Kern EB. Nasal valve physiology: implications in nasal surgery. Otolaryngol Clin North Am 1987;20(4):699–719.
8. Chu CT, Lebowitz RA, Jacobs JB. An analysis of sites of disease in revision endoscopic sinus surgery. Am J Rhinol 1997;11(4):287–91.
9. Ulusoy B, Arbag H, Sari O, et al. Evaluation of the effects of nasal septal deviation and its surgery on nasal mucociliary clearance in both nasal cavities. Am J Rhinol 2007;21(2):180–3.
10. Perić A, Sotirović J, Baletić N, et al. Concha bullosa and the nasal middle meatus obstructive syndrome. Vojnosanit Pregl 2008;65(3):255–8.
11. Bolger WE, Butzin CA, Parson DS. Paranasal sinus bony anatomic variations and mucosal abnormalities: CT analysis for endoscopic sinus surgery. Laryngoscope 1991;101:56–64.
12. Rodrigo TJP, Alvarez AI, Casas RC, et al. A giant bilateral concha bullosa causing nasal obstruction. Acta Otorrinolaringol Esp 1999;50(6):490–2.
13. Stallman JS, Lobo JN, Som PM. The incidence of concha bullosa and its relationship to nasal septal deviation and paranasal sinus disease. AJNR Am J Neuroradiol 2004;25:1613–8.
14. Lang C, Grutzenmacher S, Mlynski B, et al. Investigating the nasal cycle using endoscopy, rhinoresistometry, and acoustic rhinometry. Laryngoscope 2003;113(2):284–9.
15. Portugal LG, Mehta RH, Smith BE, et al. Objective assessment of the breatheright device during exercise in adult males. Am J Rhinol 1997;11(5):393–7.
16. Boccieri A, Macro C, Pascali M. The use of spreader grafts in primary rhinoplasty. Ann Plast Surg 2005;55(2):127–31.

17. Vaiman M, Shlamkovich N, Eviatar E, et al. Treatment of nasal valve collapse with transcutaneous and intranasal electric stimulation. Ear Nose Throat J 2004; 83(11):757–62, 764.

18. Vaiman M, Shlamkovick N, Kessler A, et al. Biofeedback training of nasal muscles using internal and external surface electromyography of the nose. Am J Otol 2005;26(5):302–7.

19. The Allergy Report. American Academy of Allergy Asthma and Immunology. Available at: http://www.theallergyreport.com/reportindex.html. Accessed October 27, 2008.

20. Roithmann R, Demeneghi P, Faggiano R, et al. Effects of posture change on nasal patency. Rev Bras Otorrinolaringol 2005;71(4):478–84.

21. Schumacher MJ. Rhinomanometry. J Allergy Clin Immunol 1989;83(4):711–8.

22. Ciprandi G, Cirillo I, Pistorio A, et al. Relationship between rhinitis duration and worsening of nasal function. Otolaryngol Head Neck Surg 2008;138(6): 725–9.

23. Shimojo N, Suzuki S, Tomiita M, et al. Allergic rhinitis in children: association with asthma. Clin Exp Allergy Rev 2004;4(1):21–5.

24. Rosenfeld RM, Andes D, Bhattacharyya N. Clinical practice guideline: adult sinusitis. Otolaryngol Head Neck Surg 2007;137(3 Suppl):S1–31.

25. Knipping S, Holzhausen HJ, Goetze G, et al. Rhinitis medicamentosa: electron microscopic changes of human nasal mucosa. Otolaryngol Head Neck Surg 2007;136(1):57–61.

26. Chavanne L. Secretion nasale et glande thyroide. Otorhinolaryngol Int 1936;20: 653–64.

27. Gupta OP, Bhatia PL, Agarwal MK, et al. Nasal, pharyngeal, and laryngeal manifestations of hypothyroidism. Ear Nose Throat J 1977;56(9):349–56.

28. Mabry RL. Rhinitis medicamentosa: the forgotten factor in nasal obstruction. Southampt Med J 1982;75(7):817–9.

29. Hillman EJ. Otolaryngologic manifestations of pregnancy. Available at: http://www.bcm.edu/oto/grand/2295.html.

30. Toppozada H, Michaels L, Toppozada M, et al. The human respiratory nasal mucosa in pregnancy. An electron microscopic and histochemical study. J Laryngol Otol 1982;96:613–26.

31. Bowser C, Riederer A. Detection of progesterone receptors in connective tissue cells of the lower nasal turbinates in women. Laryngorhinootologie 2001;80(4): 182–6.

32. Wostenholme CR, Philpott CM, Oloto EJ. Does the use of the combined oral contraceptive pill cause changes in the nasal physiology in young women? Am J Rhinol 2006;20(2):238–40.

33. Moore EJ, Kern EB. Atrophic rhinitis: a review of 242 cases. Am J Rhinol 2001; 15(6):355–61.

34. Hulett KJ, Stankiewicz JA. Primary sinus surgery. In: Cummings CW, Haughey BH, Regan Thomas J, et al, editors. Cummings: otolaryngology head & neck surgery. 4th edition. St. Louis (MO): Mosby; 2005.

35. Hyams VJ. Papillomas of the nasal cavity and paranasal sinuses: a clinicopathologic study of 315 cases. Ann Otol Rhinol Laryngol 1971;80:192–206.

36. Myers EN, Fernau JL, Johnson JT, et al. Management of inverted papilloma. Laryngoscope 1990;100:481–90.

37. Tami TA. Granulomatous diseases and chronic rhinosinusitis. Otolaryngol Clin North Am 2005;38(6):1267–78.

38. Gurney TA, Murr AH. Otolaryngologic manifestations of human immunodeficiency virus infection. Otolaryngol clin North Am 2003;36:607–24.
39. Kridel RWH, Kelly PE, MacGregor AR. The nasal septum. In: Cummings: otolaryngology, head and neck surgery. 4th edition. St. Louis (MO): Mosby; 2005.
40. Corey JP. A comparison of the nasal cross-sectional areas and volumes obtained with acoustic rhinometry and magnetic resonance imaging. Otolaryngol Head Neck Surg 1997;117:349.
41. Lanfranchi PV, Steiger J, Soprano A, et al. Diagnostic and surgical endoscopy in functional rhinoplasty. Facial Plast Surg 2004;20:207–15.
42. Malm L. Rhinomanometric assessment for rhinologic surgery. Ear Nose Throat J 1992;71:11.
43. Hilberg O, Jackson AC, Swift DL, et al. Acoustic rhinometry: evaluation of nasal cavity geometry by acoustic reflection. J Appl Phys 1989;66:295–303.
44. Lund VJ. Objective assessment of nasal obstruction. Otolaryngol Clin North Am 1989;22(2):279–90.
45. Schumacher MJ. Nasal congestion and airway obstruction: the validity of available objective and subjective measures. Curr Allergy Asthma Rep 2002;2(3):245–51.
46. Bermuller C, Kirsche H, Rettinger G, et al. Diagnostic accuracy of peak nasal inspiratory flow and rhinomanometry in functional rhinosurgery. Laryngoscope 2008;118(4):605–10.
47. Dastidar P, Numminen J, Heinonen T, et al. Nasal airway volumetric measurement using segmented HRCT images and acoustic rhinometry. Am J Rhinol 1999; 13(2):97–103.
48. Roithmann R, Chapnik J, Zamel N, et al. Acoustic rhinometric assessment of the nasal valve. Am J Rhinol 1997;11(5):379–85.
49. Zeiders J, Pallanch JF, McCaffrey TV. Evaluation of nasal breathing function with objective airway testing. In: Cummings: otolaryngology, head and neck surgery. 4th edition. St. Louis (MO): Mosby; 2005.
50. Lal D, Corey JP. Acoustic rhinometry and its uses in rhinology and diagnosis of nasal obstruction. Facial Plast Surg Clin North Am 2004;12(4):397–405.
51. Corey JP, Gungor A, Nelson R, et al. Normative standards for nasal cross sectional areas by race as measured by acoustic rhinometry. Otolaryngol Head Neck Surg 1998;119(4):389–93.
52. Millqvist E, Bende M. Reference values for acoustic rhinometry in subjects without nasal symptoms. Am J Rhinol 1998;12:341–3.
53. Hilberg O, Jensen FT, Pederson OF. Nasal airway geometry: comparison between acoustic reflections and magnetic resonance scanning. J Appl Phys 1993;75(6):2811–9.
54. Min YG, Jang YJ. Measurements of cross-sectional area of the nasal cavity by acoustic rhinometry and CT scanning. Laryngoscope 1995;105:757–9.
55. Hilberg O. Objective measurement of nasal airway dimensions using acoustic rhinometry: methodological and clinical aspects. Allergy 2002;57(Suppl 70):5–39.
56. Tahamiler R, Edizer DT, Canakcioglus S, et al. Odiosoft-Rhino versus rhinomanometry in healthy subjects. Acta Otolaryngol 2008;128(2):181–5.
57. Seren F. Frequency spectra of normal expiratory nasal sound. Am J Rhinol 2005; 19:257–61.
58. Tahamiler R, Edizer DT, Canakcioglu S, et al. Nasal sound analysis: a new method for evaluating nasal obstruction in allergic rhinitis. Laryngoscope 2006;116(11): 2050–4.

59. Hasegawa M, Kern EB. The effect of breath holding, hyperventilation, and exercise on nasal resistance. Rhinology 1978;16(4):243–9.
60. Cole P, Forsyth R, Haight JS. Effects of cold air and exercise on nasal patency. Ann Otol Rhinol Laryngol 1983;92(2 Pt 1):196–8.
61. Haight JS, Cole P. Unilateral nasal resistance and asymmetrical body pressure. J Otolaryngol 1986;15(Suppl 16):3.
62. Jones AS, Lancer JM, Moir AA, et al. Effect of aspirin on nasal resistance to airflow. Br Med J 1985;290:1171–3.
63. Dessi P, Sambuc R, Moulin G, et al. Effect of heavy smoking on nasal resistance. Acta Otolaryngol 1994;114(3):305–10.
64. Ohki M, Naito K, Cole P. Dimensions and resistances of the human nose: racial differences. Laryngoscope 1991;101(3):276–8.
65. Morgan NJ, MacGregor FB, Birchall MA, et al. Racial differences in nasal fossa dimensions determined by acoustic rhinometry. Rhinology 1995;33(4):224–8.
66. Kern EB. Committee report on standardization of rhinomanometry. Rhinology 1981;19(4):231–6.
67. Clement PA, Gordts F. Standardization Committee on Objective Assessment of the Nasal Airway, IRS, and ERS. Consensus report on acoustic rhinometry and rhinomanometry. Rhinology 2005;43(3):169–79.
68. Roithmann R, Cole P, Chapnik J, et al. Acoustic rhinometry, rhinomanometry, and the sensation of nasal patency: a correlative study. J Otolaryngol 1994;23(6): 454–8.
69. Scadding GK, Darby YC, Austin CE. Acoustic rhinometry compared with anterior rhinomanometry in the assessment of the response to nasal allergen challenge. Clin Otolaryngol Allied Sci 1994;19(5):451–4.
70. Passali D, Mezzedimi C, Passali GC, et al. The role of rhinomanometry, acoustic rhinometry, and mucociliary transport time in the assessment of nasal patency. Ear Nose Throat J 2000;79(5):397–400.
71. Corey JP. Acoustic rhinometry: should we be using it? Curr Opin Otolaryngol Head Neck Surg 2006;14(1):29–34.
72. Tomkinson A, Eccles R. Comparison of the relative abilities of acoustic rhinometry, rhinomanometry and the visual analog scale in detecting change in the nasal cavity in a healthy adult population. Am J Rhinol 1996;10:161–5.
73. Gordon AS, McCaffrey TV, Kern EB, et al. Rhinomanometry for preoperative and postoperative assessment of nasal obstruction. Otolaryngol Head Neck Surg 1989;101:20–6.

Endoscopic Sinus Surgery in the Management of Nasal Obstruction

Bruce K. Tan, MD, Andrew P. Lane, MD*

KEYWORDS

- Endoscopic sinus surgery • Nasal obstruction
- Nasal congestion • Outcomes • Chronic rhinosinusitis

NASAL OBSTRUCTION AMONG PATIENTS WHO HAVE CHRONIC RHINOSINUSITIS

Nasal obstruction is the most common and severe complaint among patients who have chronic rhinosinusitis (CRS).[1–3] The prevalence of nasal obstruction among patients undergoing functional endoscopic sinus surgery (FESS) for CRS is reported to be between 83.5% and 98%.[4,5] When assessing individual symptoms of CRS, nasal obstruction often ranks highest in patient-reported symptom severity.[2,3,6] Furthermore, patients who have CRS with nasal polyposis seem to have a statistically higher incidence of nasal obstruction when compared with patients without nasal polyposis.[7]

Consequently, nasal obstruction is one of six major symptom criteria adopted by the 2003 American Academy of Otolaryngology–Head and Neck Surgery (AAOHNS) Rhinosinusitis Task Force (RSTF) for the diagnosis of CRS.[8] In their recent update, the 2007 AAOHNS sinusitis practice guideline continued to identify nasal obstruction as one of the major symptom criteria used to diagnose CRS with high sensitivity.[9] Given its prevalence in patients who have CRS, it also constitutes one of the specific symptoms evaluated by validated instruments developed to measure disease-specific symptoms in CRS, including the Rhinosinusitis Symptom Inventory (RSI)[10] and the Chronic Sinusitis Survey (CSS).[11]

Although studies comparing objective or subjective assessments of nasal obstruction in patients who have CRS with those of matched normal controls are still lacking, studies demonstrate subjective and objective improvements in patients who have CRS after medical[12] and surgical[5,13–15] therapy.

The authors have no financial interests in the studies mentioned in this article, the subject matter, or materials discussed in this article.

Department of Otolaryngology–Head and Neck Surgery, Johns Hopkins University School of Medicine, 601 North Caroline Street, Baltimore, MD 21287, USA

* Corresponding author.

E-mail address: alane3@jhmi.edu (A.P. Lane).

Otolaryngol Clin N Am 42 (2009) 227–240

doi:10.1016/j.otc.2009.01.012

0030-6665/09/$ – see front matter © 2009 Elsevier Inc. All rights reserved.

SENSATION OF NASAL AIRFLOW

The mechanisms used by the nasal airway to perceive nasal airflow still remain under investigation. The sensation of airflow is thought to be mediated by tactile and thermoreceptors located in the skin of the nasal vestibule and the mucosa of the nasal cavum. The sensitivity of these receptors has been shown to decrease in an anterior-to-posterior direction, with a minimum detected airflow velocity of 6.5 ms^{-1} at the nasal vestibule and 19.2 ms^{-1} in the posterior nose.[16] These receptors are thought to originate from ophthalmic and maxillary branches of the trigeminal nerve, because topical anesthesia of these branches results in the sensation of nasal obstruction.[17]

Although the exact receptor for nasal airflow sensation is still unknown, the effect of menthol or other volatile oils provides us with some insight on the molecular events that mediate the ability to perceive nasal airflow. When applied to the nose, menthol causes a well-known cooling sensation resulting in the perception of decongestion. This perception does not correlate with an increase in nasal airflow or a decrease in total nasal airway resistance (TNAR).[18] The mechanism of menthol's action on thermoreceptors was recently elucidated by two independent studies, which showed that menthol's cooling effect was mediated by its being an agonist for TRPM8—a cool, temperature-activated, cationic channel.[19,20]

MEASURING NASAL OBSTRUCTION

Rhinomanometry is the traditional method for measuring nasal airway resistance and nasal patency. This invasive technique requires simultaneous pressure measurements in the anterior and posterior parts of the nasal airway so as to calculate a transnasal pressure gradient. The ratio of the transnasal pressure gradient and the measured rate of nasal airflow allows an estimate of the TNAR.[21] Among normal subjects, total resistance of the nasal passage has been reported, with a range of 0.15 to 0.39 Pa/cc/s.[22] The major limitation of rhinomanometry is its inability to measure nasal resistance in instances of total nasal obstruction.

Acoustic rhinometry uses reflected sound waves to calculate the patent cross-sectional area at any point in the nasal passage to identify anatomically obstructed portions of the nasal airway. Because the cross-sectional area of any point within the nasal airway can be measured, the summation of these individual slices can be used to calculate a total nasal cavity volume. These measures of cross-sectional area and total nasal cavity volume have been validated against other anatomic measures, such CT,[23] MRI,[24] and nasal endoscopy.[25] Given the correlation between acoustic rhinometry and these various imaging modalities, CT- and MRI-generated measurements of patent nasal airway have also been advocated as means of noninvasively evaluating the patency of the nasal airway.

Nasal spirometry, typically reported as the nasal inspiratory peak flow (NIPF) rate, provides a noninvasive physiologic measure of nasal patency by asking patients to inspire forcefully while attached to a specially designed nasal flow meter mask. The peak airflow achieved is measured in liters per minute and has been validated against rhinomanometry as a valid measure of nasal patency.[26,27]

CORRELATION BETWEEN OBJECTIVE MEASUREMENTS OF NASAL PATENCY AND PATIENT-REPORTED NASAL OBSTRUCTION

Unfortunately, objective measurements of nasal obstruction and patient-reported symptoms of nasal obstruction correlate poorly. A study of 250 subjects compared TNAR, as determined by rhinomanometry, with assessments of total nasal obstruction, as reported by a visual analog scale (VAS) and failed to show any correlation between the two parameters.[17] Conversely, rhinomanometric studies investigating unilateral nasal resistance[28] in 60 participants who had the common cold found that patients could correctly identify acute unilateral nasal obstruction in approximately 77% of cases. When the level of airflow asymmetry exceeded 100 cm^3/s, the same study found that a subject's ability to identify the more obstructed side increased to 95%. The investigators concluded that subjects would be unable to discriminate unilateral nasal obstruction if the airflow difference was less than 50 cm^3/s.

Recently, Kjaergaard and colleagues[29] reported a cross-sectional study evaluating 2523 consecutive otolaryngology patients using acoustic rhinometry and peak nasal inspiratory flow and correlated these measurements with subject-reported nasal obstruction. This study found that the minimum cross-sectional area of the posterior and entire nasal passage, the nasal cavity volume of the anterior and posterior nasal passage, and the peak nasal inspiratory flow rate were significantly correlated with subject VAS-reported ratings of nasal obstruction. Interestingly, the study showed that the minimum cross-sectional area of the anterior nasal passage (defined in this study as the first 3 cm of the nasal cavity), which includes the nasal vestibule and nasal valve, was not significantly correlated with the sensation of nasal obstruction. Unlike the findings of this study, a separate investigation prospectively examined 290 nonrhinologic patients using similar subjective and objective measures of a VAS, acoustic rhinometry, and peak nasal inspiratory flow[30] and failed to show any significant correlation between objective and subjective measures of nasal obstruction.

Together, these findings suggest that despite the high sensitivity of receptors located within the nasal vestibule, narrowing within the region of the nasal airway containing the turbinates results in a higher perception of nasal obstruction. Perhaps the formation of a functional nasal valve outside the anticipated position in the anterior nasal cavity results in a perception of nasal obstruction. Another theme seems to be that studies consisting of predominantly rhinologic patients show better correlation between perceived and objectively measured nasal obstruction than those examining normal subjects. Hence, by inference, the presence of obstruction induced by pathologic findings, such as CRS, would heighten the perceptibility of nasal obstruction. These findings highlight the challenges in designing and analyzing studies examining nasal obstruction before and after FESS.

INFLUENCE OF FUNCTIONAL ENDOSCOPIC SINUS SURGERY ON PATIENT-REPORTED NASAL OBSTRUCTION

After treatment with maximal medical therapy, FESS is the preferred modality of treatment for refractory CRS. Although nasal obstruction is one of the most prevalent and severe symptoms of CRS, it was specifically studied in only 42% of the 131 FESS outcome studies identified in an extensive search of English-language studies including 10 or more patients.[31] The studies examining patient-reported changes in nasal obstruction also show significant variability in study design, ranging from retrospective patient experiences after surgery to prospectively recruited patient cohorts with pre- and postsurgical questionnaires. Some of the patient-reported symptom-specific data use validated measures, such as patient reported pre- and postoperative VAS scoring and Likert scale scoring. **Table 1** summarizes some of the studies that specifically address the symptom of nasal obstruction in assessing outcomes after FESS.

Table 1
Selected studies examining effects of functional endoscopic sinus surgery on subjective outcome measures of nasal obstruction

Article	No. Patients	Instrument	Preoperative Score (Mean)	Postoperative Score (Mean)	Follow-up (Months)	Assigned P Value	Comments
Retrospective							
Kennedy, 1992[32]	120	Subjective rating of improvement (25%, 50%, 75%, or 100%)	—	56%	18	NR	—
Senior et al, 1998[33]	72	Subjective rating of improvement (25%, 50%, 75%, or 100%)	—	60%	93.6	NR	—
Prospective							
Damm et al, 2002[2]	279	Likert ranking scales from 0 (mild) to 5 (intolerable)	2.8 ± 1.2	0.59 ±1.1	31.7	<.001	—
Bhattacharyya, 2004[1]	100	Likert ranking scales from 0 (mild) to 5 (severe)	3.5	1.2	19	<.001	—
Lund and Scadding, 1994[13]	200	VAS score from 0 (none) to 10 (severe)	5.5	2.4	27.6	<.05	—
Sipila et al, 1996[15]	51	VAS score from 0 (none) to 100 (severe)	23.3	6.2	3	<.001	—

(continued on next page)

Table 1
(continued)

Article	No. Patients	Instrument	Preoperative Score (Mean)	Postoperative Score (Mean)	Follow-up (Months)	Assigned P Value	Comments
Giger et al, 2003[5]	61	VAS score from 0 (none) to 5 (severe)	4.3	1	24	<.001	Estimated from provided figures
Ling and Kountakis, 2007[4]	158	VAS score from 0 (none) to 10 (severe)	5.7 ± 0.3	0.4 ± 0.1	12	<.001	
Young et al, 2007[36]	82	VAS score from 0 (none) to 10 (severe)	7.97 ± 2.27	2.19 ± 2.82	36	NR	Patients with reported seasonal allergies
			3.23 ± 2.74	36	NR		Patients who have asthma
		7.58 ± 2.20	3.25 ± 3.89	36	NR		Patients with Samter's triad
		7.66 ± 2.54					
Poetker et al, 2007[40]	43	VAS score from 0 (none) to 10 (severe)	7.5 ± 2.3	3.6 ± 2.8	16	<.0001	Patients with nasal polyps
	76		5.8 ± 3.1	4.3 ± 3.0	16	<.0001	Patients without nasal polyps
Soler et al, 2008[3]	207	VAS score from 0 (none) to 10 (severe)	6.52 ± 2.84	2.81 ± 2.51	3	<.001	
				3.36 ± 2.78	6	<.001	
				3.76 ± 2.92	12	<.001	
				4.25 ± 3.02	18	<.001	

Abbreviations: NR, not reported; NS, nonsignificant.

Several retrospective studies have examined outcomes after FESS with specific attention paid to patient-reported symptoms of nasal obstruction. In a study published in 1992, Kennedy[32] reported on the outcomes in 120 patients who had inflammatory sinus disease, with a mean follow-up of 1.5 years; subsequently, Senior and colleagues[33] reported outcomes of the same cohort at 7.8 years. This cohort was surveyed after surgery using categoric responses, with patients asked to estimate the level of improvement of nasal obstruction after endoscopic sinus surgery (eg, improvement of 25%, 50%, 75%, or 100%). Their responses in the dimension of nasal obstruction indicated an average of 66% improvement at 1.5 years after surgery and 65% improvement at 7.8 years after surgery. The overall percentage of patients reporting some improvement after surgery at 7.8 years after surgery was 97.1%. These results were generally supported in a study by Chambers and colleagues,[34] which showed a similar large improvement in subjective nasal obstruction.

To address the inherent problems of retrospective data, several prospective studies have since evaluated the effectiveness of FESS in relieving symptoms specific to CRS. Bhattacharyya[1] prospectively examined 100 consecutive adult patients undergoing primary FESS with mean follow-up at 12.4 months and showed that post-FESS nasal obstruction severity decreased by the largest magnitude when compared with all other symptoms in the RSTF diagnostic criteria. The effectiveness of FESS on relieving patient-reported nasal obstruction persisted in a separate group of 21 patients who underwent revision FESS for refractory disease.[35] A separate study involving 82 prospectively enrolled patients demonstrated that the relief of nasal obstruction was durable at 3 years after surgery. These researchers noted that patients with Samter's triad had significantly more nasal obstruction at their 24-month and 36-month follow-ups.[36]

More recently, Damm and colleagues[2] prospectively evaluated the impact of FESS on CRS-specific symptoms using pre-FESS and post-FESS questionnaires utilizing a Likert-scale like instrument (eg, 0 [no symptoms]–4 [intolerable]) that was completed by the 279 patients in their study. At a mean follow-up of 31.7 months, patients reported that their nasal obstruction severity had decreased from a mean score of 2.8 to a mean score of 0.59 ($P<.001$). When compared with patient-reported overall quality of life (QOL), improvement in nasal obstruction showed the highest correlation with increased QOL ($r = 0.59$) compared with the other symptom parameters evaluated in this study. A separate study by Ling and Kountakis[4] examined this issue of symptom correlation to QOL using VAS-reported RSTF symptom criteria to evaluate its relation to the Sinonasal Outcome Test-20 (SNOT-20), a validated broader measure that summarizes disease-specific symptoms and QOL into a single mean item score. At 1 year after FESS for CRS, their study involving 158 patients showed that postsurgical nasal obstruction decreased in prevalence (20.9% versus 83.5%) and severity (0.4 versus 5.9) on VAS-reported nasal obstruction when compared with preoperative scores. Unlike the findings of Damm and colleagues,[2] however, the RSTF reported that scores failed to correlate with the SNOT-20, which includes measures of overall QOL.

Soler and colleagues[3] published a series of 279 prospectively enrolled patients with a comprehensive evaluation of individual patient symptoms before surgery and with detailed postoperative follow-up to 18 months. Their study once again reiterated the high prevalence and severity of nasal obstruction among their patients, while also identifying nasal congestion as one of the most disabling aspects of CRS after headache and facial pain. Their study demonstrated significant and durable relief of nasal obstruction after FESS, but their results also suggested that the relief from nasal obstruction was maximal 3 months after surgery and tended to increase slowly with time.

In an effort to compare medical and surgical management of CRS, Ragab and colleagues[37] prospectively randomized 90 patients who had failed medical therapy consisting of nasal douching and a nasal steroid spray to FESS or further medical therapy consisting of low-dose macrolide therapy, intranasal or oral steroid therapy, and nasal douching. Although specific data are not provided in the report of this study, these investigators state that nasal obstruction was specifically studied as a parameter and that significant (P<.01) reductions were noted in the medical and surgical groups. With the sample size in their study, no significant differences were noted comparing nasal obstruction in patients managed using medical or surgical therapy.

INFLUENCE OF FUNCTIONAL ENDOSCOPIC SINUS SURGERY ON OBJECTIVE MEASURES OF NASAL OBSTRUCTION

Unlike the studies examining patient-reported nasal obstruction, published studies using objective measures of nasal obstruction seem to show a more equivocal benefit of FESS. Furthermore, most studies using objective measures of nasal obstruction are also limited by smaller study sizes, variations in the techniques and equipment used to measure nasal obstruction, and variations in the extent of FESS used in the studies. **Table 2** summarizes some of the published results using objective measures, such as rhinomanometry, acoustic rhinometry, and nasal spirometry.

In 1994, Lund and Scadding[13] reported results on 200 patients who underwent FESS for treatment of CRS. Of the 200 patients, 58% had previously undergone nasal surgery, including prior sinus surgery. Of these 200 patients, pre- and post-FESS NIPF and TNAR were recorded in 50 patients. The article did not note the time interval after FESS at which these objective data were collected or whether decongestion was used at the time of recording. The study found that although VAS-reported CRS symptoms decreased significantly after FESS, no significant differences were found in NIPF or TNAR. A separate study examined rhinomanometry measurements in 16 patients before and after an endoscopic uncinectomy and also found no improvement in rhinomanometric measurements or any correlation between patient-reported nasal obstruction and nasal resistance.[38]

Sipila and colleagues[15] examined a group of 51 patients who had sinusitis or polyposis before and 3 months after FESS (which was limited to uncinectomy, maxillary antrostomy, ethmoidectomy, and appropriate polypectomy) using patient-reported VAS scores of nasal obstruction and active anterior rhinomanometry recorded before and after nasal decongestion. They separated their patients into two groups based on the presence or absence of nasal polyposis. Among patients without nasal polyposis, a statistically significant reduction in resistance was found only in the more obstructed nostril before nasal decongestion and before surgery. Among patients with nasal polyposis, they found statistically significant reductions in resistance in unilateral and TNAR, despite having only 8 patients in this group. These findings were significant only before applying topical nasal decongestion. The patient-reported subjective improvements in symptoms of nasal obstruction were all highly significant. Similar to the study by Sipila and colleagues,[15] Giger and colleagues[5] examined 61 patients using anterior active rhinomanometry and VAS-reported symptoms of nasal obstruction before FESS and at 4 months and 2 years after FESS. Unlike Sipila and colleagues,[15] they found that mean TNAR was reduced from 0.35 Pa/cm^3 to 0.21 Pa/cm^3 at 4 months after FESS and to 0.25 Pa/cm^3 at 2 years after FESS (P<.001 at both time points). Their data also seemed to suggest that the effect of topical decongestion on decreasing TNAR decreased in patients after FESS, suggesting that overall mucosal inflammation decreased after FESS. A limitation to this study

Table 2
Selected studies examining effects of functional endoscopic sinus surgery on objective outcome measures of nasal obstruction

Article	No. Patients	Preoperative Score (Mean)	Postoperative Score (Mean)	Change	Assigned P Value	Comments
Anterior rhinomanometry (results reported in Pa/cc/s)						
Lund and Scadding, 1994[13]	50	0.27	0.26	−0.01	NS	—
Sipila et al, 1995[15]	43	0.13	0.08	−0.05	.016	Polyposis
	8	0.42	0.13	−0.29	—	No polyps
Numminen et al, 2004[14]	11	1.00	0.20	−0.80	NR	Ethmoidectomy
	—	0.78	0.19	−0.59	NR	Middle meatal antrostomy
Giger et al, 2003[5]	61	0.35	0.21 (4 months)	−0.14	<.05	—
	—	—	0.25 (2 years)	−0.10	<.05	—
Acoustic rhinometry (cm^3)						
de Paula Santos, et al, 2006[39]	40	39.7	45.2	5.5	.006	—
Lund and Scadding, 1994[13]	26	NR	NR	4.3	<.005	—
Nasal spirometry (L/min)						
Lund and Scadding, 1994[13]	50	155	150	−5	NS	—

Abbreviations: NR, not reported; NS, nonsignificant.

was that, interestingly, all their patients underwent concurrent septoplasty and partial middle turbinectomy as part of their FESS, possibly contributing to the significant changes in TNAR with or without decongestion that were not seen in previous studies.

Using acoustic rhinometry, several studies have measured the changes in nasal cavity volume as an objective measure of nasal obstruction. In the study by Lund and Scadding,[13] 26 patients underwent acoustic rhinometric evaluation. After decongestion, a mean increase in total nasal volume of 3.5 cm^3 was seen after FESS when the nasal cavity was measured between 6.9 cm^3 and 14.1 cm^3. Supporting these findings was a separate study by de Paula Santos and colleagues[39] that used acoustic rhinometry to examine 40 patients undergoing FESS and found a 5.4-cm^3 increase in total nasal cavity volume. In both these studies, the increase in nasal cavity volume after FESS showed a high variance.

Together, these studies suggest that although some conflicting data exist in the literature, patients who undergo endoscopic ethmoidectomy and appropriate polypectomy experience a substantial relief in subjective nasal obstruction. This reduction in the subjective sensation of nasal obstruction is associated with a measurable decrease in nasal airway resistance and increase in nasal cavity volume. The large magnitude of the subjective relief from FESS is associated with more modest and variable changes in nasal aerodynamics, however.

EFFECT OF NASAL POLYPOSIS AFTER FUNCTIONAL ENDOSCOPIC SINUS SURGERY IMPROVEMENTS IN NASAL OBSTRUCTION

CRS with polyposis represents a subset of patients who have CRS and also have inflammatory polyps that can obliterate the sinus ostia, sinuses, and, in advanced cases, the entire nasal cavity. The exact mechanisms driving the mucosal pathologic changes have not been fully elucidated and are under active investigation. Given the bulky obstructive nature of this disease, it would be logical that nasal obstruction would be more prevalent in CRS with polyposis, and several studies have directly examined this issue.

Poetker and colleagues[40] prospectively enrolled a cohort of 43 consecutively enrolled patients with polyposis and 76 patients without polyposis undergoing FESS for management of CRS. As expected, they found that patients with nasal polyposis had higher average preoperative VAS-reported (0–10 scale) scores of nasal obstruction than patients without polyposis (7.5 versus 5.8, respectively; $P = .002$). Although having average higher scores of nasal obstruction, patients with nasal polyposis had lower levels of facial pain and headaches than patients without polyposis, indicating a more prominent role for nasal obstruction in polyposis symptomatology. With a mean postoperative follow-up of 1.4 years, patients with polyposis reported similar mean levels of nasal obstruction as patients without polyposis (3.6 versus 4.3, respectively; $P = .205$). Because of higher levels of preoperative nasal obstruction, however, patients with nasal polyps showed a greater mean improvement in nasal obstruction when compared with patients without polyposis (3.9 versus 1.6; $P = .003$). The other two VAS-measured symptoms specifically examined in this study, headaches and facial pain, did not show significantly different improvements between patients with and without polyposis and polyposis.

A separate study examined 21 patients with nasal polyposis using active anterior rhinomanometry and acoustic rhinometry before and 4 to 8 months after FESS with appropriate polypectomy.[41] They showed that nasal airflow increased from 136 cm^3/s before surgery to 286 cm^3/s after surgery ($P<.001$). Nasal cavity volumes also increased from 3.11 to 4.71 cm^3 (P = .006) after surgery, demonstrating that FESS results in objectively measurable improvements in nasal obstruction.

Using a unique study design, Blomqvist and colleagues[42] randomized 32 patients with nasal polyposis and symmetrical nasal airways to unilateral FESS with postoperative topical budesonide therapy or topical budesonide only. After a 12-month follow-up period, both groups reported improvements in VAS-reported sense of smell, nasal obstruction, sinus pressure, nasal secretions, and headaches when compared with pretreatment scores. Patients receiving the unilateral FESS showed statistically significant improvements ($P<.05$) in nasal obstruction, nasal secretions, and sinus pressure, however. Twenty-five percent of patients in both study groups elected for further FESS at the end of the study period, although the study did not analyze whether patients receiving unilateral FESS were more likely to seek FESS than medically treated patients.

Together, these data show that nasal obstruction plays a more prominent role in the symptomatology of CRS with polyposis. FESS shows efficacy in relieving nasal obstruction in CRS with polyposis even at intermediate-length follow-up after surgery. Compared with patients receiving conservative medical management of nasal polyposis, FESS shows significant efficacy in improving nasal obstruction in particular. The improvements after FESS for CRS with nasal polyposis are significant in patient-reported and objectively measured nasal obstruction.

NASAL OBSTRUCTION IN CHILDREN UNDERGOING FUNCTIONAL ENDOSCOPIC SINUS SURGERY

Although ample data demonstrating symptomatic and objective improvements in nasal obstruction among adult patients undergoing FESS exist, data examining FESS in children are limited. The challenges to studying FESS in children include the relative efficacy of medical management and adenoidectomy in treating CRS in children, persistent concerns about the implications of FESS on facial development, the inability for children to participate in self-reported patient surveys, and the lack of existing validated instruments to study CRS in children.

Despite these challenges, Parsons and Phillips[43] retrospectively interviewed parents of 52 children who had undergone FESS for medically refractory sinusitis at an average of 7.4 years after surgery. They found that nasal obstruction was present in almost all patients before surgery and had improved in 79% of patients, with 54% reporting complete resolution. Another study retrospectively examined postoperative parental questionnaires in children receiving adenoidectomy or FESS for management of medically refractory CRS.[44] Nasal obstruction was the most prevalent symptom reported before surgery (84%) and showed improvements in the adenoidectomy and FESS groups. Parents in this study were asked to rate the degree of improvement after FESS retrospectively, and the adenoidectomy group reported a 47% improvement compared with a 57% improvement in the FESS group. No direct statistics were available in either of these studies to assess the significance of these findings with regard to nasal obstruction.

A more recent study retrospectively compared an age-matched cohort study of young (aged 2–5 years) children who had CRS and were treated with FESS (n = 37) with those treated conservatively with medical management alone (n = 7).[45] The patients who received FESS had higher baseline CT findings but similar symptom severity scores. Given the differences in the two groups, the investigators had to adjust for baseline symptom severity and CT severity to demonstrate a slightly lower nasal obstruction symptom severity score that achieved statistical significance (P = .04).

These data suggest that like adult CRS, nasal obstruction is a prevalent problem among children who have CRS. Although all the studies examined were limited by recall bias, lack of validated measures of nasal obstruction, and power to detect, they are suggestive of durable symptomatic improvements among children receiving FESS.

NASAL AIRFLOW MODELING AND THE INFLUENCE OF FUNCTIONAL ENDOSCOPIC SINUS SURGERY ON INTRANASAL AIRFLOW

The nasal cavity serves to warm, filter, and humidify inspired air. Several studies have used cast or imaging-guided scale models to study the nature of airflow within the nasal passage.[46,47] These scale models generally show a laminar airflow pattern, with highest velocities attained in the regions of the nasal valve and the inferior nasal airway. Relatively low flow rates are seen within the olfactory regions and the nasal meatuses. More recently, studies using computational fluid dynamics (CFD) of nasal airflow have largely confirmed these same findings.[48,49]

Recently, CFD techniques have been applied to analyzing three-dimensional numeric reconstructions of individual CT scans of the nasal airway. This has permitted computational simulations of nasal airflow distribution patterns to visualize changes between pre- and postsurgical patients. Zhao and colleagues[50] applied CFD simulations to pre- and postsurgical CT scans of a patient who had CRS with nasal polyposis and underwent a bilateral total ethmoidectomy, maxillary antrostomy, sphenoidotomy, and nasal polypectomy. These researchers found that in the presurgical model, streamlines were constricted toward the floor of the nasal cavity. The postsurgical model showed redistribution of airflow toward the middle and upper portions of the nasal cavity. The surgically enlarged sphenoid and maxillary ostia did not significantly change the airflow distribution, and increased airflow was particularly noted in the anterior superior portion of the nasal cavity in the vicinity of the olfactory epithelium.

SUMMARY

Nasal obstruction is among the most prevalent and severe symptoms experienced by patients who have CRS. The discomfort and annoyance of nasal obstruction are also highly associated with the disability and accompanying morbidity of the disease. Patients with nasal polyposis particularly experience nasal obstruction relative to other CRS-specific symptoms. FESS is highly successful in reducing the symptom severity of nasal obstruction, with durable long-term results. Although not as dramatic, the improvement in subjective symptom severity after FESS is associated with measurable decreases in nasal airway resistance and increases in nasal patency and airflow. These findings seem to hold true among pediatric patients, although further study is needed, particularly in the area of symptom-specific outcomes. The changes after FESS enable a more widespread distribution of airflow within the nasal passage and contact of inspired air with the olfactory epithelium. Given the prevalence, relevance, and defining nature of nasal obstruction in patients who have CRS, nasal obstruction should be specifically investigated in future FESS outcome studies.

REFERENCES

1. Bhattacharyya N. Symptom outcomes after endoscopic sinus surgery for chronic rhinosinusitis. Arch Otolaryngol Head Neck Surg 2004;130(3):329–33.

2. Damm M, Quante G, Jungehuelsing M, et al. Impact of functional endoscopic sinus surgery on symptoms and quality of life in chronic rhinosinusitis. Laryngoscope 2002;112(2):310–5.

3. Soler ZM, Mace J, Smith TL. Symptom-based presentation of chronic rhinosinusitis and symptom-specific outcomes after endoscopic sinus surgery. Am J Rhinol 2008;22(3):297–301.

4. Ling FT, Kountakis SE. Important clinical symptoms in patients undergoing functional endoscopic sinus surgery for chronic rhinosinusitis. Laryngoscope 2007; 117(6):1090–3.

5. Giger R, Landis BN, Zheng C, et al. Objective and subjective evaluation of endoscopic nasal surgery outcomes. Am J Rhinol 2003;17(6):327–33.

6. Bhattacharyya N. Clinical and symptom criteria for the accurate diagnosis of chronic rhinosinusitis. Laryngoscope 2006;116(7 Pt 2 Suppl 110):1–22.

7. Banerji A, Piccirillo JF, Thawley SE, et al. Chronic rhinosinusitis patients with polyps or polypoid mucosa have a greater burden of illness. Am J Rhinol 2007; 21(1):19–26.

8. Lanza DC, Kennedy DW. Adult rhinosinusitis defined. Otolaryngol Head Neck Surg 1997;117(3 Pt 2):S1–7.

9. Rosenfeld RM, Andes D, Bhattacharyya N, et al. Clinical practice guideline: adult sinusitis. Otolaryngol Head Neck Surg 2007;137(3 Suppl):S1–31.

10. Bhattacharyya T, Piccirillo J, Wippold FJ 2nd. Relationship between patient-based descriptions of sinusitis and paranasal sinus computed tomographic findings. Arch Otolaryngol Head Neck Surg 1997;123(11):1189–92.

11. Gliklich RE, Metson R. Techniques for outcomes research in chronic sinusitis. Laryngoscope 1995;105(4 Pt 1):387–90.

12. Lund VJ, Flood J, Sykes AP, et al. Effect of fluticasone in severe polyposis. Arch Otolaryngol Head Neck Surg 1998;124(5):513–8.

13. Lund VJ, Scadding GK. Objective assessment of endoscopic sinus surgery in the management of chronic rhinosinusitis: an update. J Laryngol Otol 1994;108(9): 749–53.

14. Numminen J, Dastidar P, Rautiainen M. Influence of sinus surgery in rhinometric measurements. J Otolaryngol 2004;33(2):98–103.

15. Sipila J, Antila J, Suonpaa J. Pre- and postoperative evaluation of patients with nasal obstruction undergoing endoscopic sinus surgery. Eur Arch Otorhinolaryngol 1996;253(4–5):237–9.

16. Clarke RW, Jones AS. The distribution of nasal airflow sensitivity in normal subjects. J Laryngol Otol 1994;108(12):1045–7.

17. Jones AS, Willatt DJ, Durham LM. Nasal airflow: resistance and sensation. J Laryngol Otol 1989;103(10):909–11.

18. Eccles R, Jones AS. The effect of menthol on nasal resistance to air flow. J Laryngol Otol 1983;97(8):705–9.

19. McKemy DD, Neuhausser WM, Julius D. Identification of a cold receptor reveals a general role for TRP channels in thermosensation. Nature 2002; 416(6876):52–8.

20. Peier AM, Moqrich A, Hergarden AC, et al. A TRP channel that senses cold stimuli and menthol. Cellule 2002;108(5):705–15.

21. Schumacher MJ. Rhinomanometry. J Allergy Clin Immunol 1989;83(4):711–8.

22. Eccles R. Nasal airflow in health and disease. Acta Otolaryngol 2000;120(5): 580–95.

23. Min YG, Jang YJ. Measurements of cross-sectional area of the nasal cavity by acoustic rhinometry and CT scanning. Laryngoscope 1995;105(7 Pt 1):757–9.

24. Corey JP, Gungor A, Nelson R, et al. A comparison of the nasal cross-sectional areas and volumes obtained with acoustic rhinometry and magnetic resonance imaging. Otolaryngol Head Neck Surg 1997;117(4):349–54.
25. Corey JP, Nalbone VP, Ng BA. Anatomic correlates of acoustic rhinometry as measured by rigid nasal endoscopy. Otolaryngol Head Neck Surg 1999;121(5): 572–6.
26. Holmstrom M, Scadding GK, Lund VJ, et al. Assessment of nasal obstruction. A comparison between rhinomanometry and nasal inspiratory peak flow. Rhinology 1990;28(3):191–6.
27. Wihl JA, Malm L. Rhinomanometry and nasal peak expiratory and inspiratory flow rate. Ann Allergy 1988;61(1):50–5.
28. Clarke JD, Hopkins ML, Eccles R. How good are patients at determining which side of the nose is more obstructed? A study on the limits of discrimination of the subjective assessment of unilateral nasal obstruction. Am J Rhinol 2006;20(1):20–4.
29. Kjaergaard T, Cvancarova M, Steinsvag SK. Does nasal obstruction mean that the nose is obstructed? Laryngoscope 2008;118(8):1476–81.
30. Lam DJ, James KT, Weaver EM. Comparison of anatomic, physiological, and subjective measures of the nasal airway. Am J Rhinol 2006;20(5):463–70.
31. Chester AC, Sindwani R. Symptom outcomes in endoscopic sinus surgery: a systematic review of measurement methods. Laryngoscope 2007;117(12): 2239–43.
32. Kennedy DW. Prognostic factors, outcomes and staging in ethmoid sinus surgery. Laryngoscope 1992;102(12 Pt 2 Suppl 57):1–18.
33. Senior BA, Kennedy DW, Tanabodee J, et al. Long-term results of functional endoscopic sinus surgery. Laryngoscope 1998;108(2):151–7.
34. Chambers DW, Davis WE, Cook PR, et al. Long-term outcome analysis of functional endoscopic sinus surgery: correlation of symptoms with endoscopic examination findings and potential prognostic variables. Laryngoscope 1997;107(4): 504–10.
35. Bhattacharyya N. Clinical outcomes after revision endoscopic sinus surgery. Arch Otolaryngol Head Neck Surg 2004;130(8):975–8.
36. Young J, Frenkiel S, Tewfik MA, et al. Long-term outcome analysis of endoscopic sinus surgery for chronic sinusitis. Am J Rhinol 2007;21(6):743–7.
37. Ragab SM, Lund VJ, Scadding G. Evaluation of the medical and surgical treatment of chronic rhinosinusitis: a prospective, randomised, controlled trial. Laryngoscope 2004;114(5):923–30.
38. Yaniv E, Hadar T, Shvero J, et al. Objective and subjective nasal airflow. Am J Otol 1997;18(1):29–32.
39. de Paula Santos R, Habermann W, Hofmann T, et al. Pre and post functional endoscopic sinus surgery nasal cavity volume assessment by acoustic rhinometry. Braz J Otorhinolaryngol 2006;72(4):549–53.
40. Poetker DM, Mendolia-Loffredo S, Smith TL. Outcomes of endoscopic sinus surgery for chronic rhinosinusitis associated with sinonasal polyposis. Am J Rhinol 2007;21(1):84–8.
41. Kappe T, Papp J, Rozsasi A, et al. Nasal conditioning after endonasal surgery in chronic rhinosinusitis with nasal polyps. Am J Rhinol 2008;22(1):89–94.
42. Blomqvist EH, Lundblad L, Anggard A, et al. A randomized controlled study evaluating medical treatment versus surgical treatment in addition to medical treatment of nasal polyposis. J Allergy Clin Immunol 2001;107(2):224–8.
43. Parsons DS, Phillips SE. Functional endoscopic surgery in children: a retrospective analysis of results. Laryngoscope 1993;103(8):899–903.

44. Ramadan HH. Adenoidectomy vs endoscopic sinus surgery for the treatment of pediatric sinusitis. Arch Otolaryngol Head Neck Surg 1999;125(11):1208–11.
45. Lusk RP, Bothwell MR, Piccirillo J. Long-term follow-up for children treated with surgical intervention for chronic rhinosinusitis. Laryngoscope 2006;116(12): 2099–107.
46. Kelly JT, Prasad AK, Wexler AS. Detailed flow patterns in the nasal cavity. J Appl Phys 2000;89(1):323–37.
47. Hornung DE, Leopold DA, Youngentob SL, et al. Airflow patterns in a human nasal model. Arch Otolaryngol Head Neck Surg 1987;113(2):169–72.
48. Kimbell JS, Subramaniam RP. Use of computational fluid dynamics models for dosimetry of inhaled gases in the nasal passages. Inhal Toxicol 2001;13(5): 325–34.
49. Zhao K, Scherer PW, Hajiloo SA, et al. Effect of anatomy on human nasal air flow and odorant transport patterns: implications for olfaction. Chem Senses 2004; 29(5):365–79.
50. Zhao K, Pribitkin EA, Cowart BJ, et al. Numerical modeling of nasal obstruction and endoscopic surgical intervention: outcome to airflow and olfaction. Am J Rhinol 2006;20(3):308–16.

Surgical Management of the Deviated Septum: Techniques in Septoplasty

Nicholas Fettman, MD, Thomas Sanford, MD, Raj Sindwani, MD*

KEYWORDS

- Septoplasty • Nasal obstruction • Surgery
- Submucous resection • Septal deviation
- Technique • Open septoplasty

The nasal septum is a central support structure for the nose. When significantly deformed, the septum may cause dysfunction and cosmetic deformity, potentially having an impact on the many functions of the nasal cavity.

Nasal obstruction is the most common complaint in an average rhinologic practice,[1] and a deviated nasal septum is the most common cause of nasal obstruction. It has been estimated that as many as one third of the population has some nasal obstruction, and as many as one quarter of these patients pursue surgical treatment.[2] Often, the patient provides a history of trauma to the nose; however, many times, there is no clear history of an inciting event. The initial insult to the nasal septum may have been caused by birth trauma or by microfractures occurring early in life that have led to asymmetric growth of the septal cartilage.[3]

The evaluation of a septal deviation causing nasal obstruction depends heavily on physical examination and, possibly, imaging. Interestingly, studies[4] have shown that the degree of septal deviation has little correlation with subjective ratings of nasal obstruction. Once a septal deviation is diagnosed, however, medical management targeting the nasal mucosa is typically attempted first with topical nasal steroids, antihistamines, and decongestants as tolerated. If the patient fails medical therapy, a surgical intervention to correct the underlying septal deformity is considered.

Apart from nasal obstruction, a significantly deviated nasal septum has been implicated in epistaxis, sinusitis, obstructive sleep apnea, and headaches attributable to contact points with structures of the lateral nasal wall. These conditions are also

Department of Otolaryngology–Head and Neck Surgery, St. Louis University, 3635 Vista Avenue, 6th Floor, FDT, St. Louis, MO 63110, USA
* Corresponding author. Department of Otolaryngology–Head and Neck Surgery, St. Louis University Hospital, 3635 Vista Avenue, 6th Floor, FDT, St. Louis, MO 63110.
E-mail address: sindwani@slu.edu (R. Sindwani).

Otolaryngol Clin N Am 42 (2009) 241–252
doi:10.1016/j.otc.2009.01.005
0030-6665/09/$ – see front matter © 2009 Elsevier Inc. All rights reserved.

accepted indications for septoplasty, although some, such as facial pain or headache, may be controversial. Additionally, if the deviated nasal septum impairs access to the middle meatus, which is necessary to perform effective sinus surgery or endoscopic orbital procedures (eg, dacryocystorhinostomy, orbital decompression), or if a transseptal transsphenoidal hypophysectomy is pursued, a septoplasty may be advantageous as well.[5,6]

EMBRYOLOGY AND ANATOMY OF THE NASAL SEPTUM

During development of the face, five facial prominences form the nose:

1. Frontal prominence
2. Paired medial prominences
3. Paired lateral prominences

The nasal septum begins as a downward growth of the frontal prominence.[7] As the primary and secondary palatal shelves join, the descending septum fuses with the palate to separate the nasal cavity into two distinct nasal passages.[8]

The nasal septum consists of a membranous component anteriorly, a cartilaginous component, and an osseus component posteriorly. The membranous septum is located between the columellar lower lateral cartilages and the quadrangular cartilage posteriorly. It is composed of fibrofatty tissue. The septal cartilage, also known as the quadrangular cartilage for its geometry, is located just posterior to the membranous portion of the septum. Posteriorly, the nasal septum becomes osseus and consists of the perpendicular plate of ethmoid, the nasal crest of palatine and maxillary bones, and the vomer dividing the posterior choanae (**Fig. 1**). The lateral surfaces of the septal cartilage and bones are invested with the mucoperichondrium and mucoperiosteum, respectively. There is a decussation of fibers from these investing layers, which is particularly thick and densely adherent inferiorly, where the quadrangular cartilage meets the maxillary crest. The mucosa of the septum is composed of a pseudostratified columnar respiratory epithelium along the inferior two thirds and often contains olfactory epithelium along the superior one third.

The arterial supply of the nasal septum stems from the internal carotid and external carotid systems. The anterior and posterior ethmoidal arteries, which are branches of

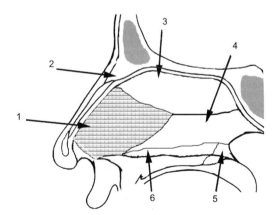

Fig. 1. Anatomy of nasal septum: 1, quadrangular cartilage; 2, nasal process of frontal bone; 3, perpendicular plate of ethmoid bone; 4, vomer; 5, palatine bone; 6, maxillary crest.

the ophthalmic artery, comprise the internal carotid component. The sphenopalatine artery, the terminal branch of the internal maxillary artery, and the superior labial artery (a branch of the facial artery) comprise the external carotid component. These arterial branches create an extensive plexus along the septum bilaterally that is especially evident during periods of epistaxis, which most commonly occurs along the anterior nasal septum in a region known as Kiesselbach's plexus. This rich anastomotic network is also responsible for the excellent healing properties of the mucoperichondrium or mucoperiosteum.

The nervous supply to the nasal septum originates from the trigeminal nerve (CN V). The posteroinferior half of nasal mucosa is innervated by the nasopalatine nerve, a branch of the maxillary nerve (CN V2). The superoanterior half of nasal mucosa is innervated by anterior ethmoidal nerves, branches of the nasociliary nerve from the ophthalmic nerve (CN V1). Superiorly, the mucosa is innervated by the olfactory nerve (CN I), with nerve endings traversing the cribriform plate through multiple tiny foramina.

Functionally, the internal nasal valve is of great significance. This region is the narrowest point of the upper airway and is defined by a two-dimensional plane slicing through the caudal end of the upper lateral cartilages superiorly; the alae laterally, along with the head of the inferior turbinate; and the bony nasal floor inferiorly. The septum defines the medial aspect of the internal nasal valve. The internal nasal valve is a point at which small changes in the nasal septal structure can have significant effects on airflow resistance and the sensation of obstruction.

HISTORY OF SEPTOPLASTY

Written accounts describing correction of nasal septal deformities date back to the beginning of medical literature in the Egyptian papyri. The Edwin Smith papyrus suggests treating the broken nose by placing two plugs of linen coated with grease within each nostril and then applying stiff rolls of linen externally to fix the fracture. In the late 19th century, the Bosworth operation was the most common procedure to correct septal deviation.[9] This procedure required the surgeon to amputate the deviation, along with the mucosa of the convex side. It was recognized at that time that the contralateral mucosa needed to be preserved; nonetheless, this technique resulted in frequent perforations. Around this period, Adams[10] and Asch[11] advocated fracturing the septum, followed by splinting. Asch[11] additionally suggested using full-thickness cruciate incisions to eliminate the resilient memory of the septal cartilage. Shortly thereafter, Killian[12] and Freer[13] published a technique involving raising the subperichondrial flaps and resecting the septal cartilage while leaving the overlying mucosa intact.

They emphasized that an L-shaped cartilaginous strut must be left dorsally and caudally for nasal support. This technique is known as the submucous resection (SMR) and is still widely used today. In 1929, Metzenbaum[14] addressed the issue of the caudal septal deviation. He used a vertical incision to mobilize the caudal strip of cartilage back to the maxillary crest in the midline, where it was fixed with suture. Several years later, Peer[15] recommended modifying this procedure when the caudal segment was curved or fractured. In this situation, Peer[15] advised to resect the caudal segment and to graft a separate piece of septal cartilage in its place. In 1948, Cottle and Loring[16] described conservative resections of deflected septal cartilage as well. Complications of significant cartilage resection and the SMR procedure, including large septal perforations and saddle nose deformity, were encountered, and a more conservative approach eventually gained popularity.

These developments provide the foundation of modern nasal septal surgery. Newer innovations, such as endoscopic septal surgery and extracorporeal septoplasty (in which a portion of the septal cartilage is removed, modified, and replaced), have built on the established tenets of intact flap elevation and careful reapproximation, preservation of dorsal and caudal support mechanisms, conservative resection, and meticulous surgical technique. With the proliferation of endoscopic techniques, the use of the endoscope to examine the nasal cavity and septum closely and also to correct deformities successfully has been gaining acceptance as a sound alternative for pathologic conditions not involving the anterocaudal septum. In its varied forms, septoplasty has grown to become one of the most commonly performed procedures in otolaryngology.

SUBMUCOUS RESECTION

The textbook and surgical atlas descriptions of SMR have not varied significantly in the past 50 years (**Table 1**). The basic procedure removes most of the quadrangular cartilage, leaving an inverted L-shaped strut for structural support (**Fig. 2**). Bony portions of the septum that are significantly deformed are also resected. The SMR procedure can leave a large defect in the cartilage and osseous portions of the septum. These large defects have been associated with increased risk for complications. Other researchers have made the point that removal of most of the quadrangular cartilage decreases the need for repeat surgery. Most surgeons now blend SMR and septoplasty techniques to address the unique deformities encountered in each patient.

Anesthesia

SMR can be performed under local or general anesthesia. In either case, the septum is anesthetized with a hemostatic agent, such as 1% lidocaine with 1/100,000 epinephrine. This solution is injected subperichondrially and is used not only as a hemostatic agent but for hydrodissection, with the pressure lifting the mucosa and perichondrium from the cartilage. This is usually performed in an anterior-to-posterior direction, and the mucosa should blanch as the injection proceeds. The injection should extend posterior to the deviation. The agent is injected bilaterally.

Incision

After the injection, an incision is made using a number 15 blade. The side of septum that the incision is placed in is the choice of the surgeon but can be dictated by nature

| Table 1 ||||
| Textbook and surgical atlas descriptions of nasal septal surgery ||||
Source Title	Editor	Year	Page
Atlas of Head and Neck Surgery	Lore JM	1962	90–102
Scott Brown's Otolaryngology, 5th Edition	Kerr AG	1987	154–169
Principles and Practice of Rhinology	Goldman J	1987	385–394
Atlas of Head and Neck Surgery	Johns ME	1990	109–120
Atlas of Head and Neck Surgery–Otolaryngology	Bailey BJ	1996	828–831
Operative Otolaryngology–Head and Neck Surgery	Myers E	1997	21–37
Otolaryngology Head and Neck Surgery, 3rd Edition	Cummings CW	1998	921–948
Otolaryngology–Head and Neck Surgery, 4th Edition	Bailey BJ	2006	307–334

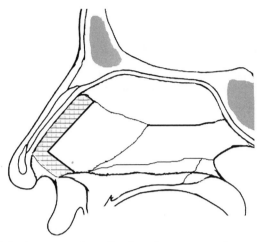

Fig. 2. Diagram of the SMR procedure. Shading demonstrates the area of L-shaped strut cartilage preserved.

of the deviation. The exact location and type of incision used are dictated by the caudal extent and nature of the deformity. A Killian type incision is placed 1 cm or more behind the caudal edge of the septum in the region of the mucosquamous junction. The incision should extend through the mucosa and perichondrium but spare the cartilage itself.

Flap Elevation

A gently curved elevator is then used to elevate the perichondrium and mucosa from the cartilage as an intact flap. It is advocated that a sharp elevator, such as the Cottle elevator, be used initially, because a sharp edge greatly facilitates breaking the fibrous attachments of the perichondrium to the underlying cartilage. After the elevation has started, a blunter elevator, such as the Freer elevator, may then be used to continue the dissection posteriorly. The nasal speculum can also be inserted carefully into the subperichondrial space itself to provide adequate visualization of the dissection. Care must be taken during flap elevation along the deviation or over any sharp septal spurs, because the mucosa tears easily at these sites. Broad flap elevation continuing over and under the septal deformity is advised initially because this provides some laxity to the flap as the dissection proceeds toward the apex of the septal spur, which mitigates against the creation of a tear.

Once this flap has been elevated, a contralateral flap must also be elevated. To begin the contralateral flap elevation, an incision through the cartilage at the initial mucosal incision site is made. An adequate 1-cm (or wider) strut is left intact and undisturbed with the Killian incision approach. The caudal strut of cartilage that is preserved is critical in preventing any columellar collapse with resultant tip ptosis. Care must be taken not to incise through the contralateral mucosa during cartilage incision, or contralateral flap elevation as septal perforation may occur. If the contralateral mucosa is inadvertently incised, it may be repaired using suture. After incising the cartilage, the Cottle elevator is inserted through the initial mucosal incision and the cartilaginous incision to begin elevating. As with the ipsilateral flap, a Freer elevator can replace the Cottle elevator to elevate more posteriorly.

Excision

Once both mucoperichondrial flaps are widely elevated and the deformed cartilage is exposed, a Ballenger swivel knife is used to excise the bent cartilage. Scissors may be used to make a cut posteriorly at the dorsal point of the initial cartilage incision. The Ballenger swivel knife is then placed into this dorsal cut and pushed posteriorly to the bony septum. Care must be taken to preserve a 1-cm strut of cartilage dorsally to prevent a saddle deformity. The swivel knife can then be advanced caudally to the nasal floor and anteriorly back to the caudal septum. This maneuver completes the excision of septal cartilage, which can then be removed with a bayonet or a non-specific instrument type. True-cut forceps or Jansen-Middleton forceps can then be used to remove any portions of the bony septum that are also deviated.

Suture and Packing

Once the deformity is resected, the flaps are placed back to their anatomic positions and the nasal cavities are examined. The mucosal incision is closed using an absorbable suture, such as chromic or plain gut, and many surgeons place a few tacking sutures more posteriorly to reapproximate the mucoperichondrial flaps. Nasal packing in the form of silastic splints or other nonabsorbable material is then placed on each side of the septum to compress the flaps together. Splints can secured in place using a 2-0 silk or Prolene horizontal mattress suture through the membranous septum. Packing or splints are removed in the clinic 2 to 5 days after surgery. An antibiotic with adequate coverage for *Staphylococcus aureus* infection (toxic shock syndrome secondary to nasal packing) should be instituted.

SEPTOPLASTY

Perhaps more commonly performed than the classically described SMR is the septoplasty, which is a more conservative procedure. Septoplasty identifies the specific area of septal deviation and targets that area for resection. The techniques are similar to the SMR, but far less cartilage is removed. In addition, a septoplasty often includes septal cartilage modification or placement of a cartilage graft in place of cartilage resection.

Anesthesia

As with the SMR, the nose is decongested with oxymetazoline (0.05%)-soaked pledgets bilaterally. The septum is injected with 1% lidocaine with epinephrine bilaterally.

Incision and Flap Elevation

Either the Killian or hemitransfixion incision can be used. The hemitransfixion is used when the caudal portion of the septum is involved and requires exposure (**Fig. 3**). If a septal spur is encountered, it is beneficial to elevate superiorly and inferiorly with the Freer elevator, and then to encroach on the spur carefully with a Cottle elevator to avoid perforating the mucosa.

Once the ipsilateral flap is elevated, the Cottle elevator can be used to incise the septum anterior to the deviation, and the contralateral flap can then be elevated. At this point, a Cottle elevator can be used to incise the septal cartilage inferior and superior to the deviation, or True-cut forceps or Jansen-Middleton forceps can be used to resect a small amount of cartilage over and under the deviation. This move isolates the deviated portion of septum and allows the surgeon to grasp this isolated segment with

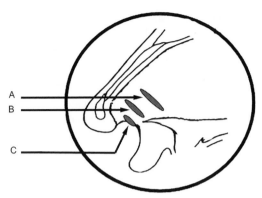

Fig. 3. Schematic of incisions used during septal surgery: A, Killian incision; B, hemitransfixion; C, external rhinoplasty incision.

Takahashi forceps. Using a rotational movement about an anterior-posterior axis, the isolated segment can then be fractured from its remaining posterior attachment.

There are two potential pitfalls associated with this technique that deserve attention:

1. Potential for perforation in the mucosa
2. Fracture of cribriform and resulting cerebrospinal fluid leak

The first pitfall, the potential for perforation in the mucosa, can occur if the Takahashi forceps accidentally grasp the flap in addition to the septal cartilage. Care must be taken to ensure that the mucosa is not damaged. The second potential pitfall involves being overly aggressive with maneuvering the isolated fragment with the Takahashi forceps. There should be no pulling movement or twisting motion outside of the anterior-posterior axis. These movements could fracture the cribriform plate, theoretically causing a cerebrospinal fluid leak.

If the deviated portion of cartilage or bone of the septum is large, modification of cartilage may be used to minimize the extent of the septal cartilage resected. Cartilaginous scoring or weakening incisions can affect the shape and strength of the septum, which helps it to assume a more desirable shape. The location and extent of these releasing incisions have been debated. The cartilage can also be removed and morselized and then placed back into the mucoperichondrial flap. The results of septal modification can be unpredictable because of cartilage memory and reabsorption. Some have advocated for a variety of suturing techniques to encourage "straighter" more reliable healing of the septum after surgery for severe cases.

After removing or modifying the cartilaginous portion of deviated nasal septum, any remaining posterior osseus deviation can then be resected using True-cut forceps or Jansen-Middleton forceps. The mucosal flaps are then reapproximated as in the SMR technique, the incision is closed using absorbable suture, and splints or packs are placed bilaterally for optimum healing.

CAUDAL DEVIATIONS

Caudal septal deviations are unique in that they cause not only nasal obstruction but an aesthetic abnormality. A caudal deviation may cause the nares to appear asymmetric and the columella to appear widened. Simply resecting the caudal segment of nasal septum violates the L-shaped strut principle and would result in a significant loss of nasal tip support and shortening of the columella leading to collapse. Metzenbaum[14] recognized the importance of the caudal nasal septum and developed the innovative "swinging door" procedure to correct the caudal deviation while preserving the cartilage for tip support.

Swinging Door Procedure

The swinging door procedure has undergone modifications since Metzenbaum's original description;[14] however, the general concept remains the same.

Incision

Caudal septal pathologic findings are approached by means of a hemitransfixion incision that is placed at the caudal tip of the quadrangular septum, thereby providing access and exposure to the entirety of the septum. The caudal edge of the septum is usually identified deflected into one side of the nasal vestibule. An incision is made vertically with a number 15 blade.

Flap Elevation and Cartilage Work

Once the incision is carried through the mucoperichondrium, the caudal septum is exposed by bilateral subperichondrial flap elevation. Because this dissection is performed anteriorly in the nasal vestibule, skin hooks are often used to help retract the flap as it is elevated initially.

Flaps are then elevated widely. Superior and inferior "tunnels" on both sides of the inferior septum over and under the maxillary crest are created and then connected. Flaps are raised bilaterally until all the deformity is exposed and well visualized. Next, the septum must be mobilized from three of its four attachments areas. The cartilage is first disarticulated from its posterior bony attachments, and it is then elevated (posterior to anterior) from its groove within the maxillary crest. A Cottle elevator works well for this technique. Lastly, the cartilage is freed from its attachment to the anterior nasal spine, leaving only its superior attachment intact. This allows it to be repositioned and "swung" into more of a midline position and then sutured into place at the nasal spine using absorbable suture, such as 3-0 chromic. Adequate mobilization and repositioning may require excision of a triangular strip of cartilage along the anteroinferior border so that a "better fit" is achieved with the cartilage and the maxillary crest in the midline. Any prominent spurs or projections from the maxillary crest can also be resected.

The most caudal tip of the cartilage is addressed by creating a small pocket in a retrograde fashion in the columella into which the caudal septum is sutured using septocolumellar sutures. This repositions the anterior edge of the cartilage in a more favorable midline position. Kridel and colleagues[17] advocate a retrograde dissection between the medial crura with subsequent suturing of the caudal septum to the crura themselves for additional stabilization. Surgery on the anterior septum by means of a hemitransfixion incision does disrupt some important nasal tip support mechanisms, and great care is necessary to ensure adequate support. As highlighted previously, maintaining the integrity of the caudal 1 cm of the septum is of paramount importance if a major cosmetic deformity is to be avoided.

As with SMR, the septoplasty procedure is concluded by closing the incision with interrupted dissolving sutures and tacking the mucoperichondrial flaps together at a few selected locations. Splints are placed for a few days after surgery.

Despite caudal septoplasty being a more technically challenging procedure than traditional septoplasty to perform, its benefits have been well established. In a retrospective review performed by Sedwick and colleagues[18] exploring the efficacy of caudal septoplasty in relieving nasal obstruction, 62 of 62 patients reported an improvement. Fifty-one of these patients (82%) thought they had no nasal obstruction at all after surgery. The technique used is nearly identical to the swinging door technique described previously.

OPEN SEPTOPLASTY

Often, the deviation of the nasal septum is one component of a larger nasal deformity. The deformity may involve the nasal tip, dorsum, and nasal bones. An intranasal approach to such deformities may not be adequate. In these situations, an open septorhinoplasty approach is best. Here, the authors focus their discussion on the management of the severely deviated septum using the open septorhinoplasty approach and elaborate on two techniques commonly implemented. The open septoplasty is approached through a rhinoplasty incision, which is made at the midcolumella. An irregular line (eg, W-shaped) incision works well in camouflaging this well-healing scar.

Extracorporeal septoplasty is a technique that has been described to address these severe cases. This technique involves removing the entire nasal septum and straightening the septum using various techniques, followed by reimplantation. Often, the external nose appears twisted in addition to symptomatic nasal obstruction, and extracorporeal septoplasty may help to correct this deformity as well.

Gubisch[19] describes a retrospective experience of 2119 patients undergoing extracorporeal septoplasty. An open approach is used if there is an external nasal deformity to be corrected. Using a closed approach, a hemitransfixion incision is extended into an intercartilaginous incision. A mucosal flap is then elevated to allow separation of dorsal septum from the upper lateral cartilages. The flap is then extended to allow fracture along the premaxilla and vertically as far posterior as possible. The septum is then removed.

At this point, the septum needs to be straightened, and there are various techniques that can be used. The graft may be drilled, or partial-thickness releasing incisions can be scored into the concave side. Also, the lamina perpendicularis of ethmoid or spreader grafts may be sutured to the cartilaginous septum. In a posttraumatic comminuted septum, multiple straight fragments may be compacted in a polydioxane (PDS) foil and sutured together for septal reconstruction. In the previously operated nose, there may be little to no cartilaginous septum remaining; in these cases, it may be possible to use just the osseus septum, with or without filing, with holes drilled for subsequent suture fixation.

Gubisch[19] then describes reimplantation, which may require reorientation of the septum to provide maximal dorsal and caudal support. The reimplanted septum is then sutured to the lateral cartilages, and the caudal septum is sutured to the nasal spine.

Most[20] describes an alternative to the extracorporeal septoplasty in which the dorsal strut of septal cartilage is retained, thus attempting to avoid the complication of an irregular nasal dorsum. The procedure, which he calls anterior septal reconstruction, is indicated for the patient with a severely deviated anterocaudal nasal septum. Deviations of the posterior dorsal septum thus would not be addressed using this technique. Most[20] highlights that the extracorporeal septoplasty technique requires fixation of the reimplanted septum to the nasal bones, labeled (referred to as) the keystone area, and that any disruption of this point results in notching or saddling of the dorsum. By maintaining the dorsal strut, this complication is avoided.

OUTCOMES

It is expected that once the septal deviation is corrected, the complaint of nasal obstruction should be significantly improved. In a frequently cited study known as the Nasal Obstruction Septoplasty Effectiveness (NOSE) study,[4] the outcomes after nasal septoplasty were examined. Fifty-nine patients with chronic nasal obstruction who had failed medical management were enrolled and underwent a septoplasty, with or without turbinate reduction, for a deviated nasal septum. The primary outcome measure was disease-specific quality of life at 3 and 6 months after surgery. The investigators used a validated NOSE scale to measure subjective nasal obstruction on a scale from 0 to 100, with individual items using a score of 0 indicating no problem and a score of 4 indicating a severe problem. Results from the NOSE study indicated that there was a significant improvement in subjective nasal obstruction from an average baseline score of 67.5 to a 3-month score of 23.1. Stability of the improvement was demonstrated by a 6-month score of 26.6.

In another study by Konstantinidis and colleagues[1] exploring long-term patient satisfaction after 51 patients underwent septoplasty by a modified Cottle approach, the outcomes were not as successful. This study evaluated subjective nasal obstruction using the Fairley nasal questionnaire (FNQ), which is a validated measure of nasal symptoms, and the Glasgow benefit inventory (GBI), which assesses patient perception of the success of surgery, the influence of surgery on the patient's health, and psychosocial function and social interaction. Patients were evaluated 2 to 3 years after surgery, with FNQ results showing 45% of patients having a persistent improvement in nasal obstruction. Surprisingly, the findings from the GBI suggest that patients had low satisfaction from their procedure and did not exhibit a significantly improved quality of life, even when analyzing the subset of patients who did show a significant improvement in nasal symptoms. This study demonstrates that perhaps some septoplasty procedures are being performed unnecessarily and also that patients tend to view the impact of their septal surgery less positively over time, which is consistent with other studies.

The results of these studies pose the interesting question of which patients are likely to benefit the most from septoplasty. The study by Konstantinidis and colleagues[1] also correlated a significant association between the location of septal deviation and postoperative improvement in nasal obstruction. Patients with an anterior deviation had a greater postoperative improvement than those with a posterior obstruction. It is logical to conclude that the location of the narrow internal nasal valve, lying along the anterior portion of the nasal septum, plays a major role in anteriorly based obstructions and that correction of the anterior deviation results in greater relief than correction of posteriorly located deviations.

It is widely accepted that the sensations of nasal obstruction and nasal patency are highly subjective and do not correlate well with the degree of septal deflection. This important but unintuitive concept should be openly discussed during the informed consent process before surgery to avoid disappointment. The etiology of nasal obstruction is also multifactorial many times. The presence of concomitant allergic rhinitis, inferior turbinate hypertrophy, or chronic rhinosinusitis can further confound the clinical picture. These possibilities should be fully considered and evaluated as necessary before embarking on any surgical intervention involving the nasal septum.

COMPLICATIONS

There are three main complications with septoplasty and SMR surgery. In descending rate of occurrence, they are incomplete correction with persistent symptoms, septal perforation, and external nasal deformity. Intranasal scarring and epistaxis may also occur. Other more rare complications can include nasal septal cyst formation, unilateral blindness, cerebrospinal fluid leak, septal abscess formation, and death.[21] Incomplete repair is usually associated with severe deviations, requiring a more aggressive open approach to the nasal tip and dorsum. Septal perforation is less likely to occur if mucosal flaps are elevated intact. Processes like postoperative hematoma formation can lead to vascular compromise of the mucosa resulting in perforation as well, however. Packing or nasal septal stents are thought to decrease the risk for bleeding and hematoma formation. Suturing of the nasal septum with quilting stitches has also been shown to be effective at decreasing postoperative bleeding and perforation. Nasal dorsal defects or saddle nose deformity is usually the result of excessive resection of the dorsal aspect of the septal cartilage. Maintenance of a good dorsal strut during surgery, along with supportive sutures, serves to decrease the risk for this major complication.

SUMMARY

Septoplasty is an effective and well-tolerated procedure. This procedure has a long history with multiple variations, but the core principles have remained unchanged for decades. A thorough history and physical examination evaluating for other conditions that may also be contributing to the complaint of nasal obstruction are important in selecting candidates for surgery. An intimate understanding of the anatomy, physiology, and key support mechanisms of the nose is necessary to avoid complications.

REFERENCES

1. Konstantinidis I, Triaridis S, Triaridis A, et al. Long term results following nasal septal surgery, focus on patient satisfaction. Auris Nasus Larynx 2005;32:369–74.
2. Bateman ND, Woolford TJ. Informed consent for septal surgery: the evidence-base. J Laryngol Otol 2003;117(3):186–9.
3. Holt GR. Biomechanics of nasal septal trauma. Otolaryngol Clin North Am 1999; 32(4):615–9.
4. Stewart M, Smith T, Weaver E, et al. Outcomes after nasal septoplasty: results from the Nasal Septoplasty Effectiveness (NOSE) study. Otolaryngol Head Neck Surg 2004;130:283–90.
5. Pletcher S, Sindwani R, Metson R. Endoscopic orbital and optic nerve decompression. Otolaryngol Clin North Am Oct 2006;39(5):943–58.
6. Woog JJ, Sindwani R. Endoscopic dacryocystorhinostomy and conjunctivodacryocystorhinostomy. Otolaryngol Clin North Am Oct 2006;39(5):1001–17.
7. Sadler TW. Langman's medical embryology. 8th edition. Baltimore (MD): Lippincott Williams & Wilkins; 2000.
8. Beck JC, Sie KCY. The growth and development of the nasal airway. Facial Plast Surg Clin North Am 1999;7:257–62.
9. Bailey B. Nasal septal surgery 1896–1899: transition and controversy. Laryngoscope 1997;107(1):10–6.
10. Adams W. The treatment of the broken nose by forcible straightening and mechanical apparatus. BMJ 1875;2:421–2.
11. Asch M. Treatment of nasal stenosis due to deflective septum with and without thickening of the convex side. Laryngoscope 1899;6:340–61.
12. Killian G. Die submucöse fensterresektion der nasenscheidewand. Archiv Für Laryngologie und Rhinologie 1904;16:362–87.

13. Freer OT. The correction of deflections of the nasal septum with a minimum of traumatism. JAMA 1902;38:636–42.
14. Metzenbaum M. Replacement of the lower end of the dislocated septal cartilage versus submucous resection of the dislocated end of the septal cartilage. Arch Otolaryngol 1929;9:282–92.
15. Peer LA. An operation to repair lateral displacement of the lower border of the septal cartilage. Arch Otolaryngol 1929;9:282–96.
16. Cottle MH, Loring RM. Newer concepts of septum surgery: present status. Eye Ear Nose Throat Mon 1948;27:403–29.
17. Kridel RW, Scott BA, Foda HM. The tongue in groove technique in septorhino-plasty: a 10-year experience. Arch Facial Plast Surg 1999;1:246–56.
18. Sedwick JD, Lopez AB, Gajewski BJ, et al. Caudal septoplasty for treatment of septal deviation: aesthetic and functional correction of the nasal base. Arch Facial Plast Surg 2005;7:158–62.
19. Gubisch W. Extracorporeal septoplasty for the markedly deviated septum. Arch Facial Plast Surg 2005;7:218–26.
20. Most S. Anterior septal reconstruction: outcomes after a modified extracorporeal septoplasty technique. Arch Facial Plast Surg 2006;8:202–7.
21. Mlynski G. Surgery of the nasal septum. Facial Plast Surg 2006;22(4):223–9.

Endoscopic Septoplasty

Nathan B. Sautter, MD*, Timothy L. Smith, MD, MPH

KEYWORDS

- Nasal obstruction • Minimally invasive • Technique
- Caudal septum • Septal spur • Revision septoplasty

Septoplasty is one of the most common procedures performed in otolaryngology. Modern septoplasty techniques were initially described by Killian and Freer[1,2] in the early twentieth century. Indications for septoplasty are broad, and include correction of septal deviation resulting in nasal obstruction, the need for improved access during endoscopic sinus surgery (ESS) or endoscopic dacrocystorhinotomy, and treatment of facial pain/headaches associated with septal spurs contacting the lateral nasal wall. Septoplasty is classically performed under direct visualization using a headlight and nasal speculum. However, a newer technique using endoscopic visualization and instrumentation has gained widespread popularity and acceptance following several reports of favorable outcomes.[3–8]

Endoscopic septoplasty was initially described by Lanza and colleagues[3] and Stammberger[4] in 1991. Early reports of endoscopic septoplasty describe several advantages associated with the technique. For example, the technique makes it easier for surgeons to see tissue planes. Also, because the technique is minimally invasive, it offers a better way to treat isolated septal spurs. Furthermore, the technique gives surgeons improved access to a deviation that is posterior to a septal perforation. Additionally, the endoscopic approach makes it possible for many people to simultaneously observe the procedure on a monitor, making the approach useful in a teaching setting. Nasal endoscopy is a valuable tool for initial assessment of the relationship of the septum to the middle turbinates, which allows the surgeon to judge whether or not the position of the septum will limit access during ESS. Even in the absence of subjective nasal obstruction or gross septal deviation, septoplasty may be necessary to maximize access to the middle meatus during ESS, such as in the setting of a narrow nasal cavity with a prominent septal body (**Fig. 1**). Nasal endoscopy is an excellent tool for outpatient surveillance following septoplasty during the initial postoperative healing period and beyond.

NASAL SEPTUM FUNCTION AND ANATOMY

The nasal septum lies in the sagittal plane and separates the nasal cavity into two sides. In most cases, the bony or cartilaginous septum deviates to some degree

Oregon Sinus Center Division of Rhinology & Sinus Surgery, Department of Otolaryngology—Head and Neck Surgery, Oregon Health & Science University, 3181 SW Sam Jackson Park Rd. PV-01, Portland, OR 97239, USA
* Corresponding author.
E-mail address: sauttern@ohsu.edu (N.B. Sautter).

Otolaryngol Clin N Am 42 (2009) 253–260
doi:10.1016/j.otc.2009.01.010
0030-6665/09/$ – see front matter © 2009 Elsevier Inc. All rights reserved.

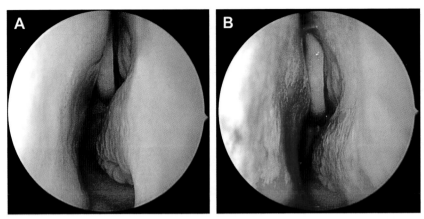

Fig.1. (*A*) Endoscopic view of the left middle meatus demonstrating a prominent septal body resulting in suboptimal view of the middle turbinate and middle meatus. (*B*) Following endoscopic septoplasty, visualization of the middle meatus is greatly improved.

from the midline. Such deviations may be congenital or acquired. Septal deviations may be broad and convex (often termed *bowing*) or sharp and acute (often termed *spurring*). The septal mucosa often becomes very thin over the apex of a spur, which is an important consideration during septoplasty. The cartilaginous septum is formed by the quadrangular cartilage anteriorly, while the bony septum comprises vomer posteriorly and the perpendicular plate of the ethmoid posterosuperiorly. The septum sits atop the midline crest of the maxilla anteriorly and the palatine bone posteriorly. The septum is bordered anterosuperiorly by the paired nasal bones and upper/lower lateral nasal cartilages, superiorly by the cribriform plate and floor of the frontal sinus, and posterosuperiorly by the face of the sphenoid. The vomer thickens considerably at the posterior aspect of the septum, where it terminates at the junction with the nasopharynx.

The nasal septum is lined with ciliated columnar respiratory epithelium, which transitions to squamous epithelium within several millimeters of the collumella. The vascular supply to the septum is robust, and is provided by branches of the sphenopalatine, anterior ethmoid, posterior ethmoid, greater palatine, and superior labial arteries. The septum works in conjunction with other structures within the nasal cavity to warm and humidify inspired air, while directing air and mucus posteriorly toward the nasopharynx.

TECHNIQUE
Drawbacks of Traditional Septoplasty

Traditional septoplasty is performed under direct visualization using headlight illumination and a nasal speculum. Visualization is limited with this technique, and the relation of the nasal septum to the lateral nasal wall structures is difficult to determine. The posterior septum is particularly difficult to visualize with this technique because of the narrow field of view and limited illumination. However, instrumentation is relatively simple, and a surgeon experienced in the technique can perform it rapidly.

Advantages of Endoscopic Septoplasty

Endoscopic septoplasty is associated with several distinct advantages over traditional septoplasty. The endoscopic technique provides the benefit of magnification, which the traditional headlight technique does not offer. In addition, illumination and visualization is better with the endoscopic technique than with the headlight technique. With the endoscope, it is possible to see the separation of collagenous fibers connecting the perichondrium and periostium to underlying bone and cartilage during surgical dissection. Mucosal disruptions are recognized immediately, and their size may be controlled using careful and meticulous dissection. Bleeding is minimized using injection of lidocaine with epinephrine, and optimal visualization is obtained with use of a suction Freer elevator. Endoscopic views of the nasal cavity are more natural than with the traditional headlight/speculum technique, since the nasal speculum causes some distortion of normal nasal anatomy.

One distinct advantage of the endoscopic approach is that it enables many people to observe the procedure on a monitor. This is very useful in a teaching setting, where it offers a convenient way for residents and students to directly observe the procedure, and a useful tool for a teaching surgeon to closely observe a resident. Operating room personnel may also observe the procedure and more accurately predict the next step in the case.

Endoscopic septoplasty may be performed using traditional ESS instrumentation. Because of this and because both endoscopic septoplasty and ESS involve the same field, endoscopic septoplasty can be performed in conjunction with ESS. This is important because concomitant septoplasty during sinus surgery may be necessary to provide the best access to the middle meatus. Suboptimal access during ESS leads to poor visualization, thereby increasing the likelihood of surgical complications or poor surgical outcomes. In some cases, uncorrected septal deviation increases the likelihood of middle turbinate lateralization and may lead to poor visualization during postoperative endoscopic examination.

Description of Endoscopic Septoplasty Technique

Little additional instrumentation is required when endoscopic septoplasty is performed in conjunction with ESS (**Fig. 2**). Before the procedure, the nasal mucosa is decongested with topical epinephrine, oxymetazoline, or cocaine. The nasal cavity is examined using a 0° endoscope. The location and degree of septal deflection or spurring is noted. If ESS is planned, the position of the septum to the middle turbinates is noted. A useful landmark is the axilla of the middle turbinate where it attaches anteriorly and superiorly to the lateral nasal wall. If the axilla is not easily visualized, the surgeon may have difficulty with access and visualization during ESS or in the postoperative period. In a narrow nasal cavity, the septal mucosal flaps may be "retracted"

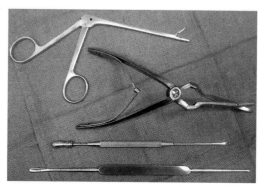

Fig. 2. Common instrumentation for endoscopic septoplasty. (*Top to bottom*) Takahashi forceps, Jansen-Middleton punch, suction Freer elevator, and Cottle elevator.

following septoplasty, allowing for improved endoscopic access and visualization (**Fig. 3**). An additional consideration is the superior aspect of the septum and septal body. While not usually deviated, this portion of the septum tends to be thicker than other parts of the septum, thus narrowing the nasal cavity and limiting access to the middle meatus.

One-percent lidocaine with 1:100,000 units of epinephrine is injected along both sides of the septum in a subperichondrial plane. A Killian incision is made on the left side of the caudal septum at the mucocutaneous junction. A Cottle elevator is then used to develop a submucoperichondrial plane along the left side of the septum. Further dissection in a posterior direction is performed using the suction Freer elevator (**Fig. 4**). When elevating the mucosa over spurs, care is taken to prevent mucosal tears due to thinning of the mucosa. The septal cartilage is then sharply scored and incised, leaving at least 1 cm of caudal and dorsal septum for nasal tip support (**Fig. 5**). A submucoperichondrial plane is then developed on the opposite side of the septum. Once the septal cartilage and bone is isolated from the mucosa, the Jansen-Middleton punch is used to incise the septum in an anterior to posterior manner (**Fig. 6**). The Takahashi forceps are then used to remove all deviated portions of the bone and cartilage in a twisting motion. The endoscope is used throughout the procedure, and may be placed between the mucosal flaps or within the nasal cavity to ensure correction of all septal deformities. The mucosal flaps are reapproximated and the Killian incision is closed using a 4-0 chromic gut suture. A 4-0 Vicryl rapide suture is used to further reapproximate the flaps in a quilting fashion. If a perforation is not present in one of the mucosal flaps, a drainage port is created posteriorly and inferiorly to allow for dependent drainage and to avoid development of a septal hematoma. Nasal packing and splints are used only in special cases (see **Fig. 3**).

SPECIAL CONSIDERATIONS
Directed Septoplasty

A directed endoscopic septoplasty approach is useful for treatment of isolated septal spurs in the absence of larger septal deviations (**Fig. 7**).[9] A directed approach results in limited dissection and quicker postoperative healing. With this technique, a horizontal

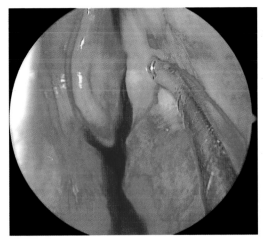

Fig. 3. The suction Freer elevator is used to retract the septal mucosa following endoscopic septoplasty, optimizing visualization of the middle meatus in preparation for ESS.

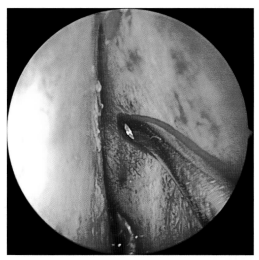

Fig. 4. Dissection in a submucoperichondrial plane is performed using the suction Freer.

incision is made over the apex of the spur, and mucosal flaps are elevated in a superior and inferior direction. The spur may then be incised with a microdebrider, with a sharp through-cutting instrument, or by a traditional septal transfixion with resection of the spurring cartilage/bone. The flaps are then redraped to minimize exposure of raw mucosa.

Septal Perforation

As with directed septal spur resection, a minimally invasive approach is useful in the presence of a previously existing septal perforation. Endoscopic visualization allows the surgeon to easily make a mucosal incision posterior to a septal perforation. When revision surgery becomes necessary, use of this technique may help prevent enlargement of pre-existing septal perforations.

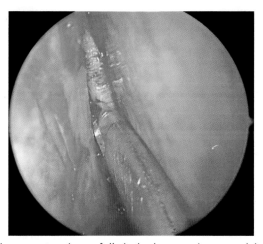

Fig. 5. The cartilaginous septum is carefully incised, preserving a caudal septal strut.

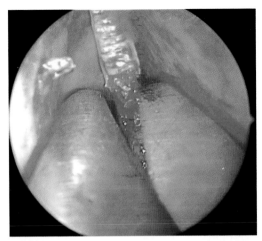

Fig. 6. Once the mucosal flaps have been raised, the Jansen-Middleton punch is used to sharply incise the septal bone and cartilage in an anterior to posterior fashion.

Revision Septoplasty

The endoscopic approach is quite useful during revision septoplasty. In these cases, scarring from previous septal surgery obscures normal tissue planes, resulting in increased risk of mucosal tearing with resulting septal perforation. Endoscopic

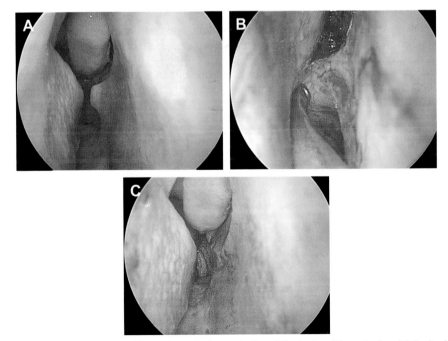

Fig. 7. An isolated posterior septal spur is shown before (*A*), during (*B*), and after (*C*) limited endoscopic septoplasty.

techniques provide optimal visualization of tissue planes, minimizing the risk of mucosal and septal perforation by allowing the surgeon to immediately recognize the presence of a mucosal rent, thus preventing enlargement of the tear.[5] In addition, previously dissected areas can be avoided, and a directed septoplasty approach can be used that addresses the remaining deflection, which is often high or posterior.

COMPLICATIONS

Complications of endoscopic septoplasty are identical to those following traditional headlight septoplasty. Major complications following septoplasty are rare. Minor complications include epistaxis, septal hematoma, injury to the nasopalatine nerve with subsequent dental numbness, scarring, septal perforation, cerebrospinal fluid leak, and persistent nasal obstruction.

Severe epistaxis following septoplasty is rare. Patients are advised to avoid perioperative use of medications that may interfere with blood clotting, such as aspirin and nonsteroidal anti-inflammatory drugs. Patients are also advised to avoid strenuous activities and heavy lifting during the first two postoperative weeks to minimize the risk of epistaxis.

Patients should be counseled regarding the risk of dental numbness following septoplasty. Temporary dental numbness is common, and usually resolves within several weeks or months. Permanent numbness is less common; avoiding extensive undermining of the anterior septal and nasal floor mucosa may help minimize this risk.

During the initial postoperative visit, the use of nasal endoscopy easily detects the presence of a septal hematoma. If present, the hematoma should be drained to prevent permanent nasal deformity. Quilting sutures in conjunction with posterior/inferior septal incisions allowing for dependent drainage may help minimize risk of septal hematoma.

Cerebrospinal fluid leak is a rare complication of septoplasty. If the dissection is taken too high, the cribriform plate injury with cerebrospinal fluid leak may occur. It is important to maintain proper orientation during dissection, and occasional reorientation by placing the scope within the nasal cavity may be helpful.

In a report of 116 patients undergoing endoscopic septoplasty, 4.3% of patients reported transient dental pain or hypesthesia, while less than 1% of patients suffered from epistaxis or septal hematoma following surgery.[10]

SUMMARY

Endoscopic septoplasty is a useful technique well suited to ESS. It provides optimal illumination and visualization of tissue planes, and allows the surgeon to more accurately assess nasal anatomy without the distortion of a nasal speculum. Through the use of a monitor, the technique enables many observers to watch the procedure, which is useful in a teaching setting. Endoscopic septoplasty is not associated with higher complication rates and does not significantly lengthen operative time compared with traditional septoplasty techniques. Regular postoperative nasal endoscopy is a useful tool to ensure optimal healing following surgery.

REFERENCES

1. Freer OT. The correction of deflections of the nasal septum with minimal traumatism. JAMA 1902;38:636–42.
2. Killian G. The submucous window resection of the nasal septum. Ann Otol Rhinol Laryngol 1905;14:363–93.

3. Lanza DC, Kennedy DW, Zinreich SJ. Nasal endoscopy and its surgical applications. In: Lee KJ, editor. Essential otolaryngology: head and neck surgery. 5th edition. New York: Medical Examination; 1991. p. 373–87.

4. Stammberger H. Special problems. In: Hawke M, editor. Functional endoscopic sinus surgery: the Messerklinger technique. Philadelphia: BC Decker; 1991. p. 432–3.

5. Hwang PH, McLaughlin RB, Lanza DC, et al. Endoscopic septoplasty: indications, technique and results. Otolaryngol Head Neck Surg 1999;120:678–82.

6. Giles WC, Gross CW, Abram AC, et al. Endoscopic septoplasty. Laryngoscope 1994;104:1507–9.

7. Cantrell H. Limited septoplasty for endoscopic sinus surgery. Otolaryngol Head Neck Surg 1997;116(2):274–7.

8. Sindwani R, Wright ED. Role of endoscopic septoplasty in the treatment of atypical facial pain. J Otolaryngol 2003;32:77–80.

9. Lanza DC, Farb Rosin D, Kennedy DW. Endoscopic septal spur resection. Am J Rhinol 1993;7:213–6.

10. Chung BJ, Batra PS, Citardi MJ, et al. Endoscopic septoplasty: revisitation of the technique, indications and outcomes. Am J Rhinol 2007;21:307–11.

Revision Septoplasty

Michael J. Sillers, MD, FACS[a],*, Artemus J. Cox III, MD[b], Brian Kulbersh, MD[c]

KEYWORDS

- Septoplasty • Endocopic septoplasty • Nasal valve
- Inferior turbinate • Septal deformity • Swinging door
- Extracorporeal septoplasty • Septal spur

Septoplasty, turbinoplasty, and nasal valve surgery are all done in an effort to improve patients' complaints of nasal airway obstruction. Septoplasty for nasal airway obstruction is perhaps the most common of these procedures performed by otolaryngologists in their adult patient population. It can be a challenging and complex procedure to do well, as evidenced by numerous contributions to the literature of different mechanisms to correct nasal airway obstruction brought about by a deviated septum. Efforts to improve the nasal airway by manipulating the septum began with Ingalls[1] in 1882 and Freer[2] and Killian[3] in 1902 and 1904, respectively. Some of the most famous names in surgery—Metzenbaum, Cottle, Goldman, Converse—and still others are credited with describing and improving septoplasty techniques. Despite advances and techniques that include closed, open, and endoscopic approaches, septoplasty is not always successful. In 2002, Dinis and Haider[4] found by questionnaire that only 42% of septoplasty patients thought they had a good to excellent result. A moderately successful result was found in 35%; a poor to mediocre result in 23%. A study recently published by Becker and colleagues[5] found that lack of improvement after primary septoplasty was often due to factors that affect the airway other than the septum, such as the nasal valve.

The purpose of this article is to address the challenge of persistent nasal airway obstruction following septoplasty, specifically as it relates to revision septoplasty. This article divides revision surgery into two categories: surgery involving the cartilaginous septum and surgery involving the bony septum, because the evaluation and management of these areas are distinct.

A revision septoplasty is usually spawned by the patient's feeling that he or she is still not breathing as well as possible. Sometimes this is noticed in the first several months after surgery by the surgeon or by the patient. Usually, however, the request for a revision septoplasty occurs well over a year after the initial surgery, oftentimes

[a] Alabama Nasal and Sinus Center, 7191 Cahaba Valley Road, Birmingham, AL 35242, USA
[b] Facial Plastic and Reconstructive Surgery, The University of Alabama–Birmingham, BDB 563, 1530 3rd Avenue So., Birmingham, AL 35294-0012, USA
[c] Division of Otolaryngology, Otolaryngology–Head and Neck Surgery, The University of Alabama–Birmingham, BDB 563, 1530 3rd Avenue So., Birmingham, AL 35294-0012, USA
* Corresponding author.
E-mail address: michaelsillers@charter.net (M.J. Sillers).

Otolaryngol Clin N Am 42 (2009) 261–278
doi:10.1016/j.otc.2009.01.014
0030-6665/09/$ – see front matter. Published by Elsevier Inc.

oto.theclinics.com

following a period in which the patient had felt significant initial improvement in their nasal airway. Septoplasty may also unmask tension in the nose that then allows an unexpected change in appearance to occur long after the initial surgery (**Fig. 1**).

When a patient complains of nasal obstruction following septoplasty, it is incumbent on the surgeon to determine whether this is a medical or surgical issue. Patients who have anatomic nasal obstruction may also have underlying inflammatory disease (allergic, infectious, or both) that is not being adequately treated. Revision surgery may not be effective, even when there are residual anatomic abnormalities, unless concomitant medical therapy is optimized (**Fig. 2**).

Airflow dynamics are complicated, and air does not travel through the nose in a laminar pattern. Airflow generally occurs in an arc-wise fashion, with creation of turbulent, eddy currents that likely are responsible for the "sensation" of airflow. When air passes through the nasal valve (the flow-limiting anatomic region of the nasal cavity), it arcs superiorly over the anterior end of the inferior turbinate toward the head of the middle turbinate. Air passes medial and lateral to the middle turbinate and subsequently through the posterior choanae (**Fig. 3**).[6] Therefore, evaluation of the inferior and middle turbinates and the nasal valve is essential because these structures often are additional sources of airflow obstruction.

There are several means by which to objectively assess nasal volume and patency. Acoustic rhinometry and CT can give static measures of nasal volume, whereas anterior active rhinomanometry provides information on dynamic airflow. These techniques have been shown in some studies to correlate well with findings on physical examination, including nasal endoscopy, and can document improvement in objective measures following treatment, whether medical or surgical.[7–11] One must exert caution, however, in the interpretation of cross-sectional minima with acoustic rhinometry, because these do not always correlate to specific anatomic structures.[12] After the determination is made that anatomic nasal obstruction involving the septum exists, revision septoplasty can be considered.

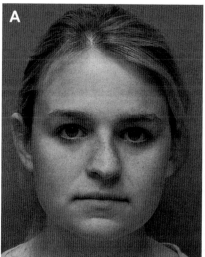
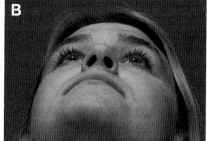

Fig. 1. (*A, B*) Six months following initial septoplasty, with subsequent deviation of the nose and caudal septal deflection.

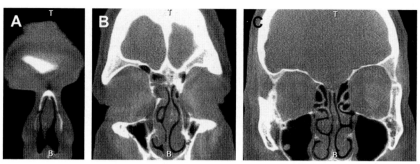

Fig. 2. (A–C) Prior septoplasty with anterior septal perforation, residual leftward septal deviation, and inferior turbinate hypertrophy. The patient has untreated allergic rhinitis.

In general, there are several challenges in revision septoplasty. Patients are often frustrated and want to know why the initial surgery did not work. This question is always important to answer, as is the question of what will be done differently in a subsequent procedure. Further, a more challenging dissection in compromised tissue with an unknown amount of cartilage or bone present must be done, and done in a fashion so as not to create unanticipated external changes or a subsequent perforation. The surgeon must also accept the responsibility of exposing the patient to another anesthetic along with similar risks inherent to the initial operation.

The etiology of a persistent airway blockage by the septum following an initial surgery is commonly multifactorial. Perhaps there was simply incomplete resection of the bony or cartilaginous septum that was not obvious at the time of surgery. Especially in the traumatic nose, initial resection of the septum may be adequate, but release of tension previously caused by the traumatized septum, allows another portion of the septum and possibly the external nose to reposition in a non-anatomically favorable direction (**Fig. 4**). Of course, there is the possibility of re-injury in a nose that is less well supported due to resection of septal cartilage and bone. Tension may also be created by inappropriate or varying planes of dissection that are noted only after healing. And, certainly, the patient's airway complaints may have initially been due to more than simply the septal deviation and, despite a successful septoplasty,

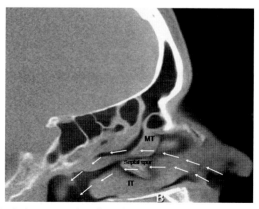

Fig. 3. Sagittal CT depicting general airflow direction through the nasal cavity; a septal spur impacts the inferior turbinate (IT). MT, middle turbinate.

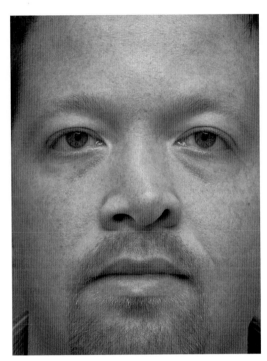

Fig. 4. Years following nasal trauma and initial septoplasty.

airway obstruction persists. This etiology is the most common reason for patient visits to the authors' office asking for a revision.

A common reason for an initially corrected septal deviation to "redeviate" is failure of the primary surgeon to realize that "the cartilage always wins" (Tom Wang, MD, personal communication, 1999). Multiple techniques have been fostered to change the shape of a curved piece of cartilage, including scoring, sutures, repositioning, and bolstering. Sometimes these techniques can work, but if the memory of the cartilage is not altered sufficiently, it often returns over time to its initial curvature and "wins." Breaking this memory commonly demands a much more invasive operation, sometimes including complete autotransplantation and perhaps challenging the skill set of the general otolaryngologist.

A closer analysis of the anatomy in a revision case is imperative. One must evaluate whether the septum is still a cause of airway obstruction or a cause of a change in the external appearance of the nose. The examination must include the external nose as well as the internal nose.

Is the problem due to the bony or cartilaginous septum?
Is the caudal septum blocking the airway in the dorsal or ventral direction and causing the tip to deviate?
Is the nasal spine the culprit?
Is the patient's face simply asymmetric congenitally, creating a difference in the nostril size or position? **(Fig. 5)**
Are there also cosmetic issues as a result of the initial septoplasty?
Has the caudal septum been removed, creating tip ptosis and excessive loss of columellar show?

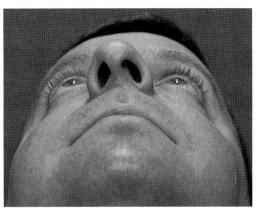

Fig. 5. Congenital asymmetry of facial platform resulting in nasal and septal deviation.

Asking these questions and making a thorough examination, including an endoscopic evaluation, are necessary to determine whether a revision may be helpful. The surgeon must be assured that no other cause of obstruction such as polyps, turbinate hypertrophy, adenoids, concha bullosa, nasal valve, or congenital deformity exists. Or, perhaps, the decision must be made that a revision septoplasty is necessary in addition to other adjunct procedures.

The quadrangular cartilage can be manipulated extensively in an effort to improve the nasal airway initially or even in a revision case. The key elements involve maintaining support with attachment at the nasal spine and an adequate "L strut" caudally and dorsally. The size of the L strut can vary depending on the inherent strength of the cartilage and the weight of the nasal skin but usually needs to be 7 to 8 mm in width.

SURGICAL APPROACHES TO CARTILAGINOUS SEPTAL DEFORMITY

The surgical approach to revising a cartilaginous septal deformity can be performed through a "closed" incision (hemitransfixion, full transfixion, or Killian) or through a standard open rhinoplastic approach, accessing the septum between the medial crura of the lower lateral cartilages. Historically, techniques of moving the nasal spine and caudal septal resection, like that advocated by Peer and colleagues,[13] were fairly effective at straightening the caudal septum initially. Rarely, however, were the needs of resupporting the nose accomplished, often resulting in loss of appropriate columellar show and other cosmetic deformities such as a pollybeak (**Fig. 6**).

"Swinging Door" Technique

Another closed technique introduced by Metzenbaum is called the "swinging door," in which a caudally deviated septum is released from the nasal spine and maxillary crest, adjustments are made to any excess of cartilage along the nasal floor, and the ventral caudal septum is "swung" to the other side of the nasal spine and sewn into place.[14] This technique can be very effective for the ventral aspect of the caudal septum but does not change the inherent twist or bow of the septum. The nasal tip may remain deviated, and again, resupporting the nasal tip must be considered in this procedure (**Fig. 7**).

Cartilage Scoring

Performed in conjunction with other techniques or separately, cartilage scoring is done to weaken the concave side of a septal deviation, to remove the inherent twist

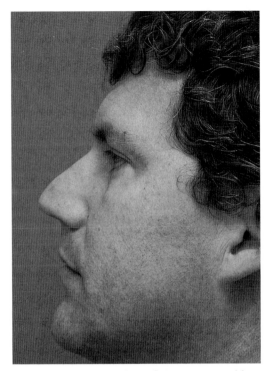

Fig. 6. Caudal septal resection resulting in loss of tip support and loss of columellar show with concomitant pollybeak deformity.

or bend, and to "allow" the cartilage to straighten. Scoring is done perpendicular to the orientation of deviation, often requiring light incisions into the cartilage in both directions and perhaps on both sides of the septum.[15] This technique has found favor historically and in the literature for primary and revision septoplasty; however, rarely

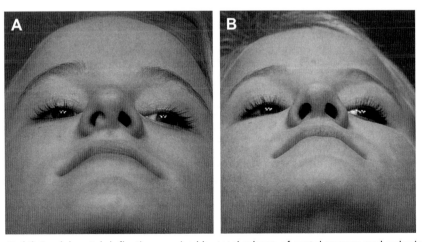

Fig. 7. (A) Caudal septal deflection repaired by total release of septal mucosa and swinging door technique. (B) Six months post surgery.

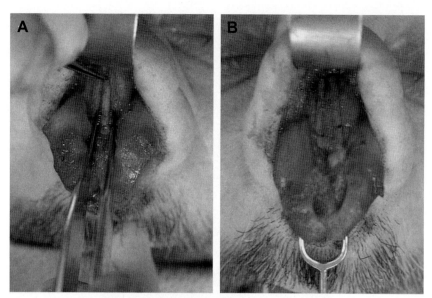

Fig. 8. (*A*) Placement of spreader grafts. (*B*) Spreader grafts in place.

can the cartilage be weakened enough to straighten and still provide the necessary support for long-term favorable results.

Open Approach

Due to the limitations of the closed approaches and the generally greater complexity in revising the cartilaginous septum, the authors primarily use the open approach. Most of the revisions they see involve the caudal septum, and the authors commonly add spreader grafts (**Fig. 8**) or make attempts to straighten the nose, which are accomplished with greater facility by the open approach. A standard inverted V transcolumellar incision (**Fig. 9**) is made, and dissection to expose the upper and lower lateral cartilages is completed. The medial crura are retracted laterally, and dissection is carried down onto the caudal septal angle. Meticulous dissection ensues to ensure

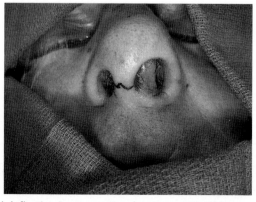

Fig. 9. Caudal septal deflection in preparation for open septoplasty approach with inverted V incision.

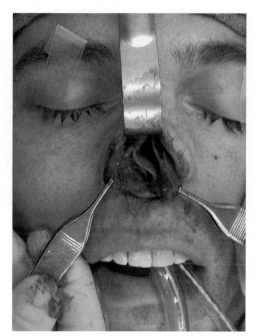

Fig. 10. Open approach to caudal septum with medial crura reflected laterally.

exposure of the cartilage in the submucoperichondrial plane. Access to the complete dorsal and ventral aspects of the caudal septum and nasal spine is achieved (**Fig. 10**).

When the dorsal septum is deviated or the nose is crooked, the upper lateral cartilages are separated from the septum. The mucoperichondria of both sides are dissected to release all forces of scarring and contraction. This is a tedious dissection but gives excellent visualization and often allows simultaneous repair of perforations that may have resulted from primary septoplasty. Not infrequently, total release of the mucoperichondrium also releases external forces created by previous healing or trauma, setting "free" the crooked cartilage to straighten automatically.

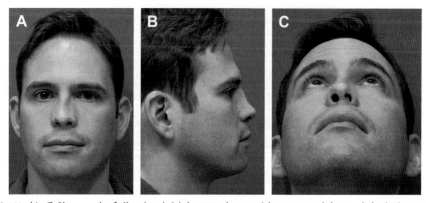

Fig. 11. (*A–C*) Six months following initial septoplasty, with new caudal septal deviation and dorsal deformity.

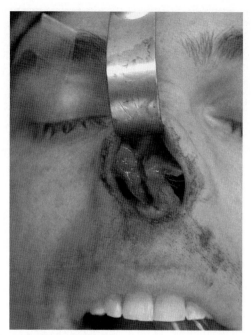

Fig. 12. Operative view of septal deviation.

This approach also gives excellent access to placing spreader grafts, batten grafts, or both to address a commonly compromised nasal valve that was not recognized initially or was caused by weakening of the septal cartilage in the initial operation.

Graduated Series of Techniques

The authors' approach for revision of the cartilaginous septum, therefore, is generally open and follows a graduated series of techniques. Any deviated portions of the quadrangular cartilage not occupying the L strut area are removed and maintained for grafting purposes. When the L strut is mildly deviated, the concave side is scored, and a straight, reinforcing graft of harvested septal cartilage is sutured across the

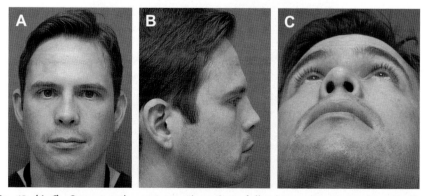

Fig. 13. (A–C) One month postoperative view following extracorporeal septoplasty augmented with Porex extended spreader grafts.

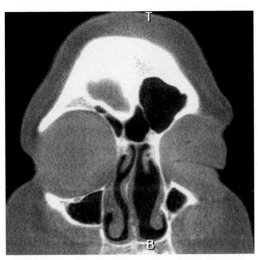

Fig.14. Coronal CT depicts residual rightward deviation of the PPE bone following septoplasty.

deviation to maintain the correction and add support. When scoring is not effective to break the cartilage's "memory," the deviation is divided at its maximum point of curvature and then grafted. The preferable graft is septal cartilage, but autologous rib, thin perpendicular plate of the ethmoid bone (PPE), donor rib, and Porex (Porex Corporation, Newnan, Georgia) may also be used. Porex is well tolerated so long as it is well covered, usually by adjacent cartilage, and not directly underlying skin.

Extracorporeal Septoplasty

A more common presentation for the authors is the patient who has a poorly supported nose and virtually no straight septal cartilage. In this case, extracorporeal septoplasty is advocated. This method involves removal of most of the septal cartilage after making careful measurements of the appropriate dorsal length and caudal

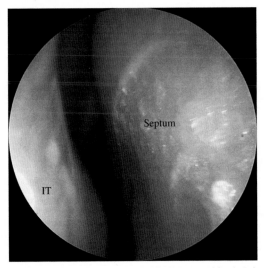

Fig. 15. Endoscopic view of the right nasal cavity showing residual rightward septal deviation. IT, inferior turbinate.

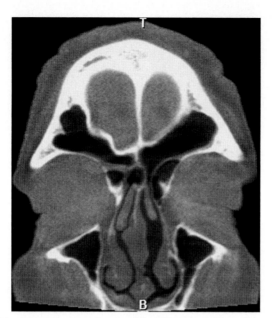

Fig.16. Coronal CT shows anterior superior septal deviation in a patient undergoing sinus surgery.

height. A portion of the dorsal septum at the junction of the nasal bones (keystone area) is left intact to have an area to which to sew.[16] The harvested cartilage is then carved and fashioned using sutures into an adequate L strut and introduced back into the nose, securing it to the keystone area and upper lateral cartilage. The configuration is made such that the caudal strut also functions as a columellar strut and is sewn to the nasal spine in addition to the medial crus of the lower lateral cartilage for tip support. In the last few years, the authors have found that a more efficient and effective variation of this method is to maintain the dorsal strut, even when crooked. Any deviations are effectively scored and then straightened by applying bilateral "extended" spreader grafts, which are then sewn to an "extended" columellar

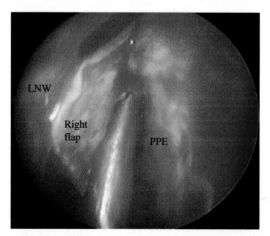

Fig. 17. Endoscopic septoplasty with incision made over residual bony deviation. LNW, lateral nasal wall.

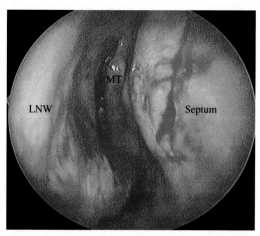

Fig. 18. After revision endoscopic septoplasty, the middle turbinate (MT) can easily be seen. LNW, left nasal wall.

strut. Commonly, a tip graft is then applied to tie the support units together even further. This process nicely straightens the dorsum, addresses the nasal valve, and re-supports the nose adequately (**Figs. 11–13**).

Of course, the extracorporeal approach and the authors' modification of it are aggressive and perhaps best performed by seasoned rhinoplastic surgeons. Although these procedures involve increased potential of operative risks, including poor healing of the transcolumellar scar, slight widening of the distal third of the nose, nasal rigidity, extra surgical time, and potential loss of skin in the multirevision patient,[17] they offer a definitive, effective, and long-lasting repair of difficult revision septoplasty in patients and have proved to be successful in the authors' hands.

TECHNIQUES FOR ADDRESSING RESIDUAL BONY OBSTRUCTION

Deviation of the PPE bone is commonly noted in patients who have residual nasal obstruction following septoplasty (**Figs. 14** and **15**). This deviation perhaps arises

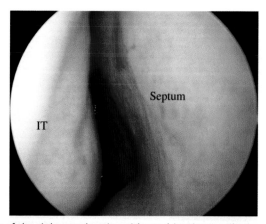

Fig. 19. Initial view of the right nasal cavity with combination cartilaginous and bony septal deformity; anterior rhinoscopy alone failed to show the posterior septal deformity. IT, inferior turbinate.

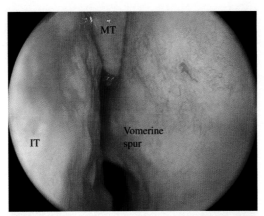

Fig. 20. After the anterior deformity was corrected, intraoperative endoscopic examination reveals a posterior vomerine spur. IT, inferior turbinate; MT, middle turbinate.

from a concern of "overdisarticulating" the bony cartilaginous junction, which may lead to dorsal deformities when the dorsal septum is separated from the nasal bones at the keystone area. Not only does PPE bone deviation lead to nasal obstruction but it can also make access to the agger nasi region, frontal recess, and frontal sinus difficult during endoscopic sinus surgery (**Figs. 16–18**).

Large vomerine spurs may be "missed" during initial septal surgery for several reasons. CTs are not routinely performed in the workup of nasal obstruction, particularly when there is no associated paranasal sinus disease. When there are more anterior cartilaginous or PPE bone deviations, vomerine spurs may be overlooked during the initial evaluation. Anterior deformities may make it difficult to pass even a flexible scope into the nose. To avoid missing a vomerine spur during initial septal surgery, nasal endoscopes are particularly helpful for assessing the nasal airway throughout the procedure, even when open rather than endoscopic septoplasty is being performed (**Figs. 19–21**).

Various approaches have been previously discussed for addressing the cartilaginous septum, and these may be used and extended to further address bony problems

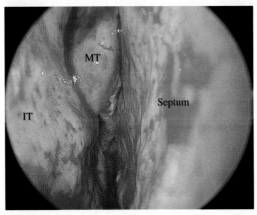

Fig. 21. Endoscopic view of the right nasal cavity after completion of septoplasty; the middle turbinate (MT) is easily seen. IT, inferior turbinate.

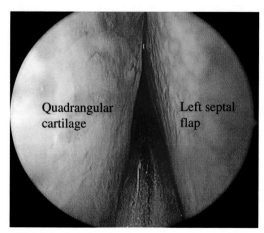

Fig. 22. Endoscopic view of the initial septal flap elevation; there appears to be a cartilaginous/bony leftward deviation.

when they exist in concert. When isolated bony abnormalities persist, endoscopic techniques are invaluable. Several investigators have described the indications and pitfalls of endoscopic septoplasty.[18–24] A common thread is that isolated spurs and deviations, including the maxillary crest, can be successfully addressed with targeted endoscopic septoplasty, eliminating the need for broad septal flap elevation, which may be problematic after prior septal surgery, particularly if quadrangular cartilage has been resected. A secondary benefit is less septal edema, which reduces postoperative morbidity and allows for easier performance of postoperative debridement when concomitant sinus surgery is performed.

The site of incision is generally chosen just anterior to the area of deviation. Infiltration with 1% lidocaine with 1:100,000 epinephrine is performed. Carefully palpating this area to ensure that there is underlying cartilage or bone is paramount. Palpation can be done with a 27-gauge needle used for injection and, when done slowly, can

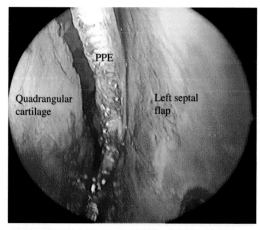

Fig. 23. After the bony–cartilaginous junction is disarticulated, the cartilage seems to take a more midline position, illustrating the influence of the PPE bone on the overall septal position.

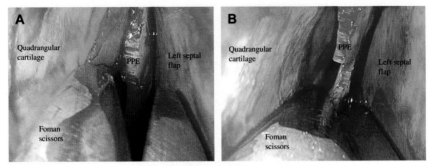

Fig. 24. Superior (*A*) and inferior (*B*) cuts are made along the PPE bone with Foman scissors.

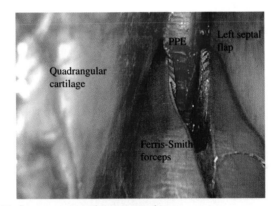

Fig. 25. Ferris-Smith forceps are used to remove bone.

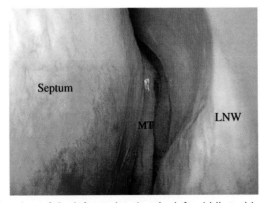

Fig. 26. Preoperative view of the left nasal cavity; the left middle turbinate (MT) is not well visualized. LNW, left nasal wall.

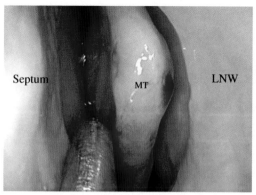

Fig. 27. Intraoperative endoscopic view of the left nasal cavity following septoplasty; the middle turbinate (MT) is seen in its entirety. LNW, left nasal wall.

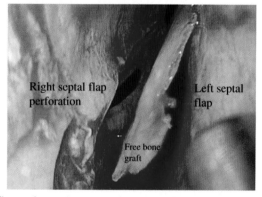

Fig. 28. Tenuous flaps after prior septoplasty may become perforated during revision septoplasty.

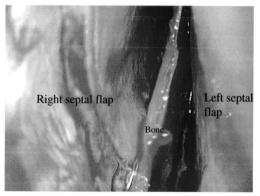

Fig. 29. Portions of the vomerine septum are replaced between the septal flaps to prevent postoperative septal perforation.

hydrodissect the initial septal flap. An incision is made with a #15 blade, and one must take care not to create a perforation at this point. After the initial flap is created, the cartilage or bone can be disarticulated to gain access to the opposite septal flap, which is subsequently elevated (**Figs. 22** and **23**). The disarticulation can be performed with specially fashioned septal burs on a microdebrider in the case of thick bony spurs. After the bony deviation is isolated, it can be cut and subsequently removed with Ferris-Smith forceps or smaller, sinus-type forceps when working through a limited incision (**Figs. 24** and **25**). When removing PPE bone, it is helpful periodically to view the nasal cavity with a 0° endoscope. In general, one should be able to see the vertical attachment of the middle turbinate to ensure that the deviation has been adequately corrected (**Figs. 26** and **27**). When removing vomerine spurs, the sphenoethmoid recess should be visible following resection. One must look carefully for perforations during revision septal surgery because the septal flaps may be somewhat tenuous. Replacing morselized cartilage or bone is helpful when small through-and-through perforations exist (**Figs. 28** and **29**). The incision is closed with a quilting stitch.

SUMMARY

Revision septoplasty is much more involved than primary septoplasty but can be done effectively and efficiently. The first key is making a complete and correct diagnosis of the problem or problems and then offering a comprehensive operative plan by way of an approach that will give adequate access. A graduated plan from simple removal of additional cartilage, to swinging doors and scoring, to potential extracorporeal septoplasty, to endoscopic techniques affords the careful surgeon an opportunity to safely and effectively improve the defects in nasal form and function resulting from a persistent septal deviation.

REFERENCES

1. Ingals E. Deflection of septum narium. Trans Am Laryngol Assoc 1882;4:61–9.
2. Freer PC. The Bureau of Government Laboratories for the Philippine Islands, and scientific positions under it. Science 1902;16:579–80.
3. Killian H, Meyer O, Sigel O. [Not Available]. Bruns Beitr Klin Chir 1947;176: 538–58.
4. Dinis PB, Haider H. Septoplasty: long-term evaluation of results. Am J Otol 2002; 23:85–90.
5. Becker SS, Dobratz EJ, Stowell N, et al. Revision septoplasty: review of sources of persistent nasal obstruction. Am J Rhinol 2008;22:440–4.
6. Stammberger H. Functional endoscopic sinus surgery. Philadelphia: B.C. Decker; 1991.
7. Grymer LF, Hilberg O, Elbrond O, et al. Acoustic rhinometry: evaluation of the nasal cavity with septal deviations, before and after septoplasty. Laryngoscope 1989;99:1180–7.
8. Kjaergaard T, Cvancarova M, Steinsvag SK. Does nasal obstruction mean that the nose is obstructed? Laryngoscope 2008;118:1476–81.
9. Lal D, Corey JP. Acoustic rhinometry and its uses in rhinology and diagnosis of nasal obstruction. Facial Plast Surg Clin North Am 2004;12:397–405, v.
10. Roithmann R, Cole P, Chapnik J, et al. Acoustic rhinometry in the evaluation of nasal obstruction. Laryngoscope 1995;105:275–81.
11. Szucs E, Clement PA. Acoustic rhinometry and rhinomanometry in the evaluation of nasal patency of patients with nasal septal deviation. Am J Rhinol 1998;12:345–52.

12. Cankurtaran M, Celik H, Coskun M, et al. Acoustic rhinometry in healthy humans: accuracy of area estimates and ability to quantify certain anatomic structures in the nasal cavity. Ann Otol Rhinol Laryngol 2007;116:906–16.
13. Peer LA, Walker JC, Van Duyn J. Progress in otolaryngology. Summaries of the bibliographic material available in the field of otolaryngology for 1947 and 1948: plastic surgery. AMA Arch Otolaryngol 1950;52:964–92.
14. Dyer WK, Kang J. Correction of severe caudal deflections with a cartilage "plating" rigid fixation graft. Arch Otolaryngol Head Neck Surg 2000;126:973–8.
15. Sedwick JD, Lopez AB, Gajewski BJ, et al. Caudal septoplasty for treatment of septal deviation: aesthetic and functional correction of the nasal base. Arch Facial Plast Surg 2005;7:158–62.
16. Most SP. Anterior septal reconstruction: outcomes after a modified extracorporeal septoplasty technique. Arch Facial Plast Surg 2006;8:202–7.
17. Gubisch W. Extracorporeal septoplasty for the markedly deviated septum. Arch Facial Plast Surg 2005;7:218–26.
18. Castelnuovo P, Pagella F, Cerniglia M, et al. Endoscopic limited septoplasty in combination with sinonasal surgery. Facial Plast Surg 1999;15:303–7.
19. Chung BJ, Batra PS, Citardi MJ, et al. Endoscopic septoplasty: revisitation of the technique, indications, and outcomes. Am J Rhinol 2007;21:307–11.
20. Dolan RW. Endoscopic septoplasty. Facial Plast Surg 2004;20:217–21.
21. Getz AE, Hwang PH. Endoscopic septoplasty. Curr Opin Otolaryngol Head Neck Surg 2008;16:26–31.
22. Hwang PH, McLaughlin RB, Lanza DC, et al. Endoscopic septoplasty: indications, technique, and results. Otolaryngol Head Neck Surg 1999;120:678–82.
23. Raynor EM. Powered endoscopic septoplasty for septal deviation and isolated spurs. Arch Facial Plast Surg 2005;7:410–2.
24. Sousa A, Iniciarte L, Levine H. Powered endoscopic nasal septal surgery. Acta Med Port 2005;18:249–55.

Postoperative Packing After Septoplasty: Is It Necessary?

Marika R. Dubin, MD*, Steven D. Pletcher, MD

KEYWORDS

- Septoplasty • Packing • Nasal splints • Morbidity
- Complications

There is a lack of consensus regarding the need for nasal packing following septoplasty. The use of postoperative packing has been proposed to minimize postoperative complications such as hemorrhage, formation of synechiae, and septal hematoma. Additionally, postoperative packing is thought to stabilize the remaining cartilaginous septum and minimize persistence or recurrence of septal deviation. Despite these theoretic advantages, evidence to support the use of postoperative packing is lacking. Additionally, nasal packing is not an innocuous procedure. The use of nasal packing carries several risks which, given the lack of firm evidence to support its efficacy, should call into question its routine application.

MORBIDITY OF NASAL PACKING

While life-threatening risks associated with nasal packing have been documented, these complications occurred primarily in the setting of posterior packing placed for the treatment of epistaxis.[1] The presumed etiology of death in these cases, the naso-pulmonary reflex,[2–5] has not been noted in the modern literature of postseptoplasty packing. The most common morbidity associated with packing in postseptoplasty patients is postoperative pain.[6–8] Additional potential complications include worsening of sleep disordered breathing[9] and postoperative infection, including reports of toxic shock syndrome due to postseptoplasty packing.[10]

Attempts have been made to limit the morbidity of nasal packing through limiting the duration of packing and altering packing materials.[11–13] Overall, the wide variety of packing materials and techniques complicates a clear assessment of the risks associated with postoperative septoplasty packing. Illum and colleagues[13] found decreased pain with removal when using fingerstall packs compared with Merocel or hydrocortisone-terramycine gauze packs with ventilation tubes. Some authors have found rehydration of foam packs with topical anesthetic to lessen discomfort

Department of Otolaryngology, Head and Neck Surgery, University of California, 400 Parnassus Avenue, Box 0342, San Francisco, CA 94143, USA
* Corresponding author.
E-mail address: mdubin@ohns.ucsf.edu (M.R. Dubin).

Otolaryngol Clin N Am 42 (2009) 279–285
doi:10.1016/j.otc.2009.01.015
0030-6665/09/$ – see front matter © 2009 Published by Elsevier Inc.

upon pack removal.[14,15] Silastic nasal splints are frequently used in place of packing and may be associated with less morbidity.

EFFICACY OF NASAL PACKING

While the morbidity and risks associated with postoperative nasal packing may be tolerated or minimized, the existence of such complications requires an evaluation of the importance of postseptoplasty nasal packing. In 1989, Guyuron published one of the few studies describing the efficacy of nasal packing in maintaining an adequate postoperative airway.[16] In this study, 50 subjects undergoing septorhinoplasty were randomized to receive packing with polysporin-impregnated gauze or placement of a quilting suture without nasal packing. Twenty-three subjects in the packed group and 22 subjects in the suture group were available for follow-up at up to 16 and 26 months, respectively. Subjective breathing improvement was found to be significantly more prevalent among the packed group. Additionally, a significantly higher percentage of persistent septal deviation was found among the unpacked group.

These findings, however, were called into question by Oneal who noted that subjects' awareness of packing as a point of study may have introduced bias into the patients' subjective assessment of breathing improvement.[17] He additionally noted that this finding, and the finding of persistent deviation as more common among the unpacked group, is weakened by the lack of preoperative assessment of degree of septal deviation. It is also important to note that this study was performed in the context of septorhinoplasty, not septoplasty alone.

Subsequent studies have failed to demonstrate a clear advantage to nasal packing while noting an increased morbidity with the use of packing. Nunez and colleagues[7] prospectively studied 59 subjects undergoing septal surgery and randomized them to packing with Vaseline gauze or no packing and placement of a septal quilting suture. Pain was recorded by a visual analog scale on postoperative day one and was found to be significantly higher in the packed group. The authors found no difference in the prevalence of adhesions, crusting/mucosal atrophy or granuloma formation between the two groups during follow-up at 6 weeks. The presence of persistent septal deviation and the extent of airway improvement were not evaluated in this study.

Von Schoenberg and colleagues[6] studied 95 subjects undergoing routine nasal surgery and randomized them to receive packing (either bismuth iodoform paraffin paste (BIPP) or Telfa) or no packing. Subjects undergoing septoplasty were further randomized to receive splints or no splints. Packs were removed at 24 hours postoperatively. Pain was recorded by visual analog scale during the first 24 hours, during pack removal, over the first week, and at the time of splint removal. Pain was significantly higher in the packed group at all points of measurement, and removal of packing proved to be the most painful event during the postoperative period, irrespective of whether splints were present. The authors found a higher rate of complications (including hemorrhage, vestibulitis and septal perforation) in the packed group, though it is not clear if this reached statistical significance. The incidence of intranasal adhesions was similar for the packed and unpacked groups, though the duration of follow-up with regard to this finding is unclear.

Additional series have demonstrated septal surgery without the use of postoperative packing to be safe. Reiter and colleagues[18] retrospectively studied 75 patients who underwent septorhinoplasty with placement of a quilting suture and no packing and identified only two cases of bleeding, both attributed to bleeding from lateral osteotomy sites. More recently, Bajaj and colleagues[19] reported a series of 78 subjects who underwent septoplasty without postoperative packing, with quilting suture used in just over a quarter of cases. They identified a 7.7% rate of postoperative hemorrhage with only half of these patients (3.8%) requiring packing to control bleeding.

Overall, the literature suggests that the use of nasal packing following septoplasty does not provide a clear advantage in improving nasal airway, nor does it appear to prevent postoperative complications. Furthermore, there is a clear increase in postoperative morbidity, specifically pain, with the use of both nasal packing following septoplasty. See **Table 1** for a summary.

EFFICACY AND MORBIDITY OF INTRANASAL SPLINTS

Intranasal (septal) splints have been used as an alternative to nasal packing to prevent intranasal adhesions and maintain septal stability. The incidence of intranasal adhesions following septoplasty is not clear, though has been reported to be as high as 31% when septal surgery is combined with inferior turbinate surgery.[20] Similar to nasal

Table 1
Efficacy of nasal packing

Author(s)	n	Procedure	Packing	Outcome
Guyuron[16]	50	Septorhinoplasty	Packing with polysporin-impregnated gauze vs quilting suture only	Subjective breathing improvement more prevalent in packed group (95.6% vs 64%, P<.01). Higher percentage of persistent septal deviation in unpacked group (41% vs 13%, P<.05).
Nunez et al[7]	59	Septal surgery	Packing with Vaseline gauze vs quilting suture only	Higher pain in packed group on postoperative day one (P<.05). No significant difference in prevalence of adhesions, crusting/mucosal atrophy, or granuloma formation between two groups
Von Schoenberg et al[6]	95	Routine nasal surgery	Packing with BIPP or Telfa vs no packing	Higher pain in packed group at 24 h, during pack removal, and over first week (P<.001 for each) Higher rate of complications in packed group[a]

[a] Indicates no statistical analysis was performed or results did not reach statistical significance.

packing, septal splints have demonstrated morbidity that calls into question their routine use.

Campbell and colleagues[21] prospectively studied 106 subjects undergoing routine nasal surgery who received splint placement in one nasal cavity at the conclusion of surgery. Pain was found to be significantly worse on the splinted side at 7 days postoperatively. The authors reported a higher incidence of adhesions among the unsplinted side, but it is not clear if this reached statistical significance, and the period of follow-up is limited at 6 weeks. Von Schoenberg and colleagues[22] prospectively studied 105 subjects undergoing septal and other routine nasal surgery who were randomized to receive or not receive nasal splints. Pain was found to be significantly higher at 7 days postoperatively among the splinted group. Three subjects developed vestibulitis and two subjects developed late septal perforations, all within the splinted group; however, these subjects were also packed with BIPP for the first 24 hours. Intranasal adhesions were assessed at 1 week and 3 months. The incidence of early intranasal adhesions (at 1 week) was higher in subjects without splints; however, there was no difference in adhesions at 3 months. The authors attribute this latter finding to the administration of nasal toilet during the first postoperative visit and conclude that the routine use of splints is not justified in light of their attendant morbidity.

Malki and colleagues[23] in a similar study of 110 subjects undergoing combined septal and inferior turbinate surgery, randomized to splints or no splints, found increased pain at 1 week postoperatively in the splinted group and no difference in adhesions at 6 weeks. The authors similarly concluded that simple nasal toilet is sufficient for the prevention of postoperative intranasal adhesions and that routine use of nasal splints is not justified.

Along with prevention of synechiae, septal splints have been postulated to improve postoperative septal stability. Cook and colleagues[24] studied 100 subjects undergoing septal surgery or septal plus inferior turbinate surgery, randomized to receive splints or no splints. Septal positioning was assessed postoperatively, characterized as straight, mild/moderate deviation, or surgically unacceptable deviation. No difference was found between the splinted or unsplinted groups with regard to this outcome. See **Table 2** for a summary of outcomes with nasal splinting.

On balance, the literature on the use of septal splints fails to demonstrate either a significant decrease in postoperative complications or a significant improvement in postoperative airway. Furthermore the use of septal splints is associated with increased postoperative pain. Overall discretion is advised in the use of surgical splints. Patients who are anticipated to be an increased risk of synechiae due to abutting mucosal injury of the septum and inferior turbinate, or those who are unlikely to perform routine post-operative nasal toilet may be appropriate candidates for postoperative splints.

ALTERNATIVES TO PACKING AND SPLINTS

Given the limited evidence to support postoperative packing and splints and the significant associated morbidity, many have come to favor alternative methods of preventing complications of septoplasty. A septal quilting suture appears be an effective means of preventing postoperative bleeding and hematoma while avoiding the morbidity of packing or splints. Lemmens and colleagues[25] evaluated the postoperative septal stability using this technique. Out of 226 subjects, only a single persistent septal deviation was noted.

Alternatively, some authors have had success with intraseptal application of fibrin glue.[26–28] Daneshrad and colleagues,[28] in their review of 100 cases of septoplasty

Author(s)	n	Procedure	Splinting	Outcome
Campbell et al[21]	106	Routine nasal surgery	One nasal cavity splinted	Pain worse on splinted side at 7 days postoperatively ($P<.05$) Higher incidence of adhesions among unsplinted side at 6 weeks (17% vs 0%)[a]
Von Schoenberg et al[22]	105	Routine nasal surgery	Splints vs no splints	Pain higher in splinted group at 7 days postoperatively ($P<.001$) Higher incidence of early nasal adhesions in unsplinted group[a] but no difference at 3 months
Malki et al[23]	110	Septal surgery + inferior turbinate surgery	Splints vs no splints	Increased pain at one week postoperatively in splinted group ($P<.0001$) No difference in adhesions at 6 weeks
Cook et al[24]	100	Septal surgery ± inferior turbinate surgery	Splints vs no splints	No difference in postoperative septal positioning

Table 2
Efficacy of intranasal splints

[a] Indicates no statistical analysis was performed or results did not reach statistical significance.

in which fibrin glue was used to approximate the septal flaps, experienced no cases of hematoma, infection, or perforation. The authors concluded that the use of fibrin glue is a rapid and reliable means to prevent complications associated with septoplasty. The cost of materials for performing this technique should be weighed against its potential advantages.

SUMMARY

The use of nasal packing following septoplasty is thought to stabilize the remaining septum and prevent complications such as bleeding, septal hematoma, and formation of synechiae. While these assertions appear intuitive, there is little evidence to support either a decrease in postoperative complications or improved surgical outcomes with the routine use of postoperative packing. Evaluation of the efficacy and rate of complications in the literature is complicated by the existence of multiple packing materials and techniques. Increased morbidity in the form of postoperative pain, however, is consistently noted with the use of nasal packing.

The use of septal splints in lieu of packing is also associated with increased postoperative pain. The routine use of splints does not appear to decrease postoperative complications or improve surgical outcomes when compared with less morbid techniques, such as septal quilting sutures and postoperative nasal douching. Therefore, placement of nasal packing or septal splints following septoplasty should be reserved for patients with increased risk of postsurgical complications.

REFERENCES

1. Fairbanks DNF. Complications of nasal packing. Otolaryngol Head Neck Surg 1986;94:412–5.
2. Angell James JE. Nasal reflexes. Proc R Soc Med 1969;62:1287–93.
3. Ogura JH, Harvey JE. Nasopulmonary mechanics – experimental evidence of the influence of the upper airway upon the lower. Acta Otolaryngol 1971;71:123–32.
4. Ogura JH, Togawa K, Dammkochler R. Nasal obstruction and the mechanics of breathing. Physiologic relationships and effects of nasal surgery. Arch Otolaryngol 1966;83:135–50.
5. Cassisi NJ, Biller HF, Ogura JH. Changes in arterial oxygen tension and pulmonary mechanics with use of posterior packing in epistaxis. Laryngoscope 1971; 81:1261–6.
6. Von Schoenberg M, Robinson P, Ryan R. Nasal packing after routine nasal surgery – is it justified? J Laryngol Otol 1993;107:902–5.
7. Nunez DA, Martin FW. An evaluation of post-operative packing in nasal septal surgery. Clin Otolaryngol 1991;16:549–50.
8. Samad I, Stevens HE, Maloney A. The efficacy of nasal septal surgery. J Otolaryngol 1992;21:88–91.
9. Taasan V, Wynne JW, Cassisi N, et al. The effect of nasal packing on sleep-disordered breathing and nocturnal oxygen desaturation. Laryngoscope 1981;91: 1163–72.
10. Toback J, Fayerman JW. Toxic shock syndrome following septorhinoplasty. Arch Otolaryngol 1983;109:627–9.
11. Lubianca-Neto JF, Sant'anna GD, Mauri M, et al. Evaluation of time of nasal packing after nasal surgery: a randomized trial. Otolaryngol Head Neck Surg 2000;122:899–901.
12. Hajiioannou JK, Bizaki A, Fragiadakis G, et al. Optimal time for nasal packing removal after septoplasty. A comparative study. Rhinology 2007;45:68–71.
13. Illum P, Grymer L, Hilberg O. Nasal packing after septoplasty. Clin Otolaryngol 1992;17:158–62.
14. Lachanas VA, Karatzias GT, Pinakas VG, et al. The use of tetracaine 0.25% solution in nasal packing removal. Am J Rhinol 2006;20:483–4.
15. Lavy JA, Small GV, Jay N, et al. A prospective randomized controlled study of 4% lignocaine solution in Merocel nasal pack removal. Rhinology 1996;34:219–21.
16. Guyuron B. Is packing after septorhinoplasty necessary? A randomized study. Plast Reconstr Surg 1989;84:41–4.
17. Oneal RM. Is packing after septorhinoplasty necessary? A randomized study. Plast Reconstr Surg 1989;84:45–6.
18. Reiter D, Alford E, Jabourian Z. Alternatives to packing in septorhinoplasty. Arch Otolaryngol Head Neck Surg 1989;115:1203–5.
19. Bajaj Y, Kanatas S, Carr N, et al. Is nasal packing really required after septoplasty? Int J Clin Pract July 2008, in press.
20. White A, Murray JAM. Intranasal adhesion formation following surgery for chronic nasal obstruction. Clin Otolaryngol 1988;13:139–43.
21. Campbell JB, Watson MG, Shenoi PM. The role of intranasal splints in the prevention of post-operative nasal adhesions. J Laryngol Otol 1987;101:1140–3.

22. Von Schoenberg M, Robinson P, Ryan R. The morbidity from nasal splints in 105 patients. Clin Otolaryngol 1992;17:528–30.
23. Malki D, Quine SM, Pfleiderer AG. Nasal splints, revisited. J Laryngol Otol 1999; 113:725–7.
24. Cook JA, Murrant NJ, Evans KL, et al. Intranasal splints and their effects on intranasal adhesions and septal stability. Clin Otolaryngol 1992;17:24–7.
25. Lemmens W, Lemkens P. Septal suturing following nasal septoplasty, a valid alternative for nasal packing? Acta Otorhinolaryngol Belg 2001;55:215–21.
26. Hayward PJ, Mackay IS. Fibrin glue in nasal septal surgery. J Laryngol Otol 1987; 101:133–8.
27. Vaiman M, Eviatar E, Segal S. The use of fibrin glue as hemostatic in endonasal operations: a prospective randomized study. Rhinology 2002;40:185–8.
28. Daneshrad P, Chin GY, Rice DH. Fibrin glue prevents complications of septal surgery: findings in a series of 100 patients. Ear Nose Throat J 2003;82:196–7.

Pediatric Septoplasty

J. Jared Christophel, MD[a], Charles W. Gross, MD, FACS[b],*

KEYWORDS

- Pediatric • Septoplasty • Facial growth • Septal repositioning
- Septal spur • Cartilage weakening

Cautionary statements regarding the effects of performing nasal surgery on the "growing nose" stretch back to the 1950s, when Gilbert and Segal published their warning against resecting the quadrilateral cartilage, referring to it as a keystone in development of the cartilaginous vault.[1] Farrior and Connolly echoed the sentiment after a review of the literature in 1970, stating that nasal surgery in children should be delayed, if possible, until growth is complete.[2]

HISTORICAL OVERVIEW: ANIMAL STUDIES

Pediatric septoplasty became the focus of multiple animal studies over the next 20 years, a few of which are landmark studies worth recognizing because they are often referred to when discussing this subject. Their results varied, and depending on which model was used, either confirmed the fears of clinicians or showed no effect on midface growth.

Sarnat and Wexler showed that moderate-size perforations in the nasal septum of young rabbits led not only to the expected saddling of the nasal dorsum, but also to significant underdevelopment of the maxilla, with resultant class III occlusion.[3] This deformity was not noticed when the same procedure was performed in adult rabbits.[4] Hartshorn repeated the procedure performed by Sarnat and Wexler on canine pups and noted a similar dramatic retardation of midface growth.[5]

Stenstrom and Thilander followed these studies by looking at the effect of septal-defect size on young guinea pigs. They found that the nasal septal cartilage was not a primary growth center in these animals, because only defects that included the bony septum resulted in skeletal deformity.[6] Fuchs' studies on the mucoperichondrium in young rabbits revealed its importance in the survival of underlying septal cartilage and its contribution to skeletal growth and deformation if it alone is resected.[7] Realizing the crucial role of the mucoperichondrium, Bernstein showed that preserving septal mucoperichondrial flaps in young pups did not result in any perceptible growth

[a] Department of Otolaryngology–Head and Neck Surgery, University of Virginia Health System, PO Box 800713, Charlottesville, VA 22908, USA
[b] Division of Rhinology, Department of Otolaryngology–Head and Neck Surgery, University of Virginia Health System, PO Box 800713, Charlottesville, VA 22908, USA
* Corresponding author.
E-mail address: cwg9u@virginia.edu (C. W. Gross).

Otolaryngol Clin N Am 42 (2009) 287–294
doi:10.1016/j.otc.2009.01.013
0030-6665/09/$ – see front matter © 2009 Published by Elsevier Inc.

oto.theclinics.com

disturbances, whether cartilaginous septum was removed or autotransplanted. Interestingly, in septums from which cartilage was removed, there was evidence of cartilage regrowth at 10 months, and in septums from which cartilage was removed and autotransplanted, the cartilage remained viable.[8]

HISTORICAL OVERVIEW: HUMAN STUDIES

With the later animal studies showing that a growing nasal septum could be altered without affecting long-term growth, longitudinal studies on children began appearing, with encouraging results.[9,10] Most of the studies were on children with a strong indication to undergo septal manipulation at a young age. McComb began performing primary rhinoplasty when repairing cleft lip nasal deformities in young children in the 1970s and noted no long-term growth effects. He performed an 18-year longitudinal study of nasal and midface growth and found no significant difference when subjects who had surgery were compared with age-matched normal subjects and age-matched control subjects with cleft lips who did not have rhinoplasty.[10]

Clinical studies became more common in the 1980s and 1990s, but the numbers were small and the statistical power inherently weak. More recently, surgeons in Toronto, Canada, began using anthropometric measurements to follow children undergoing septoplasty.[11,12] A recent study by El-Hakim and colleagues followed the anthropometric measurements of children who underwent septoplasty via an external approach with autotransplantation of the quadrilateral cartilage and compared their craniofacial development to that of age-matched control subjects. There were no deleterious effects on the development of the nose or midface.[13] However, there was a statistically significant trend in the shortening of the nasal dorsum and nasal tip protrusion, leaving the reader with a slight hesitation to call open season on the pediatric septum.

There remains a lack of a clear consensus in the literature regarding the developmental effects of septoplasty in children.[14] However, the more recent literature mentioned above shows that septoplasty can be performed safely in a selected population using mucoperichondrium- and cartilage-preserving techniques. Even with these techniques, the authors believe the indications for septoplasty in children therefore fall into a carefully selected patient population with an assured diagnosis. When done with the proper technique, the surgery can be effectively used to correct traumatic deformities, nasal airway obstruction, dermoids, septal abscesses, septal hematomas, and sleep apnea.

PREVALENCE

In contrast to the adult population, septoplasty is not a commonly performed operation in children, with most series averaging 20 patients.[13] In the authors' experience, one of the more common indications for pediatric septoplasty is severe nasal obstruction because from 7% to 12% of children snore, but less than 1% of young children have clinical obstructive sleep apnea syndrome. Even then, the majority of cases are not due to septal deviation.[15] Thus, it is important to remember that making the correct diagnosis is paramount.

EVALUATION OF THE PATIENT

The child with chronic nasal obstruction is a common referral for the otolaryngologist, and it is the exception when the cause is limited to the nasal septum. Proper evaluation of the patient and treatment of any other properly identified causes will often negate the need for septoplasty, even in patients with a tortuous septum. The clinician must always keep in mind the factors noted in **Box 1**.

Fiberoptic endoscopy is the most effective method of initial evaluation and will reveal most of the factors noted in **Box 1**. Although it is not a universal practice, the authors believe that nasal endoscopy is often indicated in the evaluation of the child with nasal obstruction and should be performed before considering septoplasty. If the diagnosis remains in question, a CT scan can be helpful, especially if there is concern for a congenital nasal mass. Only after all other causes have been ruled out or treated should one consider a septoplasty for nasal obstruction. Even then, unless the obstruction is secondary to severe septal deformity, the authors prefer to wait until the child is 5 or more years old.

INDICATIONS FOR SEPTOPLASTY

Absolute indications for performing a septoplasty in a pediatric patient include septal abscess, septal hematoma, severe deformity secondary to acute nasal fracture, dermoid cyst, and cleft lip nose (**Fig. 1**A, B). The latter two are often better addressed using an external rhinoplasty approach. Relative indications are limited to the patient with a severely deviated septum that is causing significant nasal airway obstruction or progressive distortion of the nasal dorsum.

ANATOMY

The structure of the nasal septum is well known to otolaryngologists (**Fig. 2**). The pediatric septum differs in subtle ways from that of the adult. Growth of the nasal septum

---

Box 1
Factors contributing to nasal obstruction

Congenital nasal mass

    Dermoid

    Encephalocele

    Glioma

Nasal polyp

Choanal atresia

Foreign body

Septal hematoma

Adenoid hypertrophy

Reversible obstruction

    Acute upper respiratory infection

    Chronic sinusitis

    Allergic inflammation

Deviated septum

Isolated septal spur

Turbinate hypertrophy

Midface hypoplasia

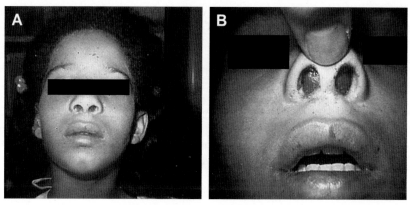

Fig. 1. (*A, B*) A young girl who presented with nasal obstruction after sustaining minor nasal trauma while playing with her siblings. Note the septal hematoma on base view.

occurs in two phases, with the cartilaginous septum reaching adult size by the time the child is 2 years old, and further enlargement due to growth of the bony septum.[16] The difference in the relative size of the quadrilateral cartilage as delineated by the osteo-cartilaginous suture lines in a 3-year-old patient and a 27-year-old patient is clearly seen when comparing sagittal sections of MRIs. (**Fig. 3**A, B) In addition to the difference in absolute size and the relative composition of the septum, the nasal vestibule is also much smaller in children compared with adults, and thus limits the exposure for septoplasty that is not done through an external approach (**Fig 4**).

SURGICAL TECHNIQUE

In the senior author's practice, the surgical approach to the pediatric patient requiring surgery on the nasal septum follows a stepwise algorithm, beginning with the least

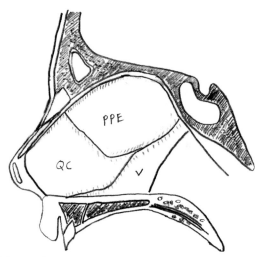

Fig. 2. Structure of the nasal septum. QC, quadrilateral cartilage; PPE, perpendicular plate of the ethmoid; V, vomer.

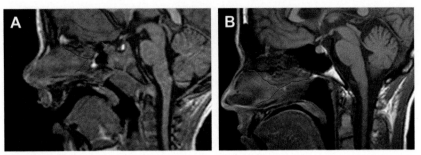

Fig. 3. Sagittal MRIs of a 3-year-old boy (*A*) and a 27-year-old man (*B*). The blue lines mark the osteochondral suture lines that delineate the different parts of the nasal septum. Note the predominance of cartilage present in the younger patient.

invasive and most conservative approach. **Box 2** summarizes some highlights and pitfalls (see later discussion) that the senior author has realized over a career of operating on children.

Closed Techniques

Closed septal repositioning

In the pediatric nose, an acutely fractured and displaced septum is rare, but it is one case that is often amenable to closed septal repositioning. This technique can also be attempted in the chronically deviated septum. Should closed repositioning correct the deviation, there is no need for further manipulation. If it is not successful, no harm has been done and the surgeon is not prevented from proceeding to more invasive procedures. If closed septal repositioning is being performed for nasal airway obstruction, it can be combined with treatment of the inferior turbinates, either with outfracture or turbinoplasty.

Although closed septal repositioning has long been regarded as outdated when addressing the adult septum, it still has application in children.[17] Unlike in adults, for

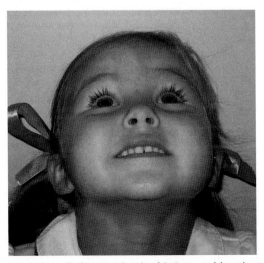

Fig. 4. Note the small nasal vestibular opening in this 3-year-old patient.

Box 2
Septoplasty pearls from Dr. Gross

- The mucoperichondrium in children is very fragile. Extreme effort is required to preserve it intact.
- Liberal use of the fiberoptic endoscope, both in the clinic for diagnosis and in the operating room, will often clarify the anatomy in these small patients.
- If operating on an acute nasal or septal fracture, and the fracture is a greenstick, the fracture must be converted to a full fracture before reduction.
- Closed reduction of the pediatric nasal septum remains a viable, noninvasive approach. Consider attempting this approach before proceeding to an open procedure.
- In addition to reimplanting resected cartilage, reimplant resected portions of the bony nasal septum in children after straightening.
- Many nonpediatric otolaryngologists are hesitant to approach the nose of children. With time and experience, one will find that the comfort level rises dramatically, and that these procedures can be performed safely and the results need not be compromised.

---

whom it is accepted that closed reduction is not efficacious in providing long-term relief of adult septal deviation, it can provide lasting results for the pediatric patient when correctly performed. The difference in the observed results in adults is likely due to the relative dominance of cartilage in the pediatric nasal septum, which is more amenable to closed repositioning. It also remains a less-invasive procedure that minimizes the risk of disrupting the mucoperichondrium and cartilage of the developing nasal septum and thus should be given consideration. In the event that there are not lasting results from closed reduction, open reduction can be attempted later.

Closed septal repositioning is performed using monitored sedation, with the occasional patient requiring general anesthesia. The patient should provide consent for a more invasive procedure should closed septal repositioning fail. The patient's nasal cavities are sprayed with oxymetazoline (or an equivalent decongestant) in the preoperative suite. Once in the operating room, the nasal cavities are packed with pledgets soaked in a decongestant and a local anesthetic. There is no need for infiltration with local anesthetic. A flat elevator of the surgeon's choice (eg, a septal displacer or another, similarly blunt, flat instrument such as Asch or Walsham forceps) is inserted into the nasal cavity that has been narrowed by the septal displacement, and the septum is reduced. Alternatively, a scalpel handle can be used. If the procedure is being performed for an acute septal fracture, one must convert a greenstick fracture to a full fracture before attempting closed repositioning. There is no need for splints or nasal packing. If the procedure is unsuccessful, proceed to a surgical septoplasty.

Targeted endoscopic resection of spurs without flap elevation

Even before Fuchs demonstrated the importance of preserving the mucoperichondrium overlying the septal cartilage, clinicians were aware that injury to this layer of tissue caused a higher rate of septal perforations after septoplasty. However, in select cases in which there is an acutely deviated spur of septal cartilage abutting a turbinate or the lateral nasal wall causing nasal airway obstruction, mucoperichondrium can be resected using powered instrumentation without the need to elevate a flap from the anterior septum. In the senior author's experience, this targeted approach using endoscopes and a microdebrider will leave only a small area of exposed cartilage at the base of the spur, which mucosalizes quickly. Also note that when using this technique great care must be taken to preserve intact the mucoperichondrial covering of the opposite side to ensure that a total perforation is not created.[18] This preservation can be achieved if resection is stopped after all of the bony spur has been removed.

Open Techniques

Targeted spur resection

Some septal spurs have a broad enough base that a targeted endoscopic resection without flap elevation would leave an unacceptable amount of exposed cartilage, placing the septum at higher risk for perforation. In these cases, it may be best to proceed with elevation of a standard submucoperichondrial flap through either a Killian or Hemitransfixion incision, though in selected cases a more limited, conservative elevation of the mucoperichondrial flap may suffice. Elevation should proceed on the ipsilateral side of the spur and include the tissue around the targeted area. A Freer or Cottle elevator is then used to make a transcartilaginous incision just anterior to the base of the spur, and a small contralateral mucoperichondrial flap is elevated opposite the spur. A Takahashi forceps can then be used to remove only the cartilage or bone causing the spur. Alternatively, a microdebrider may be used to precisely dissect the spur. This method minimizes the amount of flap elevation and thus the disruption of blood supply to the cartilaginous septum.

Cartilage weakening without resection

If the quadrilateral cartilage is deviated on a broad front, creating a convexity in the coronal and axial planes, resection would leave a large defect in the septum. Before attempting any large resections that would place the support mechanisms at risk, one can consider making incisions on the convex side of the deviation, allowing the septum to swing back to the midline. This only requires elevation of a mucoperichondrial flap on the convex side of the septal deviation.

Cartilage resection

If the more conservative techniques mentioned above do not alleviate the anatomic pathology causing the septal deviation, one can proceed with a submucoperichondrial resection of the quadrilateral cartilage in a similar fashion to that performed in the adult. As Crysdale's[13] group has shown, it is important to consider reimplantation of the cartilage after appropriate manipulations have been performed to straighten the cartilage or trim excess length that causes bowing. This also applies for bony portions of the septum that are resected.

SUMMARY

Performing a septoplasty on a pediatric patient is often viewed with fear by many practitioners. The main concern that causes hesitation is the potential for altering or stunting the growth of the nose or midface. Although the evidence pendulum appears to be swinging toward allowing the operation, which should not result in long-term sequelae if done using the proper techniques, it should still be approached with some trepidation.

The surgeon must always evaluate the child thoroughly to ensure the correct diagnosis and determine the exact location of the anatomic pathology. Absolute indications for the operation are rare, and thus the strength of the relative indications (eg, severely deviated septum) must be weighed when discussing the risks with parents.

Using the techniques described in this article and giving consideration to the varied approaches, from least to most invasive, will allow the surgeon to safely correct the patient's problem with excellent results and the least concern for affecting growth. In the senior author's experience, the surgeon's comfort level with performing pediatric septoplasty will rise dramatically with the first few cases. Once the fear of operating on the pediatric nose is overcome, the surgeon's knowledge of anatomy and comfort with patient selection will be freeing: the procedure can be done safely, and results need not be compromised.

REFERENCES

1. Gilbert JG, Segal S Jr. Growth of the nose and the septorhinoplastic problem in youth. AMA Arch Otolaryngol 1958;68:673–82.
2. Farrior RT, Connolly ME. Septorhinoplasty in children. Otolaryngol Clin North Am 1970;3:345–64.
3. Sarnat BG, Wexler MR. Growth of the face and jaws after resection of the septal cartilage in the rabbit. Am J Anat 1966;118:755–67.
4. Sarnat BG, Wexler MR. The snout after resection of nasal septum in adult rabbits. Arch Otolaryngol 1967;86:463–6.
5. Hartshorn DF. Facial growth effects of nasal septal cartilage resection in beagle pups. Iowa (IA): University of Iowa; 1970.
6. Stenstrom SJ, Thilander BL. Effects of nasal septal cartilage resections on young guinea pigs. Plast Reconstr Surg 1970;45:160–70.
7. Fuchs P. Experimental production of growth disturbance by using a caudally based vomerine flap in rabbits. Amsterdam: Excerpta Medical Foundation; 1969. p. 484–8.
8. Bernstein L. Early submucous resection of nasal septal cartilage. A pilot study in canine pups. Arch Otolaryngol 1973;97:273–8.
9. Ortiz-Monasterio F, Olmedo A. Corrective rhinoplasty before puberty: a long-term follow-up. Plast Reconstr Surg 1981;68:381–91.
10. McComb HK, Coghlan BA. Primary repair of the unilateral cleft lip nose: completion of a longitudinal study. Cleft Palate Craniofac J 1996;33:23–30 [discussion: 30–1].
11. Crysdale WS, Tatham B. External septorhinoplasty in children. Laryngoscope 1985;95:12–6.
12. Bejar I, Farkas LG, Messner AH, et al. Nasal growth after external septoplasty in children. Arch Otolaryngol Head Neck Surg 1996;122:816–21.
13. El-Hakim H, Crysdale WS, Abdollel M, et al. A study of anthropometric measures before and after external septoplasty in children: a preliminary study. Arch Otolaryngol Head Neck Surg 2001;127:1362–6.
14. Dennis SC, den Herder C, Shandilya M, et al. Open rhinoplasty in children. Facial Plast Surg 2007;23:259–66.
15. Kirk V, Kahn A, Brouillette RT. Diagnostic approach to obstructive sleep apnea in children. Sleep Med Rev 1998;2:255–69.
16. Van Loosen J, Van Zanten GA, Howard CV, et al. Growth characteristics of the human nasal septum. Rhinology 1996;34:78–82.
17. Cummings CS, Flint PW, Harker LA, et al, editors. Cummings otolaryngology head & neck surgery. Fourth edition. Philadelphia: Elsevier Mosby; 2005. p. 1010–1.
18. Giles WC, Gross CW, Abram AC, et al. Endoscopic septoplasty. Laryngoscope 1994;104:1507–9.

Surgery of the Inferior and Middle Turbinates

Leslie A. Nurse, MD*, James A. Duncavage, MD

KEYWORDS

- Turbinate • Middle • Inferior • Nasal cycle
- Frontal recess • Reduction • Resection
- Concha bullosa • Paradoxical middle turbinate
- Turbinectomy • Turbinoplasty

For over a century, surgical management of the inferior and middle turbinates has been an ongoing topic of discourse and disagreement. Treatment, either medical or surgical, of the inferior turbinate is required in cases of turbinate hypertrophy where the goals of therapy are to maximize the nasal airway, to preserve nasal mucosal function, and to minimize complications. Middle turbinate management, more controversial than inferior turbinate management, still lacks definitive consensus. This article reviews the anatomy, physiology, and pathology involving the inferior and middle turbinates. Advantages, disadvantages, complications, and controversies surrounding the surgical management of the turbinates are discussed.

INFERIOR TURBINATE

Inferior turbinate management must be considered in any discussion of sinonasal surgery because turbinate enlargement leads to obstruction of the nasal airway and limited surgical access to the paranasal sinuses in patients presenting with both sinus disease and symptomatic nasal obstruction. The inferior turbinate plays a major role in the regulation of nasal airflow and the development of nasal obstruction. Surgical turbinate reduction, either alone or as an adjunctive procedure during sinus surgery, septoplasty, or rhinoplasty, is often performed in patients after unsuccessful medical management of inferior turbinate hypertrophy. The literature describes multiple techniques of turbinate reduction, each with its associated advantages, disadvantages, and complications. In developing an understanding of which of these techniques is most effective, it is first important to discuss the anatomy and physiology of the inferior turbinate.

Inferior Turbinate Anatomy and Physiology

The nasal turbinates are important landmarks of the lateral nasal wall. The turbinate bones develop from a cartilage ossification center during the fifth intrauterine month.

Department of Otolaryngology, Vanderbilt University Medical Center, 7209 Medical Center East, South Tower, Nashville, TN 37232-8605, USA
* Corresponding author.
E-mail address: leslie.nurse@vanderbilt.edu (L. A. Nurse).

Otolaryngol Clin N Am 42 (2009) 295–309
doi:10.1016/j.otc.2009.01.009
0030-6665/09/$ – see front matter © 2009 Elsevier Inc. All rights reserved.

oto.theclinics.com

The inferior, middle, and superior turbinates are each composed of a thin bone for structural support and covered by an adherent mucoperiosteum. Stratified squamous epithelium is found on the anterior tip of the inferior turbinate, whereas pseudostratified ciliated columnar respiratory epithelium covers all other mucosal surfaces. The continually beating ciliated mucosa provides constant motion to the mucous blanket within the nose. This blanket acts as a cleaning and filtering system for the upper respiratory tract and also helps to maintain moisture within the nose.[1] The turbinates maximize the effective intranasal surface area for rapid humidification and warming of inspired air.

Similar to the rest of the upper respiratory tract, the membranes of the turbinates are composed of ciliated, pseudostratified, glandular, columnar epithelium. The cilia beat in unison to propel the mucus from the nasal cavity toward the nasopharynx, where the mucus is then swallowed. Mucociliary transport relies on mucus production and ciliary function in healthy mucosa.

Both the blood supply and the autonomic nervous system control the secretions and level of congestion of the turbinates. The autonomic nervous system provides the general innervation to the nose, with the parasympathetic nerves supplying the resting tone and controlling secretions. The nerve supply originates from the facial nerve at the inferior salivatory nucleus and follows along the distribution of the facial nerve through the sphenopalatine ganglion. Overactivity of this parasympathetic innervation or underactivity of sympathetic innervation results in nasal congestion and obstruction.[2]

The histology of the inferior turbinate deserves special consideration. Grossly, it is comprised of its epithelial mucosal layer overlying a basement membrane, an osseous layer, and an intervening lamina propria. The medial aspect of the mucosal layer is thicker and has more surface area than the lateral mucosa of the turbinate, as demonstrated by Berger and colleagues.[3]

A thin acellular basement membrane separates the mucosal epithelium from the underlying lamina propria and the periostium of turbinate bone. The composition of the lamina propria includes loose connective tissue; a superficial inflammatory cell infiltrate with lymphocytes and other immunocompetent cells; serous, mucous, and mixed glands; and a rich network of thin-walled venous sinusoids. Affecting circulation through these sinusoids is a cyclic alternating constriction and dilation of the inferior turbinate vasculature, known as the nasal cycle, which occurs approximately every 2 to 7 hours.[1]

At the core of the inferior turbinate is its central osseous layer of nonhomogeneous, cancellous, spongelike bone made of interwoven bony trabeculae separated by a labyrinth of interconnecting spaces containing fatty tissue and blood vessels.

Inferior Turbinate in Nasal Obstruction

The inferior turbinate plays a major role in the development of nasal obstruction. The nasal valve is the region of the nasal airway extending from the caudal end of the upper lateral cartilage bounded by the septum and the anterior portion of the inferior turbinate. The nasal valve provides approximately 50% of total airway resistance. As air flows through this narrow segment, it accelerates and the pressure drops, which can result in nasal valve collapse, especially if the upper lateral cartilages are anatomically weak. The erectile tissue of the nasal septum and inferior turbinate can also impinge on the nasal valve and increase resistance. Because the cross-sectional area of the nasal valve is small, even minor changes in inferior turbinate congestion can significantly decrease the total diameter and can have marked effects on resistance.

The role of the inferior turbinate in nasal obstruction is not only anatomic but may also be functional. Even in the presence of a normal radius, a sensation of obstruction can occur from turbulent airflow. Nasal airway resistance is an important parameter in nasal function. Airflow turbulence optimizes inspiratory air contact with the mucous membrane. Resistance must remain within certain limits for the perception of normal breathing. If resistance is too high or too low, a sensation of obstruction may occur.[2] The turbinate, through its participation in the nasal valve, can act as a mechanical source of nasal obstruction. Alternatively, the turbinate can also play a role in subjective nasal obstruction if there is compromise in the function of its overlying mucosa.

Some nasal disorders, such as allergic and vasomotor rhinitis, are associated with the development of permanent turbinate hypertrophy producing chronic nasal obstruction. Others are associated with anatomic bony turbinate enlargement due to progressive ossification throughout adulthood.[3] While chronic rhinitis is associated with hypertrophy of the mucosa of the entire nasal cavity, the inferior turbinates are central to the development of nasal obstruction, as they contain sinusoidal erectile tissue.[4] Medical management of these disorders includes antihistamines, sympathomimetics, anticholinergics, and steroids. These medications provide symptomatic relief but no permanent cure. When optimal medical management has been unsatisfactory in the relief of nasal obstruction, surgical intervention is warranted.

Surgical Reduction of the Inferior Turbinates

Inferior turbinate reduction can be performed by various techniques that resect, displace, or decrease the volume of the turbinate.

Turbinate resection, total or partial, was once the surgical treatment of choice for turbinate hypertrophy. However, because of concerns about postoperative crusting, bleeding, and atrophic rhinitis, the treatment fell out of favor. Although very few studies actually demonstrated the validity of these concerns, the procedure became less popular with the development of other techniques.

Outfracturing of the inferior turbinate using a blunt elevator to displace the turbinate laterally is a technique with minimal morbidity. Improvement in nasal airway is transient, however, as the turbinate eventually resumes its original position. The technique also does not address the underlying pathology of hypertrophied turbinate mucosa. Turbinate outfracture, therefore, is often performed concomitantly with another procedure.

Submucosal injection of sclerosing solutions is another intervention that has been used in an attempt to decrease turbinate engorgement by blocking vascular channels. These results are transient, however.[4]

Destructive procedures, including electrocautery, cryosurgery, laser surgery, and submucous resection, have been used to reduce the bulk of the turbinates by inducing scarring or by direct destruction. These procedures can be performed under local anesthesia in the operating room or in an outpatient office in most adult patients. Studies of some of these methods show variable long-term success and such complications as bone necrosis, synechiae, and prolonged crusting and bleeding.[5]

Total Inferior Turbinectomy

In the early 1900s, most surgeons advocated inferior turbinectomy. The procedure fell out of favor after criticisms by such prominent rhinologists as Freer[6] and because of concerns over the risks of postoperative hemorrhage, crusting, and atrophic rhinitis.

Resection of the inferior turbinate, although no longer widely performed, is still considered an option in turbinate reduction surgery. The technique involves fracture of the turbinate bone toward the midline and cutting along its lateral attachment. This can be done with the use of a nasal speculum and headlight or with endoscopic visualization.[7] Controversies regarding this procedure are related to postoperative complications, including bleeding and scar formation, and presumed loss of physiologic function leading to atrophic mucosal changes, nasal crusting, and dryness.

Although resection of the inferior turbinate results in an increase in the volume of the nasal airway and the diameter of the nasal valve, it has been shown that this increase occurs at the expense of nasal physiology with decreased humidifying activity of the nasal mucosa, excess drying of nasal secretions, and resultant crusting.[8,9] The value of inferior turbinectomy versus the risks of potential complications remains unclear. In some studies of partial or total inferior turbinectomy, complications of bleeding, crusting, and atrophic rhinitis were considered minimal, even in dry, dusty climates.[10,11]

In one of these studies, 351 patients who underwent standard total inferior turbinectomy were evaluated for subjective improvement in nasal obstruction based on a six-question survey administered at 6 and 18 months postoperatively. All but nine of the patients (97%) reported improved nasal breathing at both time intervals.[11]

In more recent comparisons of total inferior turbinectomy to other techniques, turbinectomy yielded good long-term improvement of nasal obstruction but also resulted in increased complications. In 2003, Passàli and colleagues[9] randomized 382 patients with symptomatic inferior turbinate hypertrophy into six therapeutic groups and found that patients who underwent total or near-total turbinectomy experienced good long-term relief of nasal obstruction but also had a significantly higher percentage of crusting and bleeding compared with patients who underwent laser cautery, electrocautery, cryotherapy, or submucous resection.

Many surgeons understand that, while widening of the nasal airway to reduce resistance might be an important goal, that goal must be balanced against other goals that might lead to increased nasal resistance. Such goals include the maintenance of functional nasal mucosa with normal aerodynamic contours of the lateral wall to prevent turbulence.[12]

Electrocautery

Methods of inferior turbinate electrocautery include linear surface electrocautery, bipolar electrocautery, and submucous diathermy. These may be done under local anesthesia in an operating room or clinic. The main disadvantage is that results are short-lived, but the procedure may be repeated as necessary. Additional disadvantages are postoperative pain, crusting, and scarring.

Meredith[13] reported that 31% of 81 patients treated with both surface electrocautery and outfracture subjectively noted recurrence of nasal obstruction when followed for more than 33 months. Similarly, Warwick-Brown and Marks[14] evaluated 307 patients who underwent submucosal diathermy with and without outfracture and noted that patient satisfaction with the procedure declined from 82% at 1 month postoperatively to 41% at 1 year. Edema and crusting after surface electrocautery has been shown to occur up to 3 to 6 weeks after treatment.[13] Avoidance of bone injury with appropriate needle placement is also important in preventing bone necrosis and sequestration.[4,5]

Radiofrequency Turbinate Reduction

Another technique presently in use in inferior turbinate reduction is radiofrequency volumetric tissue reduction (RFVTR), which aims at improving the nasal airway while preserving mucosal function. Radiofrequency heat is used to induce submucosal tissue destruction. The device, an electrode probe that induces ionic agitation at the cellular level, heats the turbinate tissue with little heat dissipation. Thermal injury only extends 2 to 4 mm around the active portion of electrode, thus only within the deep mucosa, sparing damage to adjacent structures or mucosal surfaces. The area of injury is replaced with scar-producing fibroblasts, as part of normal wound healing. Scar contraction leads to reduction of turbinate volume and relief of nasal obstruction. Because of the limited heat dispersal, RFVTR is different from submucous diathermy with electrocautery, where much higher tissue temperatures (up to 800°C) are thought to increase morbidities, such as crusting, pain, and bleeding, and have possible deleterious effects on mucosa.[15]

Controlled studies examining RFVTR demonstrate statistically significant long-term improvement in several parameters, including increased nasal volume and decreased nasal airway resistance, based on acoustic rhinometry and decreased subjective nasal obstruction.[16] An increase in turbinate edema may be seen in the first postoperative days. This is thought to be due to the acute tissue insult. The benefits of this procedure include preservation of nasal epithelium and mucociliary function. Also, the procedure can be performed under local anesthesia in an outpatient setting. The use of nasal packing is also generally unnecessary with this technique.

Laser Cautery

Carbon dioxide laser turbinate reduction can also be performed under local anesthesia. Use of laser turbinate reduction has gained greater favor especially because the procedure results in little blood loss and postoperative discomfort.[17,18] Disadvantages of laser turbinate reduction include eschar formation, which may cause obstruction or, rarely, hemorrhage with sloughing of the eschar.[5] Although the laser is effective at reducing hypertrophied mucosa through the induction of scarring and actual tissue removal, it is ineffective at removing turbinate bone and therefore not ideal in cases where bone reduction is necessary. Another disadvantage is that equipment for laser therapy is expensive and requires additional expertise, training, and safety precautions.

Cryosurgery

Cryoturbinectomy can be performed easily, also in an outpatient setting under local anesthesia. A typical treatment involves the application of a cryoprobe to the medial and lateral surface of the inferior turbinate, and freezing at −85°C for 60 to 75 seconds.[19]

Because of its most pronounced effect on water-laden goblet cells, cryotherapy is thought to be most effective in controlling severe rhinorrhea associated with chronic vasomotor rhinitis.[5] Although cryotherapy is considered to have relatively low associated morbidity, the duration of results is variable and usually temporary, thus requiring repeated applications.[4,20]

Submucous Resection

First described by Spielberg[21] in 1924 and further elaborated by House[22] in 1951, submucous turbinate reduction involves removal of the inferior turbinate bone while leaving overlying mucosa intact. By maintaining the mucosal flaps, normal mucosal function is preserved, reducing the likelihood of complications, such as crusting and atrophic rhinitis. After a traditional submucous resection, as described by Spielberg,[21] only minimal crusting is typically observed along the incision site. Another reported advantage of this method is very low incidence of postoperative bleeding.[5,22] The effectiveness of traditional submucous resection is even more pronounced in cases of conchal bone hypertrophy. The primary disadvantages of traditional submucous resection are the potential for mucosal shredding in inexperienced hands and the need for nasal packing postoperatively.[23]

More recently, the use of the microdebrider in submucous resection of the inferior turbinate has proven quite successful with even fewer complications of crusting and similar favorable outcomes.[24] This technique of submucous resection of the inferior turbinate is the method of choice for the senior author and is depicted in **Fig. 1**. The first turbinate is infiltrated with 1% Xylocaine and 1:100,000 epinephrine. The turbinate head is then pierced with a turbinate blade (2.9-mm microdebrider tip, Medtronic Xomed, Jacksonville, Florida), which is then inserted into the anterior face of the inferior turbinate and used to dissect a submucosal flap by tunneling along the length of the turbinate, moving anterior to posterior (see **Fig. 1A**). The microdebrider, rotating at 3000 rpm, is then run along the length of the turbinate and moved in a steady circular fashion with the intent of removing the stromal tissue from inside the turbinate. The overlying mucosa is completely preserved. In patients with significant hypertrophy of the posterior portion of the inferior turbinate, a second entry with the turbinate blade is made in the midposterior turbinate and the microdebrider is run in a similar manner. The turbinate is then outfractured using a 7-mm chisel placed at the medial aspect of the turbinate along its length, allowing for additional lateralization (see **Fig. 1B**).

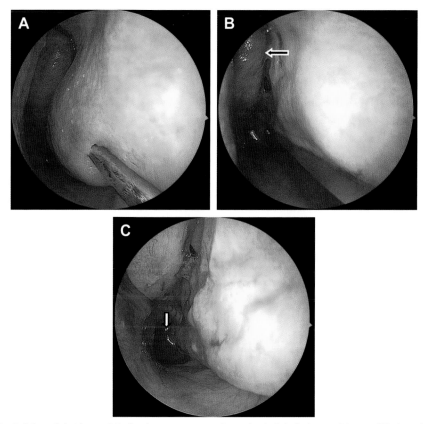

Fig. 1. Microdebrider-assisted submucous resection of a left inferior turbinate. (*A*) A turbinate blade (2.9-mm microdebrider tip; Medtronic Xomed, Jacksonville, Florida) pierces the turbinate head and is then used to dissect a submucosal flap by tunneling along the length of the turbinate moving anterior to posterior. (*B*) The turbinate is outfractured using a 7-mm chisel. The middle turbinate is exposed (*arrow*). (*C*) The turbinate has been lateralized and choana can be seen (*arrow*).

Chen and colleagues[24] compared microdebrider-assisted inferior turbinoplasty using this technique to standard submucous resection in 160 patients with inferior turbinate hypertrophy. Patients were randomly assigned to either treatment group. Outcome measures were conducted preoperatively and at 1, 2, and 3 years after surgery. These measures included anterior rhinomanometry and subjective symptom improvement. Compared to preoperative values, subjective complaints, including nasal obstruction, sneezing, rhinorrhea, and snoring, improved significantly in both groups as did rhinomanometric measures.

Each of options available in the surgical management of nasal obstruction due to inferior turbinate hypertrophy is associated with complications. Each, also, has its own advantages and disadvantage in comparison with other options, and each has proven to be effective. Most studies suggest that when any of these options is performed well, results can be favorable, albeit transient in some instances. Before undertaking surgical intervention, it is important to ensure that all medical therapy options have been fully explored as surgery may not be effective in some patients with medically treatable conditions. Ultimately, the surgeon's preference and expertise guide the selection of any particular technique. While the problem of nasal obstruction can have severe adverse effects on quality of life, treatment is almost always elective. One possible exception is severe life-threatening sleep apnea.

The best treatment is the one with minimal morbidity that yields the best response. Jackson and colleagues[5] have proposed an algorithm as a staged protocol of increasingly invasive interventions:

1. Medical management
2. Laser reduction as an initial surgical office procedure when medical management is ineffective
3. Partial anterior turbinectomy or submucosal resection, with or without microdebrider assistance, when office-based procedures fail
4. Rarely, total turbinectomy if all other treatment attempts do not succeed

Finally, other causes of nasal obstruction should be addressed in the full assessment of a patient with nasal obstruction including the need for septoplasty, nasal valve correction, and rhinoplasty.

MIDDLE TURBINATE

The middle turbinate is an important landmark in endoscopic sinus surgery. Resection of the middle turbinate remains a source of considerable debate and controversy in the surgical management of sinonasal disease. Despite the volume of literature both supporting and disparaging the removal of the middle turbinate, objective evidence either favoring or discouraging the procedure remains sparse. The current rhinology literature remains unclear regarding the best management of the middle turbinate during sinus surgery.

A great deal of controversy surrounding middle turbinate resection appears to be based on each surgeon's personal philosophy regarding nasal physiology and anatomy. The debate obviously divides those determined to preserve the middle turbinate from those who propose varying degrees of turbinate excision, from partial to near-total removal.

Historically, the practice of middle turbinate resection was condemned. Messerklinger[25] felt that, with few exceptions, the middle turbinate should be preserved. Partial removal was only to be reserved in cases of concha bullosa or paradoxical middle turbinate, and resection in these instances was always conservative. Conversely,

Wigand and colleagues[26] recommended partial or total middle turbinate resection as a routine step in virtually all endoscopic sinus surgeries. Both approaches to the middle turbinate have yielded successful outcomes, thus supporting surgeons on both sides of the issue. Yet, even with the good results seen with either approach, surgeons who either routinely resect or those who routinely preserve the middle turbinate vehemently disavow the opposing approach. Surgeons often cling to their respective positions on the issue quite passionately. Even in the face of such fervor, however, surprisingly few studies provide a hard scientific rationale in the approach to middle turbinate preservation or resection. In fact, virtually all of the literature on the subject of middle turbinate resection is based on nonrandomized retrospective data. In 2001, Clement and White[27] reviewed over 500 papers describing turbinate surgery over a period of 35 years and not one randomized controlled study was identified. Their conclusion is essentially the overarching theme regarding middle turbinate resection—there really is no conclusive evidence supporting or discrediting the procedure. For every study that appears to favor one approach, there are others that endorse the opposing view. Thus, management is largely based on personal surgical belief or anecdotal experience.

In the following sections, we review the relevant middle turbinate anatomy. The discussion includes the rationale for its resection in sinus surgery and some of the controversies and theoretical problems associated with removal of the middle turbinate. The sections specifically address the validity or actual occurrence of complications stemming from removal of the turbinate.

Middle Turbinate Development and Anatomy

The middle turbinate is embryologically derived from the ethmoid bone. Structurally, the middle turbinate can be divided into three segments.[28] The anterior third attaches superiorly and vertically to the skull base at the horizontal plate of the ethmoid bone just lateral to the cribriform plate. This attachment may be pneumatized in up to 12% of the population,[1] thus forming an aerated vertical segment of the middle turbinate, which may be referred to as the interlamellar cell. This aerated segment is subject to the same inflammatory and infectious processes as other sinonasal mucosa, thereby resulting in obstruction of drainage from the ethmoid infundibulum. The middle segment of the middle turbinate, the ground or basal lamella, inserts laterally, attaching it to the lamina papyracea. It is this attachment that divides the ethmoid sinus into anterior and a posterior compartments. The posterior segment of the middle turbinate is attached inferiorly and oriented horizontally, inserting onto the perpendicular process of the palatine bone anterior to the sphenopalatine foramen.[28] The anterior/superior portion of the middle turbinate, an important surgical landmark, forms the medial boundary of the frontal recess. Therefore, lateralization of the middle turbinate can lead to structural narrowing of the frontal sinus outflow tract and frontal sinusitis.[29] Also to be considered is the variability in the shape of the middle turbinate wherein there may be paradoxical curvature or pneumatization. Pneumatization of the head of the middle turbinate, or concha bullosa, is also a variation of special consideration in patients where this may cause nasal obstruction or obstruction of the osteomeatal unit.

Management of the Middle Turbinate

The middle turbinate debate is largely centered on one crucial question: How much of the middle turbinate can one safely resect? The effect of middle turbinate resection on normal sinus and nasal physiology remains uncertain. The nasal turbinates are thought to function collectively to direct and assist in lamination of nasal airflow, to humidify and warm inspired air, and to provide a mechanical defense against particulate matter.

In comparison with the inferior turbinate, the middle turbinate is significantly smaller, contains less vascular and erectile tissue, accounts for a negligible portion of nasal airway resistance, and is believed to have less functional significance.

Despite this evidence, as well as literature supporting the safety of middle turbinectomy, the procedure continues to provoke a considerable amount of controversy, particularly regarding lateralization of the turbinate remnant as a factor promoting postoperative frontal sinusitis. Other concerns include loss of a significant surgical landmark, development of atrophic rhinitis, postoperative hemorrhage, and anosmia. The controversy surrounding middle turbinate resection appears to be based on personal philosophy regarding nasal physiology and anatomy.

Middle Turbinate Resection

Several indications for the removal of the middle turbinates in endoscopic sinus surgery are now more generally accepted. Some cited indications for middle turbinate resection include treatment of conchae bullosa that participate in nasal obstruction or prevent access to the middle meatus in the "crowded nose,"[29] removal of disease involving the turbinate,[30] creation of surgical access to the paranasal sinuses, and treatment of headache related to the middle turbinate syndrome where contact between an enlarged middle turbinate and either the septum or lateral nasal wall leads to stimulation of the sensory portion of the trigeminal nerve.[31]

The techniques for middle turbinate resection also vary. Kennedy and Sinreich[32] describe a technique where the turbinate is split in the middle and only the lateral portion is removed, leaving the medial portion intact to function physiologically. Wigand[33] describes resecting the posterior third of the middle turbinate when performing any retrograde sphenoethmoidectomy. Morgenstein and Krieger[34] describe a technique that involves cutting the superior attachment of the middle turbinate, then snaring the anterior two thirds. Freedman and Kern[30] describe resection of the middle turbinate to within 0.5 cm of the skull base as an integral part of all headlight intranasal sphenoethmoidectomies. In the majority of patients, this maneuver addresses disease involving the turbinate (eg, polyposis or osteitis); turbinate resection is advocated regardless of the amount of pathology involving the middle turbinate.

The senior author employs a middle turbinate resection technique (**Fig. 2**) that is a modification of the techniques described by Wigand. It is performed with the use of a 0° 4-mm telescope. Initially, the middle turbinate is fractured medially toward the septum using a Freer elevator to expose its vertical, superior attachment (see **Fig. 2**A). This attachment is incised with a straight turbinate scissor at its most anterior portion (see **Fig. 2**B and C). The body of the turbinate is then grasped with straight Wilde forceps (see **Fig. 2**D) and pulled inferiorly and posteriorly, leaving at least 0.5 cm of the superior attachment and basal lamella to preserve as landmarks (see **Fig. 2**E). The most posterior attachment of the middle turbinate is then incised using through-biting forceps, thereby completing the partial resection. As prophylaxis against intraoperative or postoperative hemorrhage, the remainder of the posterior attachment is then suction-cauterized to coagulate small branches of the sphenopalatine artery (see **Fig. 2**F).

Middle Turbinate Preservation Versus Resection

Historically, the practice of middle turbinate resection has been condemned, largely because of theoretical and actual observed complications following removal. The most prominent of these concerns and complications include alteration in nasal function, such as air humidification, filtration, and airflow;[29] increased incidence of frontal sinusitis;[29] ethmoid scarring;[35] development of anosmia;[36] postoperative epistaxis;[37]

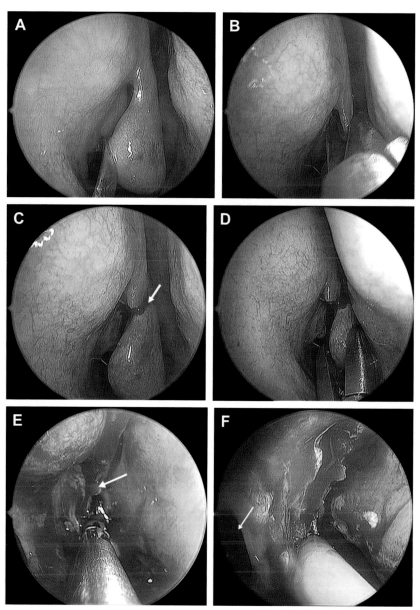

Fig. 2. Technique of endoscopic right partial middle turbinectomy. (*A*) Middle turbinate being medially fractured to expose its vertical attachment superiorly. (*B*) Vertical attachment incised with straight turbinate scissors at its most anterior part. (*C*) After this incision of the anterior, superior attachment (*arrow*), the head of the turbinate is grasped (*D*) and dissected inferiorly and posteriorly along the length of the turbinate back to the basal lamella. (*E*) Incision of the posterior turbinate attachment completes the partial resection. Arrow indicates remnants of the superior and basal lamella attachments being preserved as a landmark. (*F*) Suction cautery applied to the posterior attachment remnant to coagulate small braches of sphenopalatine artery. Arrow indicates maxillary sinus ostium.

loss of anatomic landmark for revision surgery;[29] and the development of atrophic rhinitis.[33]

Alteration in Nasal Function

If the turbinates play a role in the lamination of nasal airflow, it is quite possible that their removal may contribute to postoperative changes in nasal airflow resistance. Is there evidence of such an effect? Most recently, Brescia and colleagues[37] sought to define the effect of middle turbinate resection on nasal airflow. In this retrospective study, 23 patients with extensive sinonasal polyposis who had undergone partial resection of the middle turbinate endoscopic sinus surgery were compared with 25 polyp patients who had endoscopic sinus surgery with middle turbinate preservation. The outcomes examined included endoscopic scoring of polyposis and measurement of nasal airway resistance by computerized rhinomanometry performed at 3 months and 12 months after surgery. The findings of this study were improvement of endoscopic score and a statistically significant reduction of nasal airway resistance after both surgical techniques, with no statistically significant difference in the mean nasal airway resistance values before and after the procedure when comparing middle turbinate resection versus preservation.

Previously, Cook and colleagues[38] performed a prospective evaluation of the effect of middle turbinate resection on nasal airflow. They evaluated 31 consecutive patients who underwent endoscopic sinus surgery with partial middle turbinectomy performed as part of their surgery. They measured pre- and postoperative nasal airflow and nasal airway resistance using computerized rhinomanometry and found that all patients had significant improvement in nasal airflow ($P<.001$) and significant decrease in nasal resistance ($P<.001$) compared with preoperative measures. These findings should be considered cautiously because this study lacked a control group of patients who did not have turbinates removed.

Anosmia

It has been shown that olfactory neuroepithelium exists within the superior portions of the middle turbinate. In the late 1890s and early 1900s both Von Brunn[39] and Read[40] independently performed histologic evaluations in animals and humans and used their findings to develop schemata demonstrating the distribution of the olfactory neuroepithelium. According to these schemata, there is olfactory neuroepithelium localized to a small portion of the superior parts of the middle turbinate. The existence of this olfactory neuroepithelium would suggest the possibility of anosmia following middle turbinate resection. Because of age-related decrease in olfactory neuroepithelium, older patients especially might notice a decrease in olfaction following middle turbinate resection. Similarly, younger patients who have undergone middle turbinate resection might experience a noticeable decrease in olfaction as they age.

However, the amount of this olfactory tissue is small compared with the entire distribution of surface area available for olfaction. Thus, one could conclude that middle turbinate resection should not significantly affect olfaction, as clinical evidence seems to show. Beidlingmanger[36] reviewed the records of 110 patients undergoing 198 partial middle turbinate resections during endoscopic sinus surgery. The patients were evaluated for the complications of anosmia, bleeding, and crusting. Patients undergoing endoscopic sinus surgery with partial middle turbinate resections were evaluated by histopathologic and CT analyses. In this review of 110 patients with 198 partial turbinate resections, only one patient complained of anosmia. Also, one patient required vessel ligation for bleeding, and no patients had excessive crusting. This 0.9% incidence of anosmia is comparable to the 0.8% incidence in Wigand's series of 220 patients who underwent endoscopic sinus surgery with turbinate preservation. Similarly, in two other large series of over 1000 patients each, Lawson[41] and Freedman and Kern[30] found no increased risk of anosmia or atrophic rhinitis in patients who underwent middle turbinate resections. Similarly, Toffel,[42] who reported a large series of patients over 16 years who underwent partial middle turbinectomy, emphasizes the importance of preserving the superior rim of turbinate in which olfactory epithelium may reside in minimizing the possibility of postoperative olfactory disturbance.

Scarring and Frontal Sinusitis

Postoperative scarring can be a source of great disappointment after endoscopic sinus surgery. The incidence of scarring for all undergoing endoscopic sinus surgery ranges from 4% to 27% in the literature.[35] Such scarring may lead to recurrent symptoms and the need for further surgery. Reports of middle turbinate resection leading to lateral scarring of the middle turbinate to the nasal wall have been described.

Scarring of frontal sinus outflow secondary to middle turbinate resection is also an outcome discussed in the literature. This scarring is thought to be related to the healing process after middle turbinectomy.[29] The proposed mechanism is that a middle turbinate cut near its anterior superior attachment becomes destabilized, and the lateral aspect of the middle turbinate remnant adheres to the surgical field. Granulation tissue in the ethmoid cavity gives way to scar and gradual traction on the turbinate remnant, drawing it across the area of the frontal recess. The ensuing inadequate drainage and ventilation of the frontal sinus leads to sinusitis.

Some data support the likelihood that middle turbinate resection can cause frontal sinusitis. Other data seem to show that middle turbinate resection is unlikely to cause frontal sinusitis. In 1995, Swanson and colleagues[29] performed a retrospective review to determine if middle turbinate resection affected postoperative frontal sinus disease. They identified 110 consecutive patients with chronic or recurrent acute sinusitis. Of these patients, 69 had previous middle turbinectomy and 41 had intact middle turbinates after prior sinus surgery. In 42 patients, CT scans were scored and classified as indications of either mild-moderate or severe disease. Frontal sinusitis seen on CT scan was present in 30 of 40 (75%) of patients who had middle turbinate resection versus 45% (9 of 20) of patients who did not, and this difference was statistically significant ($P<.05$). Investigators also considered the degree of middle turbinate resection in this study by using CT scans to determine the height of middle turbinate resection in the frontal recess area. They found no statistical difference between patients with high resection and those with low resection.

The investigators discussed several potential weaknesses of their study, including its retrospective nature, the lack of information on preoperative sinus disease, and the lack of standardization of operative indications or technique. Scar formation and maxillary antrostomy patency were not addressed in this study.

Conversely, in 1998, Fortune and Duncavage[43] retrospectively reviewed 155 consecutive patients undergoing partial middle turbinate resection for either sinusitis or nasal obstruction. Their findings revealed a 10% rate of frontal sinusitis after partial middle turbinectomy and found that the development of sinusitis in these patients was largely associated with preoperative comorbidities, such as asthma, nasal polyps, and severe disease on CT or diseased middle turbinates.

SUMMARY

The role of middle turbinate resection in endoscopic sinus surgery, in spite of the myriad studies and papers on the subject, remains uncertain. Some studies emphasize and others downplay the degree to which middle turbinate resection may have deleterious effects on nasal airflow, postoperative scarring, and, with the loss of surgical landmarks, future surgery. The one prevailing theme of these studies is that none meets the standard of prospective randomized controlled evidence from which one may extrapolate a conclusion about which approach is best. Thus all we are left with are the studies of those in whose hands both methods seem to work quite well. Regardless of which side of the fence one stands, some points that must be kept in mind when approaching the turbinates. Complete removal of the middle turbinate, including its most superior attachment, is neither recommended nor necessary in the absence of malignancy or other invasive disease. The most superior attachment, if left in place, may serve as a landmark and may contain olfactory neuroepithelium whose preservation would prevent theoretical diminution in olfaction, either immediately or long term. Care should be taken to address the possibility for hemorrhage from the posterior turbinate attachment. In the hands of those familiar with their respective techniques, both yield successful outcomes.

REFERENCES

1. Amedee RG, Miller AJ. Sinus anatomy and function. In: Bailey BJ, Calhoun KH, Healy GB, et al, editors. Head and neck surgery–otolaryngology. 3rd edition. Philadelphia: Lippincott-Raven; 2001. p. 321–8.
2. Younger RAL, Denton AB. Controversies in turbinate surgery. Facial Plast Surg Clin North Am 1999;7:311–7.
3. Berger G, Balum-Azim M, Ophir D. The normal inferior turbinate: histomorphometric analysis and clinical implications. Laryngoscope 2003;113(7):1192–8.
4. Principato JJ. Chronic vasomotor rhinitis: cryogenic and other surgical modes of treatment. Laryngoscope 1979;89:619–38.
5. Jackson LE, Koch R, James MD. Controversies in the management of inferior turbinate hypertrophy: a comprehensive review. Plast Reconstr Surg 1999; 103(1):300–12.
6. Freer OT. The inferior turbinate: its longitudinal resection for chronic intumescence. Laryngoscope 1911;21:1136–44.
7. Gupta A, Mercurio E, Bielamowicz S. Endoscopic inferior turbinate reduction: an outcomes analysis. Laryngoscope 2001;111(11):1957–9.
8. Salam MA, Wengraf C. Concho-antropexy or total inferior turbinectomy for hypertrophy of the inferior turbinates: a prospective randomized study. J Laryngol Otol 1993;107:1125–8.
9. Passàli D, Passàli MF, Passàli GC, et al. Treatment of inferior turbinate hypertrophy: a randomized clinical trial. Ann Otol Rhinol Laryngol 2003;112(8):683–8.
10. Odetoyinbo O. Complications following total inferior turbinectomy: facts or myths? Clin Otolaryngol 1987;12:361–3.
11. Talmon Y, Samet A, Gilbey P. Total inferior turbinectomy: operative results and technique. Ann Otol Rhinol Laryngol 2000;109:1117–9.
12. Sulsenti G, Palma P. Tailored nasal surgery for normalization of nasal resistance. Facial Plast Surg 1996;12(4):333–45.
13. Meredith GM. Surgical reduction of hypertrophied inferior turbinates: a comparison of electrofulguration and partial resection. Plast Reconstr Surg 1988;81: 891–7.
14. Warwick-Brown NP, Marks NJ. Turbinate surgery: how effective is it? A long-term assessment. ORL J Otorhinolaryngol Relat Spec 1987;49:314–20.

15. Wiliams HOL, Fisher EW, Holding-Wood DG. Two stage turbinectomy: sequestration of the inferior turbinate following submucosal diathermy. J Laryngol Otol 1991;105:14–6.

16. Cavaliere M, Mottola G, Iemma M. Monopolar and bipolar radiofrequency thermal ablation of inferior turbinates: 20-month follow-up. Otolaryngol Head Neck Surg 2007;137:256–63.

17. Fukutake T, Yamashita T, Tomoda K, et al. Laser surgery for allergic rhinitis. Arch Otolaryngol Head Neck Surg 1986;112:1280–2.

18. Kawamura S, Fukutake T, Kubo N, et al. Subjective results of laser surgery for allergic rhinitis. Acta Otolaryngol Suppl 1993;500:109–12.

19. Elwany S, Harrison R. Inferior turbinectomy: comparison of four techniques. J Laryngol Otol 1990;104(3):206–9.

20. Rakovar Y, Rosen G. A comparison of partial inferior turbinectomy and cryosurgery for hypertrophic inferior turbinates. J Laryngol Otol 1996;110:732–5.

21. Spielberg W. The treatment of nasal obstruction by submucous resection of the inferior turbinate bone. Report of cases. Laryngoscope 1924;34:197–203.

22. House HP. Submucous resection of the inferior turbinal bone. Laryngoscope 1951;61:637–48.

23. Mabry RL. Inferior turbinoplasty: patient selection, technique, and long-term consequences. Otolaryngol Head Neck Surg 1988;98:60–6.

24. Chen YL, Tan CT, Huang HM. Long-term efficacy of microdebrider-assisted inferior turbinoplasty with lateralization for hypertrophic inferior turbinates in patients with perennial allergic rhinitis. Laryngoscope 2008;118(7):1270–4.

25. Messerklinger W. Endoscopic diagnosis and surgery of recurrent sinusitis. In: Krajira Z, editor. Advances in nose and sinus surgery. Zagreb (CR): Zagreb University; 1985.

26. Wigand ME, Steiner W, Jaumann MP. Endonasal sinus surgery with endoscopic control: from radical operation to rehabilitation of the mucosa. Endoscopy 1978;10:255–60.

27. Clement WA, White PS. Trends in turbinate surgery literature: a 35-year review. Clin Otolaryngol 2001;26:124–8.

28. Lang J. Clinical anatomy of the nose, nasal cavity, and paranasal sinuses. New York: Thieme; 1989. p.113.

29. Swanson PB, Lanza DC, Vining EM, et al. The effect of middle turbinate resection upon the frontal sinus. Am J Rhinol 1995;9:191–5.

30. Freedman HM, Kern ED. Complications of intranasal ethmoidectomy: a review of 1,000 operations. Laryngoscope 1979;89:421–34.

31. Goldsmith AJ, Zahtz GD, Stegnjajic A, et al. Middle turbinate headache syndrome. Am J Rhinol 1993;7(1):17–23.

32. Kennedy DW, Sinreich SJ. Functional endoscopic approach to inflammatory sinus disease: current perspectives and technique modifications. Am J Rhinol 1988;2:89–96.

33. Wigand ME. Endoscopic surgery of the paranasal sinuses and anterior skull base. New York: Thieme Medical Publishers; 1990. p.134–41.

34. Morgenstein KM, Krieger MK. Experiences in middle turbinectomy. Laryngoscope 1980;90:1596–603.

35. Gaskins RE. Scarring in endoscopic ethmoidectomy. Am J Rhinol 1994;8:271–4.

36. Biedlingmaier JF, Whelan P, Zoarski G, et al. Histopathology and CT analysis of partially resected middle turbinates. Laryngoscope 1996;106:102–4.

37. Brescia G, Pavin A, Giacomelli L, et al. Partial middle turbinectomy during endoscopic sinus surgery for extended sinonasal polyposis: short- and mid-term outcomes. Acta Otolaryngol 2008;128(1):73–7.
38. Cook PR, Begegni A, Bryant WC, et al. Effect of partial middle turbinectomy on nasal airflow and resistance. Otolaryngol Head Neck Surg 1995;113:413–9.
39. Von Brunn A. Contributions to the microscopic anatomy of the human nose. Arch Micr Anat 1892;39:632–51.
40. Read E. A contribution to the knowledge of the olfactory apparatus in dog, cat, and man. Am J Anat 1908;8:17–47.
41. Lawson W. The intranasal ethmoidectomy: an experience with 1,077 procedures. Laryngoscope 1991;101:367–71.
42. Toffel PH. Secure endoscopic sinus surgery with partial middle turbinate modification: a 16-year long-term outcome report and literature review. Curr Opin Otolaryngol Head Neck Surg 2003;11(1):13–8.
43. Fortune DS, Duncavage JA. Incidence of frontal sinusitis following partial middle turbinectomy. Ann Otol Rhinol Laryngol 1998;107:447–53.

The Diagnosis and Management of Empty Nose Syndrome

Nipun Chhabra, MD[a], Steven M. Houser, MD, FACS, FAAOA, FARS[a,b,*]

KEYWORDS

- Empty nose syndrome • Atrophic rhinitis
- Paradoxic nasal obstruction • Turbinectomy • Septal implant

Empty nose syndrome (ENS) is an iatrogenic disorder most often recognized for the presence of paradoxic nasal obstruction despite an objectively wide, patent nasal fossa. The term "empty nose syndrome" was initially coined to describe certain symptoms associated with tissue loss and radiographic findings of a paucity of normal anatomic structures in the nasal cavities. It has been referred to in the literature, erroneously, as a form of atrophic rhinitis. Because the understanding of ENS has progressed, it is important to appreciate its distinction from atrophic rhinitis, as well as the manifestations, diagnosis, and treatment of this debilitating disorder.

EXPLANATION OF ATROPHIC RHINITIS

Atrophic rhinitis is a chronic, degenerative condition characterized by inflammation and atrophy of the nasal and paranasal mucosa and structures.[1] It is primarily a clinical diagnosis and should be considered in patients who have chronic rhinosinusitis and significant crusting, especially subsequent to repetitive nasal trauma or injuries. The classic constellation of symptoms of atrophic rhinitis includes thick and adherent crusting, foul odor (or *fetor*), and nasal obstruction.[1,2] The hardened crusts that develop have classically been referred to as *rhinitis atrophicans cum foetore*, or *ozena*.[2] In the majority of cases, these symptoms are late sequelae of a chronic underlying inflammatory state in which much of the damage to the nasal and paranasal mucosa has already taken place. A keen clinical suspicion on the part of the otolaryngologist

[a] Department of Otolaryngology—Head and Neck Surgery, Case Western Reserve University and University Hospitals Case Medical Center, 2500 MetroHealth Drive, Cleveland, OH 44109, USA
[b] Department of Otolaryngology—Head and Neck Surgery, MetroHealth Medical Center, 2500 Metro Health Drive, Cleveland, OH 44109, USA
* Department of Otolaryngology—Head and Neck Surgery, Case Western Reserve University & University Hospitals Case Medical Center, 2500 MetroHealth Drive, Cleveland, OH 44109.
E-mail address: shouser@metrohealth.org (S.M. Houser).

Otolaryngol Clin N Am 42 (2009) 311–330
doi:10.1016/j.otc.2009.02.001
0030-6665/09/$ – see front matter © 2009 Elsevier Inc. All rights reserved.

oto.theclinics.com

aids in early diagnosis of this disease. There may be a link between infections (eg, measles, scarlet fever, and diphtheria) and atrophic rhinitis; a sharp decrease in the incidence of atrophic rhinitis has been noted in countries in which a concurrent decrease in such infections was noted, despite unchanged sanitation.[2]

It is important to note that two distinct conditions have been widely cited in the literature: primary and secondary atrophic rhinitis. Primary atrophic rhinitis is often spontaneous in onset and has a slowly progressing, debilitating course. Often, no underlying etiology is discovered, although inheritable or infectious causes are proposed mechanisms.[1,3] Although spontaneous in onset, primary atrophic rhinitis likely reflects a microvascular paucity in blood flow that has been present for a prolonged period of time.[1,3] Secondary atrophic rhinitis is much more commonly encountered and usually develops after specific insults, such as trauma, irradiation, reductive nasal surgery, or granulomatous disease.[1] In secondary entities, nasal crusting, enlarged nasal cavities, resorption of the turbinates, mucosal atrophy, and paradoxic nasal congestion are encountered. Less commonly reported symptoms include facial pain and pressure, anosmia, and intermittent epistaxis. Physical and nasal endoscopic examination will always yield abnormalities of the nasal sidewall. A retrospective review of 242 patients showed the partial and complete absence of inferior turbinate (IT) tissue in 62% and 37% of patients, respectively.[1] The absence of the middle turbinate (MT) was found in 57% of patients, and 32% of patients had either no recognizable or very small remnants of turbinate tissue. All patients had discolored (yellow, brown, or green) crusts covering the sidewalls and floor of the nose.

Histopathologic analysis of nasal mucosa may serve as confirmatory evidence of atrophic rhinitis.[1–3] Universally, atrophy of serous and mucinous glands, loss of cilia and goblet cells, and inflammatory cell infiltrates are seen. Endarteritis obliterans and dilatation of capillaries increase the fragility of the epithelium and reflect the microvascular changes present. Pathogenic organisms, most commonly *Klebsiella ozaenae*, but also *Staphylococcus aureus*, *Proteus mirabilis*, and *Escherichia coli* may be found on nasal cultures.

Computed tomography (CT) scans of the nose and paranasal sinuses may reveal characteristic findings, including:[1,4]

1. Mucosal thickening of the paranasal sinuses
2. Loss of definition of the ostiomeatal complex
3. Hyperplasia of the maxillary sinus
4. Enlargement of the nasal cavities with destruction of the lateral nasal wall
5. Bony destruction of the IT and MT.

The lack of normal anatomic turbinate tissue together with atrophic rhinitis symptoms has erroneously been termed "the empty nose" in much of the literature. The idea that the presence of these conditions indicates that a patient has ENS has been propagated by the occurrence of paradoxic nasal congestion, the most common presenting symptom of atrophic rhinitis. The cause of paradoxical nasal obstruction is unclear, but atrophy of the olfactory epithelial receptors leading to anosmia, along with atrophy of pain and temperature receptors, is likely a contributing factor.[1,5] Furthermore, the lack of anatomic nasal barriers and an adequate mucociliary elevator as the result of atrophic nasal mucosa results in substantially decreased nasal airflow.[6] Investigators believe that some degree of nasal airflow resistance is necessary to balance pulmonary inspirations.[7] The resulting lack of or offset of this balance may contribute to a subjective sense of inadequate nasal airflow, nasal breathing, and subsequent nasal congestion.

THE MANAGEMENT OF ATROPHIC RHINITIS

Atrophic rhinitis can be a crippling disease. Medical treatment has aimed at reducing symptoms and complaints to allow the afflicted patient a better quality of life. Treatment of atrophic rhinitis is not so much controversial as it is varied.[1,3] Several approaches have been used that are either primarily medical, primarily surgical, or a combination of both approaches. Aggressive nasal hygiene with regular intranasal irrigation remains the standard of conservative therapy and assists by producing minimizing crusting and restoring nasal hydration.[1] Commonly used irrigation solutions include normal saline solution, sodium bicarbonate, aminoglycoside topical therapy, and plain water. Systemic or topical antibiotic irrigations are generally reserved for patients who have atrophic rhinitis that is the result of acute infection or that is indicated by positive cultures. Such antibiotics include tetracycline, aminoglycosides, and ciprofloxacin.[1] Vasodilators and topical steroids may also provide palliative results.[2]

A variety of surgical procedures exist to address the symptoms of atrophic rhinitis. Surgical principles for atrophic rhinitis have a long and plentiful developmental history. In 1873, Rouge recommended curettage and removal of the entire atrophic mucosa in the nose. In 1900, Gersuny injected paraffin under the nasal mucosa, which heralded the era of implants. In 1948, Rethi constructed a baffle from the septum to obstruct the nasal cavities and also used transplantation of Stensen's duct, which had originally been reported by Wittmaack in 1919.[2] In 1967, Young[8] described a staged method of bilateral closure of the nostrils that had been performed in a small number of patients. This was done by raising skin flaps within the nostrils and suturing the folds together to allow effective closure of the nostril. Unilateral closure was first completed, and at the time of closure of the contralateral nostril, the opportunity was taken to re-open and examine the previously sutured nasal cavity. Young reported that crusting and purulent debris had disappeared upon such re-opening and that with time the nasal mucosa returned to a pink, healthy appearance.[8] Regeneration of ciliated epithelium and mucous glands was found on histologic examination. In 1971, Gadre and colleagues[9] reported on a modification of Young's procedure and demonstrated the disappearance of crusting at six months after such modified procedures. Serial endoscopic examinations over several years showed some mucosal regeneration when modifications of Young's original procedure were used.

A multitude of implant material has been used to augment intranasal volume. In 1923, Eckert-Mobius used macerated spongy beef bone. In 1947, Proud implanted acrylic resin in the septum and Eyries extended this technique to include the lateral nasal wall. In 1980, Chatterji[10] modified Saunders's autogenous bone-graft technique from 1958. Chatterji used a single, long piece of bone to enhance the biologic activity of the underlying nasal mucosa. The use of dermofat and placental grafts similarly is based on this theory of "biologic activation," with the underlying tissue responses reversing and rejuvenating the existing atrophic conditions of nasal cavities.[10] Goldenberg and colleagues[11] placed plastipore implants in submucosal pockets in the floor of the nose and septum in a small number of patients. They reported excellent results in the majority of their patients, with complete resolution of symptoms up to 24 months after surgery. Overall, the use of implants has been promising, but extrusion of artificial implants has been reported in up to 80% of cases.[1,12]

In general, the surgical principle of using implants in cases of atrophic rhinitis is directed at reducing the volume of the nasal fossae and, when using autogenous implantation, enhancing biologic activity of the affected nasal mucosa. The slower the absorption of the implant, as in the use of a single, long piece of graft, the greater the biologic effect.[10] The rationale of narrowing the nasal lumen is that a decreased amount of airflow will occur with inspiration, thus resulting in less drying, crusting, and subsequent damage to the nasal mucosa. The explanation further involves contributions to the shape and position of the nostrils, the valvular action of the lateral nasal cartilages, the size and function of the turbinates, and underlying mucosal changes and blood flow.[2]

THE MANIFESTATION AND SYMPTOMS OF EMPTY NOSE SYNDROME

"Empty nose syndrome," or more precisely, "the empty nose syndrome of Stenkvist," is a term first coined by Eugene Kern and Monika Stenkvist at the Mayo Clinic in 1994 to describe certain symptomatology and the type of images appearing on sinus CT scans after tissue loss. It is commonly referred to in the literature as an iatrogenic form of atrophic rhinitis, though it is important to note the two are distinct clinical entities.[5] Patients who have ENS present most commonly after undergoing IT resection. MT resection or even the presence of normal turbinate tissue and intranasal volume are also associated with ENS. There is a paucity of literature surrounding the evolution and diagnosis of this disorder, so that some otolaryngologists doubt the existence of ENS. Few patients develop ENS following turbinate resection, but this debilitating complication requires astute diagnosis and clinical suspicion on the part of the otolaryngologist.

The hallmark complaint of a patient who has been afflicted with ENS is paradoxic nasal obstruction.[5,13] On physical examination, large, patent nasal fossae may be present as the result of the lack of turbinate tissue, but patients report a subjective feeling of "stuffiness," for lack of a better descriptor. This sensation may be coupled with "emptiness," a term patients use to describe the subjective inability to sense airflow, mainly seen following total inferior turbinectomy. Another common and perplexing symptom of paradoxic nasal obstruction is shortness of breath or difficulty breathing. Patients with this symptom tend to overbreathe and often slip into hyperventilation because they feel a relentless sense of dyspnea. This condition is perhaps the most severe form of paradoxic obstruction and may worsen with strain or physical activity.

The term "paradoxic obstruction" describes the subjective feeling of poor breathing despite objective patency, which typically is overly patent. A lack of nasal resistance leads to poor pulmonary function because the body strains to sense airflow, because the nasal resistor is essential to proper pulmonary function.[14] The nasal resistor has been cited as centrally important in providing wider opening of the peripheral bronchioles and enhancing alveolar ventilation. These actions allow for better gas exchange, higher negative thoracic pressure, and overall improved venous cardiac and pulmonary backflow.[14] This claim is strengthened by clinical research that indicates that normal rates of nasal resistance to expiration help to maintain lung volumes and may indirectly determine arterial oxygenation.[15] In fact, the symptoms may be so bothersome that the patient relates a sense of suffocation. As a result, the patient who has ENS becomes preoccupied with nasal symptoms, resulting in the inability to concentrate (aprosexia nasalis), fatigue, irritability, anxiety, and depression.[5] Many times, this constellation of symptoms is overlooked because the physician does not have a clear explanation for paradoxic obstruction in the presence of a widely patent nasal cavity. Crusting and pain may be present with ENS. Dryness is a constant subjective complaint and can typically be observed objectively as well. This may lead to atrophic rhinitis, though as previously stated in this article, the two entities are separate disorders.

Although the term "empty nose syndrome" was originally coined to describe radiographic findings, the diagnosis of ENS relies heavily on clinical suspicion and physical examination. The onset of ENS's manifestations varies widely, ranging from months to years after turbinate surgery. Most commonly, ENS is encountered after IT resection; however, ENS can occur after MT resection and in patients who have seemingly normal turbinate tissue. In all cases of ENS, patients have had some type of turbinate procedure performed during their lifetimes.[13]

Overall, ENS seems most commonly associated with mucosal destructive surgeries. From personal experience and examination of the literature regarding turbinate excision, the authors estimate that approximately 20% of patients with IT resection will develop full-blown ENS and that a greater percentage suffers from at least dryness (**Table 1**). The syndrome does not occur after most turbinate procedures, even total removal. The authors are not certain why some patients develop ENS whereas others do not. One thought is that a "two hit" phenomenon that must take place, in which (1) the tissue is excised or damaged and (2) the sensory nerves to the area manage to regenerate poorly. Poor nerve growth following tissue destruction is a known risk for many forms of surgery. For example, there is a 26.4% incidence of hypoesthesia at the surgical site after inguinal herniorrhaphy.[16] Indeed, the turbinates are recognized as a source of nerve growth factor.[17] Thus, damage to turbinate tissue may predispose the nose to poor nerve regrowth and healing, leading to a significantly decreased sensation of airflow.

Another thought is that unique patient anatomy leads to varying airflow disruption. Elad[18] and Zhao[19] have elegantly demonstrated such airflow disruption after IT resection in computer modeling of airflow through the nose. In general, the turbinates define and are intimately related to the nasal meati through which air flows. The meati that are formed between the turbinates, the septum, and the nasal floor and walls are very narrow and offer a mechanism of resistance to limit the total amount of airflow. This resistance also serves to increase the velocity of airflow, ensuring a mostly laminar pattern. As a result, a maximal conductive air–mucosal interface exists, which provides maximum sensation. Loss of turbinate tissue ultimately disrupts and destroys the meatal structure, causing turbulent, less efficient, and less sensate airflow.[20,21]

The dry lining that results from a loss of physiologic humidification and heating may produce crusts that further impair the sensation of airflow. Passàli and colleagues[22] demonstrated a disruption of nasal physiology (mucociliary clearance, IgA secretion rates, and general heating and humidification capacities) in 45 patients who had total inferior turbinectomies. Naftali and colleagues and Elad and colleagues[23,24] used computational and computerized simulations to demonstrate that removal of the IT reduces overall heat and water vapor flux in the nose by 16% and that removal of the MT or removal of the IT and MT together reduces vaporization by 12% and 23%, respectively. An implant to the nose can be useful in either scenario because when the airflow is shifted toward more sensate tissue, less crusting occurs with a reduced dry air stream, and the airflow pattern is more normalized when a pseudo-turbinate created. Further research is needed to shed more light on the origin of ENS.

Because ENS is a recent area of interest and research, the literature does not elucidate a set diagnostic criterion, in particular because complaints of patients afflicted with ENS often are subjective. Houser uses the Sino-Nasal Outcome Test (SNOT-20), a validated 20-item survey that examines general nasal symptoms and can be used as a comparator before and after some type of intervention.[13] Each item is scored from zero (no symptoms) to five (severe symptoms). Houser modified the existing SNOT-20

Table 1
Spectrum of main symptoms and findings in patients after IT resection

Study	n	Resection Degree	Postoperative Complications and Patient Complaints (% of Patients)	Follow-up
Martinez et al, 1983[38]	29 of 40	Total	Crusting (6.9%) Dryness (10.35%) Epiphora (eye dryness) (3.45%)	2 months–5 years
Moore et al, 1985[39]	18[a]	Total	Dryness and crusting (89%) Malodor in nose (suspected atrophic rhinitis) (66%) Ozena (22%) Eye dryness (11.1%)	2–7 years
Ophir et al, 1985[40]	150	Total	Subjective obstruction (6.6%) Drainage (4%) Dry posterior nose (3.3%)	2.5 years (mean)
Ophir, 1990[41]	38	Total	Subjective obstruction (7.8%) Synechiae (10.5%) Crusting (8%)	2.8 years (mean)
Ophir et al, 1992[42]	186	Total	Subjective obstruction (6%) Exacerbation of asthma attacks (3%)	12 years (mean)
Courtiss and Goldwyn, 1990[43]	25	Partial	Subjective obstruction (28%) Nasal dryness (8%) Crusting (25%) Postnasal drip (28%) Epistaxis (28%)	13 years (mean)
Wight et al, 1990[35]	16[b]	Total	Subjective obstruction (20%) Felt obstruction as before surgery (18%) Crusting (30%)	14–29 months
Carrie et al, 1996[44]	14[c]	Total	Subjective obstruction (78%) Crusting (50%)	7–8 years
Salam and Wengraf, 1993[45]	20	Total	Dryness (16%) Crusting (16%)	6 months
Oburra, 1995[46]	34	Total	Synechiae (15%) Atrophic rhinitis, persistent (15%) Subjective obstruction (12%) Abnormal nasal sensation (9%) Epistaxis (6%) Infection (6% Rhinorrhea (3%)	2 years and more
Berenholz et al, 1998[47]	42	Total	Persistent obstruction (authors do not offer a cause) (33%) Facial pain and headaches (33%) Purulent rhinorrhea (52%) Opacification of the maxillary and ethmoid sinuses (31%) Suspected atrophic rhinitis (17%) Subjective significant clinical complaints of all sorts that could not be verified objectively (17%)	3–10 months

(continued on next page)

Table 1
(continued)

Study	n	Resection Degree	Postoperative Complications and Patient Complaints (% of Patients)	Follow-up
Passàli et al, 1999[22]	62	Partial, surface electrocautery	Crusting (62%) Poor MCCT + secretory IgA (56%) Synechiae (33%) Atrophy (3.2%)	1–4 years
	58	Partial, cryotherapy	Crusting (68%) Poor MCCT + IgA (62%) Synechiae (13.7%) Atrophy (5%)	1–4 years
	54	Partial, laser cautery	Crusting (74%) Poor MCCT + IgA (57.5%) Synechiae (7.5%) Atrophy (11.1%)	1–4 years
	69	Submucosal resection (−) outfracture	Crusting (10%) Poor MCCT + IgA (2.8%) Synechiae (2.8%) Atrophy (none)	1–4 years
	94	Submucosal resection (+) outfracture	Crusting (6.4%) Poor MCCT + IgA (2.1%) Synechiae (2.1%) Atrophy (none)	1–4 years
	45	Total	Crusting (75.5%) Poor MCCT + IgA (71.1%) Synechiae (31.1%) Atrophy (22.2%)	1–4 years
Gendeh, 2000[48]	15	Total	Nasal discomfort Mild (13.3%) Moderate (53.3%) Severe (33.3%) Dry throat Mild (13.3%) Moderate (46.6%) Severe (40.0%)	3–6 months
	21	Partial	Nasal discomfort Mild (52.3%) Moderate (33.3%) Severe (14.2%) Dry throat Mild (52.3%) Moderate (38.0%) Severe (9.5%)	3–6 months

Abbreviation: MCCT, mucociliary transport.

[a] According to Moore and Kern (2001), the patients in this study were 18 of the 40 patients that Martinez[38] reported on two years previously.

[b] The initial group included twenty patients. Four patients had anterior radical trimming and only later had total resection, so those four patients were excluded from the results.

[c] This study is a six-year follow-up on fourteen patients from Wight's 1990 initial study group (data also reported in this table).

to include five additional, ENS-specific questions (SNOT-25). The SNOT-25, with Houser's modifications, is shown in **Table 2**. Patients are also asked to free text or expand on their responses. The SNOT-25 is a comprehensive assessment tool to aid with recognition and diagnosis of ENS patients.

Table 2 SNOT-20 and SNOT-25 assessment for ENS						
	Scoring Range (0–5)					
SNOT-20 and SNOT-25 Nasal Symptoms	0 No Symptoms	1	2	3	4	5 Severe Symptoms
1. Need to blow nose						
2. Sneezing						
3. Runny nose						
4. Cough						
5. Postnasal discharge						
6. Thick nasal discharge						
7. Ear fullness						
8. Dizziness						
9. Ear pain						
10. Facial pain/pressure						
11. Difficulty falling asleep						
12. Waking up at night						
13. Lack of good night's sleep						
14. Waking up tired						
15. Fatigue						
16. Reduced productivity						
17. Reduced concentration						
18. Frustration/restlessness/irritability						
19. Sadness						
20. Embarrassment						
Houser Modification adds:						
21. Dryness						
22. Difficulty with nasal breathing						
23. Suffocation						
24. Nose is too open						
25. Nasal crusting						

In general, the authors recommend using a combination of the most common symptoms in making a diagnosis of ENS. These symptoms include:

- paradoxic airway obstruction
- dyspnea
- nasal and pharyngeal dryness
- hyposmia
- depression.

Nasal examination or endoscopy often demonstrates dry and pale mucosa (often indicative of underlying squamous metaplasia), occasional crusting, and a dearth of turbinate tissue (**Fig. 1**). Houser reported on the use of the "cotton test" to aid with surgical planning. This office-based procedure allows the otolaryngologist to gauge the dimensions and ideal location of potential implants. Using isotonic sodium chloride solution, cotton is moistened and placed within the nasal cavity in a region in which an implant may be feasible.[13] The cotton is kept in place for 20 to 30 minutes, and the

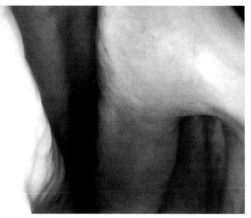

Fig. 1. Nasal endoscopic view of a patient who has ENS. Note the lack of normal IT tissue.

patient is asked to breathe comfortably and report any changes in symptoms (**Fig. 2**). Patients who report a definitive subjective improvement from the cotton test, and whose symptoms and physical examination findings seem consistent with ENS, are offered submucosal implantation.[13] Although initially the cotton test was not used as a diagnostic tool for ENS, the authors recommend its use to assist in both confirmatory diagnosis and planning of surgical intervention for patients who have ENS.

THE RELATIONSHIP BETWEEN ATROPHIC RHINITIS AND EMPTY NOSE SYNDROME

ENS has been listed erroneously in the literature as being synonymous with atrophic rhinitis. Indeed, although there are underlying similarities between these disorders, they are two separate entities arising from distinct origins. Much of the confusion results from similarities in the symptoms of ENS and atrophic rhinitis. Paradoxic congestion, dryness, and crusting may present in both disorders. However, as previously described, atrophic rhinitis may be classified as being primary or secondary, with a clear underlying cause or idiopathic in nature. Additionally, the resorption of

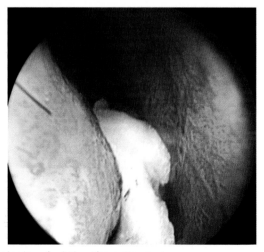

Fig. 2. An endoscopic view depicting the cotton test.

the turbinate and adjacent mucosal tissue that results from atrophic rhinitis is reflective of the underlying pathophysiology of the disease, whereas ENS is an iatrogenic disorder. This distinction is of utmost importance, because although secondary atrophic rhinitis may occur after turbinate reduction surgery, it may also be the result of a multitude of other factors, including trauma, infection, or immunologic disorders. Also, as previously stated in this article, atrophic rhinitis has clear pathogenic links to organisms isolated from nasal cultures, but as of yet, there is no pathogen associated with ENS.

The use of the term "empty nose" has been applied loosely in the literature to also suggest a paucity of intranasal structures and normal anatomy, as viewed on radiographic images. It is important to emphasize that the term "empty nose" has broader applications than the term "empty nose syndrome" and that the two should not be used interchangeably. As its name implies, ENS is a specific iatrogenic disorder that has clinical manifestations that often cause significant distress to the patient, as opposed to a single "empty nose," which may or may not have associated symptoms. Just as atrophic rhinitis has important subclassifications as primary and secondary, ENS can also be divided into several subtypes. Empty nose syndrome-inferior turbinate (ENS-IT) refers to ENS encountered after resection of IT tissue (**Fig. 3**). The most common complaints of patients who have ENS-IT are paradoxic nasal obstruction and profound dryness.[5,13] ENS-IT is the most common subtype, and these patients may also present with nasal crusting and pain on inspiration. The amount of IT tissue loss varies from patient to patient, and there is no agreed-on measure of quantifying tissue loss. The reason paradoxic obstruction occurs most commonly in the ENS-IT subtype is not well understood, although it may be a result of the physiologic function of the IT. The ITs function as pressure valves and are responsible for

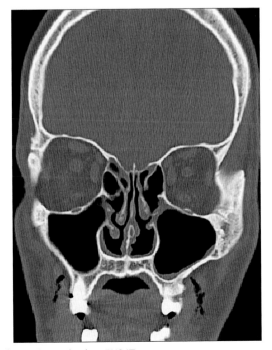

Fig. 3. A CT scan of a patient who has ENS-IT.

modulating the amount of nasal airflow and for increasing flow velocity upward. The ITs direct approximately 60% of airflow upward through the middle (50%) and superior (10%) meati during regular steady nasal respiration.[21]

Empty nose syndrome-middle turbinate (ENS-MT) is a controversial topic; it is the authors' experience that in addition to breathing dysfunction, a symptom commonly encountered with this subtype is pain associated with breathing.[5] Nasal crusting, if at all present, is not as extensive as that seen with ENS-IT. The sensation of pain may be caused by the effect of turbulent airflow striking exposed mucosa overlying the sphenopalatine ganglion.[5] The designation of "ENS-type" is used to refer to the condition in a select group of patients who seem to have adequate turbinate tissue, yet their symptoms seem to fully emulate ENS.[5] These patients improve when the cotton test is used and all of them have undergone some type of turbinate procedure in the past. The term "ENS-both," as its name implies, refers to the condition in patients who have had a resection of both IT and MT tissue. This is the most severe form of ENS, and the patient's symptoms are often crippling. Depression rates are higher with this subtype, and hyposmia or anosmia may result from alteration in airflow patterns and subsequent delivery of odorant particles to the olfactory cleft.[5]

THE CONTROVERSY SURROUNDING TURBINATE RESECTION

The authors believe they are obliged to ask whether turbinate excision deserves more consideration in light of ENS. It has been demonstrated that turbinate resection enhances antral patency and augments functional endoscopic sinus surgery.[25,26] Still, given the debilitating effects of ENS on a patient's quality of life, controversy exists as to whether physicians have become too cavalier in resecting turbinate tissue. Atrophic rhinitis and ENS are feared late complications of turbinate tissue resection. Cook and colleagues[25] used anterior rhinomanometry to conclude that partial middle turbinectomy does not impair nasal function and that partial frontoinferior turbinectomy improves nasal airflow and resistance. However, they followed patients up to a maximum of 10 months in the postoperative period. Lamear and colleagues[26] reported on a series of 298 patients who underwent partial endoscopic middle turbinectomy and were followed for up to 36 months, and they described a cumulative patency rate of 92.5% without any complications, including the development of atrophic rhinitis. On the other hand, Ramadan and Allen[27] reported on a series of 337 patients, comparing the rate of synechia formation between patients who underwent partial MT resection and those who did not. The difference in synechia formation was not statistically significant. Swanson and colleagues[28] concluded that MT resection during sinus surgery may be a risk factor for development of postoperative frontal sinus disease, and Passàli and colleagues[22] reported a 22.2% incidence of atrophy following inferior turbinectomy. Stewart[29] performed an extensive review of the literature and concluded that a randomized, controlled clinical trial may not resolve the controversy that exists regarding MT resection. Kennedy[30] argued against routine resection of MT tissue, except in the presence of clearly traumatized or inflamed mucosa. Kennedy described the protective and physiologic functions of the MT, concluding that physicians should strive toward conservation whenever possible. Indeed, the authors resect turbinate tissue only when it is deemed necessary, such as in cases of severe trauma, bony exposure, or involvement of neoplastic processes.

The authors have demonstrated that substantial controversy is present in the literature and that no gold standard recommendation exists regarding the resection of turbinates. They believe that the decision for and surgical approach to turbinate resection should be left to individual surgeon preference. The authors do recommend a cautious and judicious approach to resecting turbinates and that before undertaking turbinate resection of any kind, one should keep in mind that ENS is an iatrogenic disorder resulting from the loss of turbinate tissue. Those patients undergoing turbinate resection should be followed closely in the postoperative period, and any symptoms that relate to ENS should be given credence and taken seriously. Newer techniques of turbinate reduction (eg, submucosal resection that preserves the mucosa above) are likely safer alternatives that can avoid the possibility of ENS. Passàli's[22] study demonstrates that more destructive techniques produce more patient complaints. The author (S.H.) has only needed to treat patients who had undergone turbinectomy or had surgery involving mucosal-damaging techniques (eg, laser ablation, aggressive cautery).

UNDERSTANDING NASAL AIRFLOW SENSATION TO GUIDE IMPLANT THERAPY FOR EMPTY NOSE SYNDROME

Over the past decade, there has been increased interest and research into quantifying the degree of nasal obstruction in terms of nasal airflow models. Biomedical models, rhinomanometry, and physical resistance computational formulas have served to increase the understanding of the passage of air through the nasal conduit. Although it is still somewhat controversial, there is evidence to suggest a physiologic relationship between the respiratory center and nasal airflow sensation. A full review of various computational models and biometrics is beyond the scope of this paper; however, it is important to appreciate the role of the nasal cavity in paradoxic obstruction as a means to guiding implant therapy for patients who have ENS.

Clarke and colleagues[31] reported on the distribution of nasal airflow sensitivity as determined by delivering a pulse of air at varying velocities to different nasal sites. The endpoint was the minimum air velocity at each stimulated site needed to produce a tactile, subjective sensation in the nose. Their findings suggest that the nasal vestibule is substantially more sensitive to airflow than the mucosa of the nasal cavum and that the sensitivity of airflow is more prominent at the anterior ends of the lateral nasal wall. One would expect the greatest concentration of nasal receptors to be present at the entrance to the entire system, thus allowing ample opportunity for the respiratory–nasal reflex arc to adjust accordingly in a dynamic flow system. However, Clarke's conclusions do not explain the subjective obstruction that patients report after undergoing inferior turbinectomy because such patients have dramatically increased nasal airflow, including at the nasal vestibule. Wrobel and colleagues[32,33] also reported that the skin-lined nasal vestibule is much more sensitive to air-jet stimulation than the nasal cavity mucosa, with the inferior meatus being more sensitive than the middle meatus. Yaniv and colleagues[34] found that patients who underwent surgical uncinectomy demonstrated no difference in nasal airway resistance, yet significant subjective improvement in airflow was reported.

Wight and colleagues[35] reported that radical trimming might provoke turbulent airflow, especially over the anterior portion of the middle meatus. This trimming may in turn stimulate drying of the MT, in which other airflow receptors may exist, ultimately leading to a sensation of nasal obstruction. These studies highlight the middle meatal region as an important component of nasal airflow sensation. Overall, however, it is not known which area of the nose is most important for subjective sensation of nasal patency and airflow.

Indeed, many studies in the literature do not take into account nasal airflow sensation and instead rely predominantly on objective measures of nasal airflow, such as patterns and velocity. The sensation of nasal airflow is of central important in clinical practice. The authors emphasize that it is the sensation of nasal obstruction, rather than a quantifiable change in nasal airway resistance, that most frequently results in symptoms for the patient. This may explain why the literature has not yielded a strong correlation between turbinate resection and decreased nasal airflow and resistance. Eccles[36] emphasized the importance of this lack of correlation more than a decade ago; he understood that nasal obstruction as a symptom is primarily related to changes in the sensation of nasal airflow rather than a quantifiable or functional change in the ability to breathe through the nose. This alteration of sensation is central to understanding and appreciating ENS.

It is well known that although significantly more effort is required to breathe through the nose than the mouth, nasal breathing is far more satisfying and effective.[18] The nasal turbinates function to provide respiratory resistance in the nasal cavity, and by resection of these structures, the patient suffers the loss of a more effective and efficient method of breathing. According to Niinimaa and colleagues,[37] the vast majority of humans are predominantly nose breathers who switch to oral breathing only at high levels of physical strain.

Because ENS is a recently recognized entity, definitive treatment is still being explored. Often, patients who have ENS have failed conservative medical management and have been misdiagnosed as having atrophic rhinitis. Aggressive nasal hygiene and nasal moisturizers may be of limited palliative benefit, and as previously discussed in this article, the cotton test alludes to benefit through surgical implantation. Houser[13] published a study reporting on eight patients who had ENS of varied subtypes who underwent surgical submucosal implantation using acellular dermis. All of the patients reported subjective improvement in symptoms, including the qualitative sense of smell, although breathing dysfunction and dryness were the symptoms most successfully quelled. In addition, no new symptoms or complaints developed in the postoperative period, which varied from 6 months to 4 years. Houser used acellular dermal grafts because of their gradual incorporation with patient tissue (estimated by the authors to take approximately 3 to 6 months, depending on the size of the graft) and their stable size for years after implantation. The cotton test was used preoperatively to assist with surgical planning and determining the ideal placement of the graft.

To restore adequate nasal sensation for patients who have ENS, the placement of the implant should ideally simulate the natural airflow in the nose. Additionally, preoperative planning should be targeted at alleviating symptoms and is best done by performing an in-office cotton test. Patients who have ENS-both may benefit from a large septal implant that bridges the regions of the IT and MT. The ENS-IT subtype of patients without any residual IT tissue is a surgical challenge. In such cases, anterior septal implants may be better suited than lateral wall implants for restoration of nasal airflow. Based on the physiology of the IT, an anteriorly placed implant is likely to direct airflow up toward the middle meatus. A lateral wall implant may be in a more physiologic location, but is tethered by the nasolacrimal duct system, which limits its anterior extent.

SURGICAL TECHNIQUES OF IMPLANT THERAPY IN EMPTY NOSE SYNDROME

To rehabilitate patients who have ENS, Houser surgically implanted acellular dermis (eg, Alloderm from LifeCell, Branchburg, New Jersey, Allomax from Bard, Covington, Georgia, FlexHD from MTF, Edison, New Jersey, Graft Jacket from Wright Medical, Arlington, Tennessee, and SureDerm from HansBiomed, Seoul, Korea) into a submucoperichondrial (smpc) or submucoperiosteal (smpo) plane or into the submucous layer. The use of autologous tissue is possible as well, but Houser found acellular dermis to be reliable, predictable, and readily shaped (sutured into a configuration with chromic sutures). The implant provides additional resistance for breathing, lessening the sensation of suffocation. Most patients report some degree of benefit.[13] A multimedia video file of the procedure, performed by Houser, is available at: http://www.youtube.com/watch?v=n_VK8lmsksM.

The location of the implant is based on the patient's history, examination, CT scan findings, and the results of a cotton test in the office. As previously stated in this article, a cotton test is performed by placing cotton moistened with an isotonic sodium chloride solution into the nose. Usually the cotton is placed in the location of the excised turbinate, either laterally or against the septum. Subjects who feel no benefit or obstruction from the cotton test are deemed poor candidates for implantation. The cotton test should be deferred if any coexisting active processes, such as allergic rhinitis or rhinosinusitis, are present.

After identifying the size and location of a cotton pledget that provides the most benefit to a patient, the authors then strive to create permanent tissue expansion to provide the same benefit. Infection of the foreign acellular dermis is a feared complication in the perioperative course, so the patient is given one gram of cefazolin preoperatively, and postoperative antibiotics (typically cephalexin 250 mg or 500 mg four times per day) are maintained for 3 weeks. The face is prepped with betadine paint and draped in a sterile fashion. One-half strength hydrogen peroxide (one-half peroxide, one-half saline solution) is used for the lavage of the nose in an effort to sterilize the area. To date, no acellular dermis infections have been documented.

To simulate an IT, the implant is placed at the septum, floor, or lateral nasal wall. One should take care to keep the graft sufficiently anterior so that it is opposite the former IT head. Septal implantation via a septoplasty incision is a challenging, "workhorse" approach (**Fig. 4**A, B). Often, the septal incision and pocket will extend somewhat onto the nasal floor. Most patients who have ENS have undergone septoplasty in the past, so raising a septal flap can be challenging. If a bloodless plane is achieved, then the operator should strive to disrupt the smpc/smpo overlying the graft to allow better ingrowth of vessels. Poor vessel ingrowth will lead to atrophy of the graft. The acellular dermis can be shaped using cutting and folding, and sutured, often to resemble a teardrop, with the narrow portion positioned anteriorly and inferiorly. The graft can be secured in place to the septum using the suture normally used for septal quilting (4-0 gut on a baby Keith needle); two sutures are fixed to the graft before final placement, passed through the septum, and tied on the opposite side (**Fig. 5**). The septal flap is closed like any hemitransfixion incision, usually with several

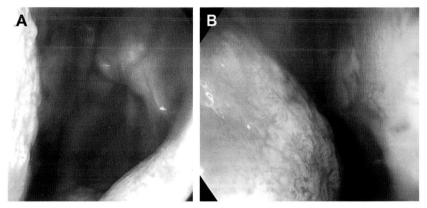

Fig. 4. (A) Left-sided, preseptal implantation for a patient who has ENS-IT. (B) Left-sided, postseptal implantation for a patient who has ENS-IT.

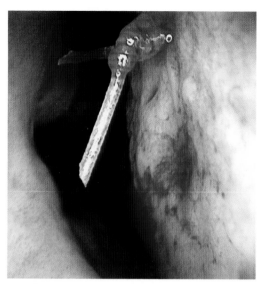

Fig. 5. Right nasal cavity showing chromic suture securing a left septal implant.

interrupted sutures. Houser has used 4-0 chromic frequently, although large grafts placed near the incision may swell postoperatively, causing suture rupture and exposure of the acellular dermis. Although these areas have healed without apparent sequela, the use of Vicryl may provide more strength to resist rupture. The volume of acellular dermis that is needed is variable, although two 2 × 4 cm–thick acellular dermis sheets are frequently used. One can expect some slight shrinkage as the tissue incorporates and the air pockets are ablated. The operator should overcorrect the area by approximately 25%.

If the graft is placed at the lateral wall, care should be taken not to obstruct the nasolacrimal duct. To date, no epiphora has been reported. The incision should either be made anterior to the limen nasi (within the nasal vestibule at the lateral nasal sill; **Fig. 6**) or just behind it. An angled knife, such as an angled beaver blade or an ophthalmologic knife, is needed to make a lateral incision behind the nasal sill. Because the

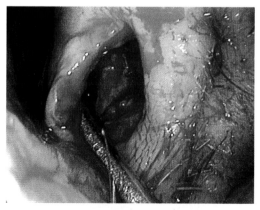

Fig. 6. Left lateral nasal wall exposure via the nasal sill. The bone of the pyriform aperture is seen within.

inferior meatus slopes laterally, the use of endoscopes may be necessary when incising and raising the flap. The smpo is then raised using a freer elevator. The issue of abrading the smpo is more of a consideration with lateral wall grafting because the tissue planes have often not been disturbed and a bloodless plane is easier to achieve. The mucosa seems to provide an excellent blood supply to support the graft and is superior to bone for this purpose. Some resorption and shrinkage of the graft is expected. Two or three of the 2 × 4 cm acellular dermis sheets are typically packed loosely into the lateral wall pocket. The graft can be expanded during a second surgery using the same approach, lifting the mucosa with the attached acellular dermis away from the underlying bone fairly readily. Regrafting should be delayed for 6 months or more to allow for the completion of healing. Consideration of using other filler materials is reasonable as well. Hydroxyapatite placed below a thickened mucosa/acellular dermal graft may provide a good platform to push the graft toward the airway. Packing, usually using strip gauze, is a consideration for hemostasis and encourages the flap to "seat" on the acellular dermis below. Although used initially, packing has not proved to be a necessity.

The treatment of ENS-MT has the least number of options because of the surrounding anatomy. The lateral nasal wall contains the drainage pathways for the paranasal sinuses. For fear of obstructing the sinuses and because of the exceedingly thin mucosa within the middle meatus, lateral implants for ENS-MT are avoided. However, the septum may be used for grafting, which simulates a "Bolgerized" MT.[5] After the septum is opened using an ipsilateral hemitransfixion incision, then the use of a 0° nasal endoscope will permit identification of the middle meatus. Acellular dermis can be positioned within the septal flap, and its proper location, which is often opposite the former MT location, is then confirmed (**Fig. 7**). The flap is raised back to the sphenoid rostrum, and there is usually some bony septum left in place, even after a prior septoplasty. The posterior end of the graft is positioned toward the ipsilateral side, over the rostrum. In patients who have ENS-MT, usually two extra-thick 1 × 2 cm pieces of acellular dermis are rolled at the tip and sutured into position using 4-0 chromic sutures (**Fig. 8**). The graft is sutured along the anterior–superior and anterior–inferior corners. After it is in the optimal position, the needles are passed through the septum and the contralateral side mucosa, and tied in place.

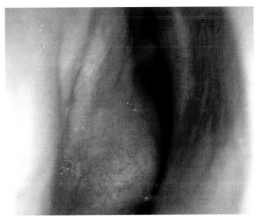

Fig. 7. Endoscopic view of an implant using acellular dermis in a patient with ENS-MT.

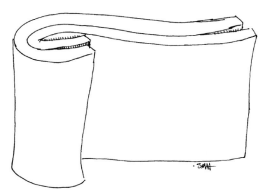

Fig. 8. Drawing of an acellular dermal graft, manually shaped before implantation.

In a patient who has ENS-both, the septum will often be the target for grafting, with a large implant spanning the region of the MT and IT. The techniques previously mentioned in this article hold true in this instance as well. A large volume of acellular dermis is required; three or more of the 2 × 4 cm–thick sheets are often required. The graft will often span the region of the IT and MT heads.

The ITs of patients designated as ENS-type can be directly expanded in a submucosal layer. A tunnel within the IT tissue can be filled with strips cut from one or two 1 × 2 cm extra-thick pieces of acellular dermis. One end of the strip is trimmed to make it somewhat sharp in appearance. The acellular dermis is only partially hydrated, so that it remains somewhat rigid. The section of acellular dermis can be easily passed into the tunnel like a spear; hence, this is dubbed the "spear technique." Multiple segments can be passed and will lie adjacent to one another. Only the anterior half of the IT is thus expanded, but this has proved sufficient. The tunnel is closed using a single 4-0 chromic suture. Packing is usually not needed.

Another method to expand an existing IT is to make an incision within the nasal sill, dissect to the edge of the pyriform using an elevator, and then raise the mucosa within the nasal cavity on the medial surface of the pyriform. This provides a larger pocket and a more anterior expansion site. The acellular dermis is packed in loosely; often a single 2 × 4 cm–thick acellular dermal sheet is used. Note that an IT can be expanded toward the septum, but usually not down toward the floor; septal/floor placement per septal incision is necessary if the cotton test suggests those sites should be expanded.

Office instillation of injectable materials is also possible. Unfortunately, the nasal mucosa is not as distensible as the external skin in which such fillers are normally employed. Excess injection will lead to mucosal rupture and leakage of filler material. The septum and floor seem especially difficult to directly inject. A prior acellular dermis graft might be expected to more readily accept an injection, but this has not proved to be the case. Injection into the IT is performed within a submucosal layer, rather than the smpo, which seems to more readily accept fillers. The author (S.H.) has used Cymetra (Lifecell), an injectable acellular dermis product, but there are a myriad of injectable products on the market. Houser is aware of subjects treated using Restalyn (Q-Med AB [publ], Uppsala, Sweden), Radiesse (BioForm Medical Inc., Franksville, Wisconsin), and injectable silicone. It has been postulated that injection of *botulinum* toxin to the lateral nasal wall musculature might narrow the airway and provide relief. An investigation of this postulate is underway at the Mayo Clinic.

SUMMARY

ENS is a poorly understood and rare iatrogenic disorder resulting from the destruction of normal nasal tissue. In severe forms, it can be debilitating, and a lack of recognition and understanding of this disease process is at the expense of the patient. In this article, the authors have elucidated the distinction between ENS and atrophic rhinitis and have provided a systematic approach to the diagnosis and management of ENS. The authors urge a judicious and cautious approach to turbinate resection, to help prevent the occurrence of ENS as a sequela of nasal surgery. When encountered in practice, patients who have ENS can be rehabilitated and their quality of life substantially improved by using nasal augmentation as a means to help restore nasal anatomy toward the premorbid state. Astute clinical suspicion, coupled with an understanding and appreciation of the pathophysiology behind ENS, can greatly benefit the otolaryngology community.

REFERENCES

1. Moore EJ, Kern EB. Atrophic rhinitis: a review of 242 cases. Am J Rhinol 2001;15: 355–61.
2. Cottle M. Nasal atrophy, atrophic rhinitis, ozena: medical and surgical treatment. J Int Coll Surg 1958;29:472–84.
3. Goodman WS, De Souza FM. Atrophic rhinitis. Otolaryngol Clin North Am 1973;6: 773–82.
4. Pace-Balzan A, Shankar L, Hawke M. Computed tomographic findings in atrophic rhinitis. J Otolaryngol 1991;20:428–32.
5. Houser SM. Empty nose syndrome associated with middle turbinate resection. Otolaryngol Head Neck Surg 2006;135:972–3.
6. Clarke RW, Jones AS. Editorial: nasal airflow sensation. Clin Otolaryngol 1995;20: 97–9.
7. Ramadan MF, Campbell IT, Linge K. The effect of nose breathing and mouth breathing on pulmonary ventilation. Clin Otolaryngol 1984;9:136.
8. Young A. Closure of the nostrils in atrophic rhinitis. J Laryngol Otol 1967;81: 515–24.
9. Gadre KC, Bhargava KB, Pradhan RY, et al. Closure of the nostrils (Young's operation) in atrophic rhinitis. J Laryngol Otol 1971;85:711–4.
10. Chatterji P. Autogenous medullary (cancellous) bone graft in ozaena. J Laryngol Otol 1980;94:737–49.
11. Goldenberg D, Danino J, Netzer A, et al. Plastipore implants in the surgical treatment of atrophic rhinitis: technique and results. Otolaryngol Head Neck Surg 2000;122:794–7.
12. Shehata M, Dogheim Y. Surgical treatment of primary chronic atrophic rhinitis— an evaluation of Silastic implants. J Laryngol Otol 1986;100:803–7.
13. Houser SM. Surgical treatment for empty nose syndrome. Arch Otolaryngol Head Neck Surg 2007;133:858–63.
14. Huizing EH, de Groot JAM. Functional reconstructive nasal surgery. Stuttgart (Germany): Thieme; 2003. p. 48.
15. Swift AC, Campbell IT, McKown TM. Oronasal obstruction, lung volumes, and arterial oxygenation. Lancet 1988;25(8600):1458–9.
16. Mikkelsen T, Werner MU, Lassen B, et al. Pain and sensory dysfunction 6 to 12 months after inguinal herniotomy. Anesth Analg 2004;99(1):146–51.

17. Wu X, Myers AC, Goldstone AC, et al. Localization of nerve growth factor and its receptors in the human nasal mucosa. J Allergy Clin Immunol 2006;118(2): 428–33.
18. Elad D, Liebenthal R, Wenig BL, et al. Analysis of airflow patters in the human nose. Med Biol Eng Comput 1993;31:585–92.
19. Zhao K, Dalton P. The way the wind blows: implications of modeling nasal airflow. Curr Allergy Asthma Rep 2007;7:117–25.
20. Elad D, Naftali S, Rosenfeld M, et al. Physical stresses at the air-wall interface of the human nasal cavity during breathing. J Appl Phys 2006;100(3): 1003–10.
21. Grützenmacher S, Lang C, Mlynski G. The combination of acoustic rhinometry, rhinoresistometry and flow simulation in noses before and after turbinate surgery: a model study. ORL J Otorhinolaryngol Relat Spec 2003;65(6):341–7.
22. Passàli D, Lauriello M, Anselmi M, et al. Treatment of the inferior turbinate: long-term results of 382 patients randomly assigned to therapy. Ann Otol Rhinol Laryngol 1999;108:569–75.
23. Naftali S, Rosenfeld M, Wolf M, et al. Pathophysiology of nasal air conditioning. In: Proceedings of the Second Joint EMBS/BMES Conference, Houston, TX, USA, October 23–26; 2002:1523–4.
24. Elad D, Wolf M, Keck T. Air-conditioning in the human nasal cavity. Respir Physiolo Neurobiol 2008;163(1–3):121–7.
25. Cook PR, Begegni A, Bryant WC, et al. Effect of partial middle turbinectomy on nasal airflow and resistance. Otolaryngol Head Neck Surg 1995;113:413–9.
26. Lamear WR, Davis WE, Templer JW, et al. Partial endoscopic middle turbinectomy augmenting functional endoscopic sinus surgery. Otolaryngol Head Neck Surg 1992;107:382–9.
27. Ramadan HH, Allen GC. Complications of endoscopic sinus surgery in a residency training program. Laryngoscope 1995;105:376–9.
28. Swanson PB, Lanza DC, Vining EM, et al. The effect of middle turbinate resection upon the frontal sinus. Am J Rhinol 1995;9:191–5.
29. Stewart MG. Middle turbinate resection. Arch Otolaryngol Head Neck Surg 1998; 124:104–6.
30. Kennedy DW. Middle turbinate resection: evaluating the issues—should we resect normal middle turbinates? Arch Otolaryngol Head Neck Surg 1998;124: 107.
31. Clarke RW, Jones AS, Charters P, et al. The role of mucosal receptors in the nasal sensation of airflow. Clin Otolaryngol 1992;17:383–7.
32. Wrobel BB, Bien AG, Holbrook EH, et al. Decreased nasal mucosal sensitivity in older subjects. Am J Otol 2006;20:364–8.
33. Wrobel BB, Leopold DA. Olfactory and sensory attributes of the nose. Otolaryngol Clin North Am 2005;38(6):1163–70.
34. Yaniv E, Hadar T, Shvero J, et al. Objective and subjective nasal airflow. Am J Otol 1997;18(1):29–32.
35. Wight RG, Jones AS, Beckingham E. Trimming of the inferior turbinates: a prospective long-term study. Clin Otolaryngol Allied Sci 1990;15(4):347–50.
36. Eccles R. Nasal airway resistance and nasal sensation of airflow. Rhinol Suppl 1992;14:86–90.
37. Niinimaa V, Cole P, Mintz S, et al. Oronasal distribution of respiratory airflow. Respir Physiol 1981;43:69–75.
38. Martinez SA, Nissen AJ, Stock CR, et al. Nasal turbinate resection for relief of nasal obstruction. Laryngoscope 1983;93(7):871–5.

39. Moore GF, Freeman TJ, Ogren FP, et al. Extended follow-up of total inferior turbinate resection for relief of chronic nasal obstruction. Laryngoscope 1985;95:1095–9.
40. Ophir D, Shapira A, Marshak G. Total inferior turbinectomy for nasal airway obstruction. Arch Otolaryngol 1985;111(2):93–5.
41. Ophir D. Resection of obstructing inferior turbinates following rhinoplasty. Plast Reconstr Surg 1990;85(5):724–7.
42. Ophir D, Schindel D, Halperin D, et al. Long-term follow-up of the effectiveness and safety of inferior turbinectomy. Plast Reconstr Surg 1992;90(6):980–7.
43. Courtiss EH, Goldwyn RM. Resection of obstructing inferior nasal turbinates: a 10-year follow-up. Plast Reconstr Surg 1990;86(1):152–4.
44. Carrie S, Wright RG, Jones AS, et al. Long-term results of trimming of the inferior turbinates. Clin Otolaryngol 1996;21:139–41.
45. Salam MA, Wengraf C. Concho-antropexy or total inferior turbinectomy for hypertrophy of the inferior turbinates? A prospective randomized study. J Laryngol Otol 1993;107:1125–8.
46. Oburra HO. Complications following bilateral turbinectomy. East Afr Med J 1995;72(2):101–2.
47. Berenholz L, Kessler A, Sarfati S, et al. Chronic sinusitis: a sequela of inferior turbinectomy. Am J Rhinol 1998;12(4):257–61.
48. Gendeh BS. Conventional versus endoscopic inferior turbinate reduction: technique and results. Med J Malaysia 2000;55(3):357–62.

Empty Nose Syndrome: What are We Really Talking About?

Spencer C. Payne, MD

KEYWORDS

- Atrophic rhinitis • Empty nose syndrome • Turbinectomy
- Inferior turbinate • Middle turbinate • Nasal obstruction

In their 2001 article on atrophic rhinitis (AR), Moore and Kern[1] state in reference to those suffering from this affliction that, "the absence of normal nasal structures is universal in these patients, and the symptoms of atrophic rhinitis coupled with a cavernous nasal airway lacking identifiable turbinate tissue has been termed 'the empty nose syndrome.'" The term "empty nose syndrome" (ENS) had been previously coined by Eugene Kern in the 1990s and used during a presentation on the same subject as his 2001 article at the spring meeting of the American Rhinologic Society in 1997.[2] Since that time, however, little has been explicitly stated about ENS and its number of direct references in the scientific literature has been few.[3–9] In his article in this issue, Dr. Houser presents his definition, proposed explanation, and suggested treatment for ENS, but just as many questions are raised as are answered, not the least of which being which definition of ENS we are to use for the purposes of this debate. Dr. Houser[3] presents ENS as a separate entity from secondary iatrogenic AR and has deemed its interchangeable use with this term as erroneous, citing only his own prior article as proof. However, it is clear from the above quotation that the broadening of the definition for ENS to include those patients who may not even be missing a turbinate is a misappropriation of the term. This is mentioned only to establish where the term originated, so that for the purposes of this article semantics can be put aside and we can remain on common ground throughout the discussion. As such, for the purposes of this article and perhaps in the medical literature to come, the term ENS should be adapted to not be considered a form of AR, but redefined as a symptom complex that, at a minimum, includes a paradoxical sense of obstruction in the face of partial or complete turbinate resection. Even still, the result of ENS or iatrogenic AR as a consequence of turbinectomy remains a controversial topic that deserves further scrutiny.

Division of Rhinology and Sinus Surgery, Department of Otolaryngology–Head & Neck Surgery, University of Virginia, P.O. Box 800713, Charlottesville, VA 22908-0713, USA
E-mail address: spencer.payne@virginia.edu

Otolaryngol Clin N Am 42 (2009) 331–337
doi:10.1016/j.otc.2009.02.002
0030-6665/09/$ – see front matter © 2009 Elsevier Inc. All rights reserved.

oto.theclinics.com

INFERIOR TURBINECTOMY

The inferior turbinate (IT) has long been recognized as a source of nasal obstruction, and seemingly every passing year brings a new technique to address this. Once medical management has failed, a plethora of options are available to reduce its size, including simple outfracture, extramural mucosal ablation (eg, superficial cautery or laser therapy), submucosal ablation (eg, intramural cautery, radiofrequency ablation, or powered resection), or partial or total resection of the turbinate. Over the years, the American literature has seen a trend toward recommending more conservative measures, so as to avoid the possibility of ENS or AR. In fact, one investigator reversed his prior recommendation of complete turbinate resection after finding, on further follow-up, that 89% of patients suffered from crusting while 39% had thick, foul-smelling secretions.[10] Given this, a panel recommendation to avoid such extensive resection was published.[9] One of the largest series of total inferior turbinectomy published within the last decade by Talmon and colleagues,[11] however, found that 97.4% (342 out of 351) of patients noted improved breathing. The investigators further stated that there were no complications of AR, despite the study being performed in "a hot, dusty climate." A comment regarding that article in a later issue also noted a lack of development of AR in 1,156 patients on whom subtotal or total inferior turbinectomy had been performed.[12] Ophir and colleagues[13] has also published a series of 186 patients in whom none developed AR after total inferior turbinectomy and, given the long-term follow-up of 10 to 15 years, it is unlikely that this represented an inability to capture a delayed presentation.

MIDDLE TURBINECTOMY

Perhaps even more controversial than IT resection is the removal of the middle turbinate (MT) during surgery. Giacchi and colleagues[14] nicely summarized many of the main issues regarding partial or complete resection of the MT in their study, looking at its effect on frontal-sinus patency, in which they found no frontal sinusitis in their resection group. They agreed with Fortune and Duncavage,[15] who felt that this specific risk was minimal after partial middle turbinectomy. Giacchi and colleagues additionally noted Lawson's[16] series of 1,077 intranasal ethmoidectomies with partial middle turbinectomies, in which none of the patients developed AR. Despite this, as noted by Houser, Kennedy[17] argues that as an important structure within the nose, the MT, should not be arbitrarily removed unless obviously damaged or involved in the disease process, and this was echoed by Rice and colleagues.[9] Several conditions in addition to tumor resection are noted, where its removal is considered appropriate by Rice, but neither investigator universally condemns its removal. Moreover, in none of the articles regarding MT resection is there any mention of the development of AR.

CONTROVERSY OR NOT?

How then can we rectify the IT data with other reports of seemingly high numbers of AR or AR-like symptoms in other studies? Why is there no apparent reporting of AR in the middle turbinectomy patients quoted in these studies? And what of ENS? Are we certain this did not occur, especially if these investigators were using its original definition as a virtual synonym of AR? Closer inspection reveals that Talmon[11] still had nine patients on follow-up who noted no improvement in their breathing. Eight and 11 patients out of 351 were also each noted to have complaints of crusting or pain/discomfort, respectively. Furthermore, Ophir[13] also acknowledged that 11 out of 186 (5.9%) patients had no readily obvious reason for their continued complaints of nasal obstruction, despite a wide, clean airway. It is uncertain if these patients would go on to suffer from AR, but it remains concerning that their persistent obstruction may have been evidence of ENS. In the middle turbinectomy patients, most of whom had resection during the course of chronic rhinosinusitis (CRS) surgery, it may have been difficult to tease out persistent obstruction in the face of this more diffuse mucosal disease process. Furthermore, it is possible that in the CRS patient, hypertrophy of the nasal septum after turbinate resection would prevent AR- or ENS-like symptoms. The author has seen this many times, especially in those patients with polypoid (CRSwNP) type disease presenting for revision surgery. In addition, if mucosal inflammation and glandular hypertrophy were to continue after surgery, any crusting might be assumed to be secondary to the disease process.

ATROPHIC RHINITIS VERSUS EMPTY NOSE SYNDROME

In Dr. Houser's discussion in this issue, as well as his two prior publications on the subject,[3,4] he discusses the significant differences which he has been able to elucidate between AR and ENS. He divides ENS into three subtypes representing and named for the turbinates that had been resected in each (either inferior, middle, or both; abbreviated as ENS-IT, ENS-MT, or ENS-both). He also characterizes a fourth entity that he dubs "ENS-type," in which patients have symptoms similar to the other subtypes but with a seemingly normal-appearing airway. In addition to the major symptom of paradoxic obstruction, he notes that patients also develop "an inability to concentrate, chronic fatigue, frustration, irritability, anger, anxiety and depression," as well as a decreasing sense of smell.[4] ENS-MT, which he states is more controversial, given the wider support for MT resection compared with IT resection, is characterized by a sense of pain with breathing and is seen less frequently than in ENS-IT. Houser theorizes that this may be secondary to circulating, cool air striking the area of the sphenopalatine ganglion, which is no longer protected by the shielding effect of the MT. ENS-both represents those who may go on to become "nasal cripples," as Kern[18] has referred to them, lacking both major turbinate structures of the nose. More controversial is Houser's ENS-type patient. These patients have undergone a partial turbinate procedure, yet present with similar symptoms of nasal obstruction despite the apparent normal airway. As the only real article to describe ENS as we are presenting it here, Dr. Houser's work is landmark. His careful evaluation of patients who were most likely ignored by their operating surgeon and his adaptation of techniques used to rehabilitate the noses of patients with AR is commendable; however, several issues are raised by his article that require addressing before we can either fully understand ENS as it is described here or plan treatment options.

First, a concern is raised regarding such a small sample of only eight patients after three were lost to follow-up among the 11 originally undergoing an operative procedure. It is not clear why of the "dozens of patients" who had undergone evaluation for ENS, that more did not undergo an operation. One would assume one of the following: (1) many resolved with medical therapy, (2) subjective improvement was not seen with the cotton test, or (3) the patients refused surgery. Those falling into the second category represent an important statistic because, if a substantial number, it would indicate that something other than airway shape or size is playing a role. Second, Houser reports a significant improvement rate in the Sino-Nasal Outcome Test (SNOT-20) scores of the eight patients involved, from a median (the more appropriate way to report a nonparametric result) of 56 to 37.5. However, SNOT-20 results, to be considered clinically significant, require an improvement of 0.6 in their indexed score (ie, total score divided by 20). Of the eight patients in the study, only four of them had an improvement greater than 12 (0.6 × 20) in their total score, indicating a failure of 50% to reach clinically significant improvement. Given this, it remains uncertain if failure to improve was a result of the size or placement of the implant or if the patients' symptoms rely on more than just the cross-sectional area of the nasal cavity. Houser does somewhat address this by discussing the possible contribution of poor nerve regeneration in the turbinate tissue after partial or complete resection of the turbinate. It would not seem logical, however, that one could then "fix" this with simply placing an implant in lieu of correcting the neurologic defect, especially at the risk of developing further neuropathy while raising the septal flap for its placement.

Neither of these two points invalidates the concept of ENS, but they do raise questions regarding what we understand, especially with what we can glean from a very limited study.

ALTERNATE EXPLANATIONS FOR THE ETIOLOGY OF ENS

Why do only some people develop AR or ENS after turbinate resection, and why does it appear from the literature that certain geographic areas may be less affected (all three articles mentioned above in the inferior turbinate section were of Israeli origin)? If what Houser provides us is only a piece of the puzzle, where else can we turn? He has already touched on concepts that may likely play a role. In dealing with such a complex topic, the airflow dynamics of the nose and how they may be affected by the internal and external nasal anatomy cannot be ignored. Significant work has already been performed to understand the effect of nasal shape on airflow.[19–22] The nasolabial angle, morphology of the nasal valve, and position of the turbinates not only affect the path of nasal airflow, but they also vary ecogeographically.[19] When the nostrils are directed anteriorly, more airflow is directed toward the floor of the nose along the inferior turbinate.[23] As the nasolabial angle decreases, the air pattern tends to be directed higher in the nose toward the middle meatus. This is further accentuated in the leptorrhine nose, where the nasal sill is often higher, acting as a baffle to direct airflow up and over the inferior turbinate.[19] The function of the nasal valve is that of a Venturi throat valve, such that the rapid expansion of cross-sectional area behind the valve results in a generator of turbulence distributing the airflow throughout the nose and allowing for more thorough contact of inspired air with the mucosal surface of the nose for conditioning purposes. As the nasal valve widens, this turbulence effect is less seen.[20] The more medially positioned the turbinate, the greater the turbulence of airflow. It is reasoned that in geographic regions where inspired air is colder and dryer, these features clump to maximize the air/surface interface, but that in warmer and more humid climates, the morphologic features that are conducive to the less energetically costly laminar airflow are favored.[19] The effect of turbinectomy on airflow can theoretically be varied. Removal of the posterior-inferior turbinate while leaving the anterior segment in place may serve to increase the turbulence of the air. This could possibly be sensed as improved or worsened airflow, depending on how turbulent it became. Removal of the IT head, however, would remove the Venturi valve phenomenom and create a more laminar column of air that, while flowing more "smoothly," would result in less mucosal contact and be sensed as decreased flow by the mucosa. As a result, it is clear that, given the significant morphologic differences already notable for aesthetic reasons between the leptorrhine (tall, thin), platyrrhine (short, broad), and mesorrhine noses, that individuals with these varied features may respond differently to adjustments in the airflow resulting from the resection of a turbinate. Furthermore, depending on the exact morphology and the extent of resection, an individual may be more susceptible to the removal of the MT instead of the IT or vice versa.

Additionally, the effect of the underlying disease process may play a role. The patient with allergic rhinitis or CRS may be less susceptible to certain symptoms because of the persistent hypertrophy of the remaining nasal tissues, even after turbinate resection. Furthermore, the differentiation of patients with CRSwNP and those without polyps (CRSsNP) may also be key. CRSwNP is typically associated with eosinophilia and an underlying "innate" mucosal inflammatory state that is not solely dependent on the obstructed drainage patterns that are opened with surgery.[24] A case of CRSsNP that is primarily the result of a protracted infectious process, however, may resolve quite readily. It may be patients in this latter group who are more likely to fair worse if the MT is removed in the course of surgery.

And what of the issue of poor regeneration of sensory nerves to the area? Quite frankly, the authors agree with Houser, in that if the turbinate is no longer present, it would be impossible for the finely tuned mechanisms that so tightly regulate that narrow air column (which amaze this author every time he evaluates a CT scan) to function properly. Or, as is suggested by Moore and Kern[1] in AR, perhaps the "wear and tear" on the mucosa under the circumstances of altered airflow leads to a disruption and degeneration of the mucosal nerve fibers. This may partly explain the ENS-type patients that Houser describes. In his study, Houser notes that two of the ENS-type patients had undergone superficial laser therapy. It could be reasoned that the destruction of the overlying mucosa, and subsequent disruption of the superficial nerve endings by extension, resulted in a decreased ability to "sense" airflow, but this remains conjecture. Without further study on the mucosa of patients with ENS, this may be an impossible question to answer, especially given the low likelihood that anyone would wish to remove even more mucosa from their noses.

UNSETTLED ISSUES—PSYCHIATRIC COMORBIDITY AND NEUROPATHY

One issue that is troubling with ENS, as it is defined by Houser, is the significant level of psychiatric findings in this patient population. One might question which disease may have given rise to the other. While the author does not mean to classify the disease as *rhinitis hystericus*, it is possible that ENS could be likened to other phenomena where there seems to be a correlation between psychosocial distress and disease tolerance, such as tinnitus.[25] Additionally, given the lack of preoperative rhinomanometry before a patient's initial turbinate surgery, it may be difficult to know to what extent they had objective nasal obstruction before surgery, especially for the ENS-type patients.

This latter point raises the possibility of a yet-to-be characterized or discovered entity, at least as far as this author is aware, akin to nasal neuropathy. Given the acceptance of neuropathic disorders of the head and neck as explanations for subjective-only complaints (eg, vagal neuropathy in the setting of globus sensation),[26] it is also possible that a certain subset of these patients could have had neuropathic issues even before their operations, which were only exacerbated by manipulation of the turbinates. While it might, literally, be a hard pill to swallow, a trial of amitriptyline or gabapentin may potentially be advantageous, especially in ENS-MT patients whose symptoms are more characterized by pain than obstruction. These patients may also benefit simply from sphenopalatine ganglion nerve blockade instead of invasive procedures, as has been advocated in Sluder's neuralgia.

SUMMARY

The problem with ENS is probably not that it does not exist, it is that we cannot adequately explain its existence by what we currently understand about the nose.

To this end, many otolaryngologists are unwilling to make a "leap of faith" and, instead of acknowledging the existence of something they do not understand, are left skeptical of it in its entirety. As a rhinologist trained in the ways of minimally invasive sinus technique,[27] the author has never removed an inferior turbinate for benign disease and recognizes only the few circumstances where partial middle turbinate resection can be beneficial. However, it is clear from the literature that not everyone undergoing a turbinectomy procedure suffers from the debilitating symptoms of either AR or ENS. It behooves us to evaluate this latter entity with a more critical eye, so that we can avoid creating future sufferers and provide relief to those who have already been afflicted.

REFERENCES

1. Moore EJ, Kern EB. Atrophic rhinitis: a review of 242 cases. Am J Rhinol 2001; 15(6):355–61.
2. Moore EJ, Kern EB. Atrophic rhinitis: a review of 222 cases. Paper presented at: American Rhinologic Society; May 1997; Scottsdale, AZ.
3. Houser SM. Empty nose syndrome associated with middle turbinate resection. Otolaryngol Head Neck Surg 2006;135(6):972–3.
4. Houser SM. Surgical treatment for empty nose syndrome. Arch Otolaryngol Head Neck Surg 2007;133(9):858–63.
5. Iqbal FR, Gendeh BS. Empty nose syndrome post radical turbinate surgery. Med J Malaysia 2007;62(4):341–2.
6. Rice DH. Rebuilding the inferior turbinate with hydroxyapatite cement. Ear Nose Throat J 2000;79(4):276–7.
7. Tichenor WS, Adinoff A, Smart B, et al. Nasal and sinus endoscopy for medical management of resistant rhinosinusitis, including postsurgical patients. J Allergy Clin Immunol 2008;121(4):917–27, e912.
8. Wang Y, Liu T, Qu Y, et al. [Empty nose syndrome]. Zhonghua Er Bi Yan Hou Ke Za Zhi 2001;36(3):203–5 [Chinese].
9. Rice DH, Kern EB, Marple BF, et al. The turbinates in nasal and sinus surgery: a consensus statement. Ear Nose Throat J 2003;82(2):82–4.
10. Moore GF, Freeman TJ, Ogren FP, et al. Extended follow-up of total inferior turbinate resection for relief of chronic nasal obstruction. Laryngoscope 1985; 95(9 Pt 1):1095–9.
11. Talmon Y, Samet A, Gilbey P. Total inferior turbinectomy: operative results and technique. Ann Otol Rhinol Laryngol 2000;109(12 Pt 1):1117–9.
12. Eliashar R. Total inferior turbinectomy: operative results and technique. Ann Otol Rhinol Laryngol 2001;110(7 Pt 1):700.
13. Ophir D, Schindel D, Halperin D, et al. Long-term follow-up of the effectiveness and safety of inferior turbinectomy. Plast Reconstr Surg 1992;90(6):980–4 [discussion: 985–87].
14. Giacchi RJ, Lebowitz RA, Jacobs JB. Middle turbinate resection: issues and controversies. Am J Rhinol 2000;14(3):193–7.
15. Fortune DS, Duncavage JA. Incidence of frontal sinusitis following partial middle turbinectomy. Ann Otol Rhinol Laryngol 1998;107(6):447–53.
16. Lawson W. The intranasal ethmoidectomy: an experience with 1,077 procedures. Laryngoscope 1991;101(4 Pt 1):367–71.
17. Kennedy DW. Middle turbinate resection: evaluating the issues–should we resect normal middle turbinates? Arch Otolaryngol Head Neck Surg 1998;124(1):107.
18. Kern EB. Nasal obstruction. In: Meyerhoff WL, Rice DH, editors. Otolaryngology—head and neck surgery. Philadelphia: Saunders; 1992. p. 496.

19. Churchill SE, Shackelford LL, Georgi JN, et al. Morphological variation and airflow dynamics in the human nose. Am J Human Biol 2004;16(6):625–38.
20. Courtiss EH, Goldwyn RM. The effects of nasal surgery on airflow. Plast Reconstr Surg 1983;72(1):9–21.
21. Simmen D, Scherrer JL, Moe K, et al. A dynamic and direct visualization model for the study of nasal airflow. Arch Otolaryngol Head Neck Surg 1999;125(9): 1015–21.
22. Weinhold I, Mlynski G. Numerical simulation of airflow in the human nose. Eur Arch Otorhinolaryngol 2004;261(8):452–5.
23. Clement PA, Gordts F. Consensus report on acoustic rhinometry and rhinomanometry. Rhinology 2005;43(3):169–79.
24. Steinke JW, Bradley D, Arango P, et al. Cysteinyl leukotriene expression in chronic hyperplastic sinusitis-nasal polyposis: importance to eosinophilia and asthma. J Allergy Clin Immunol 2003;111(2):342–9.
25. Andersson G, Westin V. Understanding tinnitus distress: introducing the concepts of moderators and mediators. Int J Audiol 2008;47(Suppl 2):S106–11.
26. Amin MR, Koufman JA. Vagal neuropathy after upper respiratory infection: a viral etiology? Am J Otol 2001;22(4):251–6.
27. Catalano PJ, Strouch M. The minimally invasive sinus technique: theory and practice. Otolaryngol Clin North Am 2004;37(2):401–9, viii.

Choanal Atresia and Choanal Stenosis

James D. Ramsden, PhD, BM, BCh, FRCS[a],*,
Paolo Campisi, MSc, MD, FRCSC, FAAP[b], Vito Forte, MD, FRCSC[b]

KEYWORDS

- Choanal atresia • CHARGE • Mitomycin • Airway
- Bilateral atresia • Neonatal airway obstruction
- Asphyxia neonatorum • Nasal stent

Congenital narrowing of the nasal airway at the posterior choanae, which can be uni- or bilateral, is an uncommon condition in pediatric patients. The surgical management of choanal atresia varies widely in different centers. This article discusses the different surgical strategies including: dilation and stenting; trans-palatal repair; and transnasal resection utilizing endoscopic sinus surgery (ESS) techniques. The merits of stents, lasers, CT-guided surgery, and the use of additional agents including mitomycin C are reviewed, as well as the particular problems associated with managing bilateral choanal atresia in neonates.

INCIDENCE

Choanal atresia is manifested by narrowing and closure of the posterior choanae of the nose. It has been recognized for more than 200 years and was first described by Roederer[1] in 1755. The reported incidence is between 1 in 5000 to 1 in 9000 live births. There may be mixed bony or membranous obstruction, but, in the majority of cases, it is bony. Original reports suggested a 90% bony stenosis and 10% membranous obstruction,[2] but more recent analysis suggests a mixed bony/membranous in 70% and pure bony in 30%.[3]

There is not just a membrane across the posterior choanae but also medialisation of the pterygoid plates and lateral wall of the nose.[4–6] The boundaries of the atretic plate are created by the undersurface of the body of the sphenoid bones superiorly, the medial pterygoid lamina laterally, the vomer medially, and the horizontal portion of the palatine bone inferiorly. The lateral wall is the principle challenge of choanal atresia surgery, as most surgical corrections tend to address the septum and atretic plate only. There may also be abnormalities of the skull base with either very thickened

[a] ENT Department, University of Oxford, John Radcliffe Hospital, Oxford OX3 9DU, UK
[b] Department of Otolaryngology–Head and Neck Surgery, Hospital for Sick Children, University of Toronto, 555 University Avenue, Toronto, Ontario M5G 1X8, Canada
* Corresponding author.
E-mail address: james.ramsden@orh.nhs.uk (J.D. Ramsden).

Otolaryngol Clin N Am 42 (2009) 339–352
doi:10.1016/j.otc.2009.01.001
0030-6665/09/$ – see front matter. Crown Copyright © 2009 Published by Elsevier Inc. All rights reserved.

oto.theclinics.com

Table 1		
Diagnostic criteria for choanal atresia		
Major	**Minor**	**Diagnosis**
1. Ocular coloboma	5. Cardiovascular	Typical CHARGE: four majors or
2. Choanal atresia	malformations	three majors and three
3. Characteristic ear	6. Genital hypoplasia	minor
abnormalities	7. Cleft lip/palate	
4. Cranial nerve	8. Tracheoesophageal fistula	
abnormalities including	9. Hypothalamo-hypophyseal	
SNHL	dysfunction	
	10. Distinctive CHARGE facies	
	11. Developmental delay	

Abbreviation: SNHL, sensory nerve hearing loss.
Adapted from Blake KD, Prasad C. CHARGE syndrome. Orphanet J Rare Dis 2006:1:34; with permission.

atretic plates or with defects in the skull base. These associated abnormalities may make surgery considerably more challenging.

There is a predominance of females over males in most series[7,8] and unilateral is more common than bilateral,[9,10] although the reported series often come from specialized centers and they may have over-representation of bilateral cases. About one half of these patients have other associated anomalies or syndromes such as CHARGE, Crouzon, Pfeiffer, Antley–Bixler, Marshall–Smith, Schinzel–Giedion, and Treacher Collins syndromes.

EMBRYOLOGY

A number of embryological models for the development of choanal atresia have been proposed, although none of them are wholly supported by convincing clinical evidence. Theories include: the persistence of the buccopharyngeal membrane from the foregut; failure of perforation of the nasobuccal membrane of Hochstetter;[1] abnormal persistence or location of mesoderm forming adhesions in the nasochoanal region; or misdirection of neural crest cell migration.[11]

MOLECULAR MODELS
Retinoic Acid

More recently other molecular pathological theories have been developed. Abnormalities in vitamin A metabolism are associated with choanal atresia. Retinoic acid is metabolized from vitamin A by retinaldehyde dehydrogenase (Raldh). Retinoic acid (RA) then transduces a cellular signal via nuclear receptors for retinoids (eg, RA receptor and 9-cis-RA receptor). This signal is indispensable for ontogenesis and homeostasis of numerous tissues. Dupe and colleagues[12] showed in mice that a Raldh3 knockout suppresses RA synthesis and causes malformations restricted to ocular and nasal regions, which are similar to those observed in vitamin A-deficient fetuses or in retinoid receptor mutants. A Raldh3 knockout mouse (unable to produce any Raldh3) notably causes choanal atresia, which is responsible for respiratory distress and death of Raldh3-null mutants at birth. Dupe suggests that choanal atresia may be caused by impaired RA down-regulation of FGF-8 expression to allow perforation of the nasobuccal membrane. Remarkably, they also showed in this knockout mouse model that choanal atresia was prevented by a simple maternal treatment with RA. Supporting a role for FGF signaling in choanal atresia is the observation that there is often choanal stenosis or atresia in human craniosynostosis syndromes resulting from constitutive activation of FGF-receptors.[13]

Thionamides and Choanal Atresia

Several case reports have associated prenatal use of thionamides (eg, methimizole or carbimizole) with choanal atresia in the offspring.[14–17] A case control study by Barbero and colleagues[18] investigated 61 children with nonsyndromic choanal atresia and found that 10 of 61 had mothers that were treated for hyperthyroidism with thionamides, compared with only two of 183 age-matched controls. This increased incidence of choanal atresia in hyperthyroid mothers treated with carbimizole is likely caused by either hyperthyroidism or the thionamides. The majority of hyperthyroid mothers have Graves' disease and elevated levels of stimulating antibody for the thyrotropin receptor. In both animal models and human studies, elevation of thyrotropin can cause altered expression of FGF, FGF receptors and angiogenic factors, which plausibly may play a role in development of choanal atresia.[19,20]

Ongoing research into the molecular mechanisms that may cause choanal atresia may reveal further insights into the pathobiology of choanal atresia.

Genetic Causes

The CHARGE association was first described in 1979 by Hall,[21] in 17 children with multiple congenital anomalies who were ascertained by choanal atresia. In the same year, Hittner and colleagues[22] reported this syndrome in 10 children with ocular colobomas and multiple congenital anomalies, hence the syndrome is also called Hall-Hittner syndrome.[23] Pagon and colleagues,[24] in 1981 first coined the acronym CHARGE association (Coloboma, Heart defect, Atresia choanae, Retarded growth and development, Genital hypoplasia, Ear anomalies/deafness). More recently an expert group defined the major (the classical four C's: Choanal atresia, Coloboma, Characteristic ears and Cranial nerve anomalies) and minor criteria of CHARGE syndrome.[25] Individuals with all four major characteristics or three major and three minor characteristics are highly likely to have CHARGE syndrome (**Table 1**).

Studies prior to the modern definition of CHARGE reported that about 30% children with choanal atresia had CHARGE syndrome, based on clinical diagnosis.[26] However, these quoted rates may change now that abnormalities in the CHD7 gene have been identified in 64% of patients diagnosed with CHARGE, allowing screening of the gene.[27] The function of the CHD7 gene is largely unknown.[28] Certainly, the presence of uni- or bilateral choanal atresia should precipitate active examination for other signs of CHARGE.[9]

PRESENTATION OF CHOANAL ATRESIA

The presentation of choanal atresia depends on three factors: whether the obstruction is unilateral, bilateral or associated with other craniofacial abnormalities.

Bilateral

The bilateral abnormalities present at birth with asphyxia neonatorum. Neonates are obligate nasal breathers and more than 50% desaturate if nasally obstructed.[29] Bilateral choanal atresia presents as a medical emergency at birth. The usual presentation is of obvious airway obstruction, stridor, and paradoxical cyanosis (where infants turn pink when crying as they begin to breathe through an open mouth). A temporizing measure, such as an oral airway, McGovern nipple, or intubation is often required prior to definitive surgical treatment.

Unilateral

These typically present later (usually 5–24 months)[8,30] and have unilateral obstruction and persistent nasal discharge. Diagnosis can rarely be delayed to adulthood and, on occasion, has been recognized after unsuccessful septal surgery.

Craniofacial Abnormalities

The children with craniofacial abnormalities make up a small but important subgroup of the choanal atresia population. They often have abnormal skull bases,with defects into the cranial cavity; intracranial injury following surgery has been reported.[31,32] Furthermore, children with craniofacial abnormalities often have very thickened pterygoid lamina rather than a simple bony partition or membranous web across the posterior choanae. It is important that other airway issues, including other sites of airway obstruction, muscle tone, associated abnormalities, requirement for tracheotomy and feeding issues are considered during the assessment and surgical planning of these complex patients.

INVESTIGATION

Bilateral choanal atresia presents early with airway compromise, but unilateral atresia typically presents later in childhood with nasal discharge, unilateral nasal obstruction, or occasionally with unilateral otitis media.[33] The clinical examination is revealing, and techniques, such as observing fogging on a cold metal speculum, movement of a wisp of cotton wool, or even detection using a tympanometer to confirm a closed cavity can raise the suspicion of atresia.[34] A fine catheter introduced through the nose which fails to pass to the pharynx can aid diagnosis, although care must be taken in patients with other craniofacial abnormalities to prevent intracranial passage of the catheter. A flexible nasendoscope may be passed through a nasal cavity prepared with a decongestant and suctioned clear; this technique may reveal the atretic plate, although the view is sometime obscured with mucus.

The definitive diagnosis is established with a CT of the paranasal sinuses and skull base, preferably after suctioning and decongestion of the nasal cavity, because it is difficult to distinguish radiologically a membranous occlusion from mucus in the unprepared nose.[3] Radiological evaluation of choanal atresia should be obtained after stabilization of the patient. CT is performed to identify the nature and severity of the anatomic deformity and to estimate the size of the nasopharynx. When the diagnosis is questionable, CT will differentiate other causes of bilateral nasal obstruction, such as pyriform aperture stenosis or bilateral nasolacrimal duct cysts from choanal atresia.

Unilateral causes of nasal obstruction, such as nasal foreign body, turbinate hypertrophy, septal deviation, antrochoanal polyp, or nasal tumor, can also be differentiated from choanal atresia by CT. CT usually shows narrowing of the posterior nasal cavity with medial bowing and thickening of the lateral wall of the nasal cavity, with impingement at the level of the anterior aspect of the pterygoid plates and enlargement of the posterior portion of the vomer, with or without a central membranous connection (**Fig. 1**). The mean width of the posterior choanal airspace in the newborn (measured from the lateral wall of the nasal cavity to the vomer) is 0.67 cm, increasing to 0.86 cm at 6 years and to 1.13 cm by 16 years of age. In patients less than 8 years of age, the vomer generally measures less than 0.23 cm in width and should not exceed 0.34 cm; in children over 8 years, the mean vomer width is 0.28 cm and should not exceed 0.55 cm.[35]

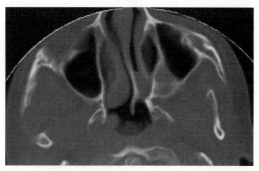

Fig. 1. CT of unilateral choanal atresia demonstrating medial bowing and thickening of the lateral wall of the nasal cavity, with impingement at the level of the anterior aspect of the pterygoid plates.

SURGICAL STRATEGIES

A variety of surgical strategies have been adopted for the treatment of choanal atresia. Johann George Roederer[1] first described CA in 1755. Adolf Otto further described the anomaly in association with the description of the deformity of the palatine bones.[36] In 1854, Carl Emmert[37] was the first to described the blind transnasal puncture of the palate using a curved trochar to establish an airway in a living infant.

Unfortunately, although more than 350 articles have since been published on the surgical management of choanal atresia, the majority of series are single surgeon or institution studies of small numbers of patients collected over a number of years, and often receiving a variety of techniques.[38] This literature makes it difficult to make firm recommendations for surgical technique. The main outcome measures are "patency" of the choanae, although there is no standard definition of patency. Other measures, such as the number of operations and duration of stenting and symptoms, are used variably by different authors. The interpretation is made more difficult as the overall development of these children, including rates of tracheotomy and difficulties with feeding and global progress, are often determined by other comorbid conditions associated with choanal atresia. Consequently, although there is a substantial literature on the treatment of choanal atresia, the optimum technique is not fully established. The choice comes down, in part, to surgical preference.

Transnasal Puncture

Transnasal puncture with Fearon dilators or urethral sounds is a long-used and safe technique to establish an airway (**Fig. 2**).[39] It is essential that the sounds are passed under direct vision with either a 120° endoscope or mirror examining the posterior aspect of the atretic plate, to ascertain that the dilators are passing into the correct position. If the plate is thick, it may be difficult to pass the dilators, and other techniques may be required, including drilling the atretic plate under direct vision. Simple transnasal puncture has a high recurrence rate of re-stenosis and it should be combined with other techniques including endoscopic resection, stenting or both. It is a very useful technique for the treatment of membranous and thin bony stenosis, and is simple to perform quickly and effectively, even in very small infants.

Gujrathi and colleagues[39] elegantly describe the use of the dilators, combined with stenting for 6 weeks, to successfully treat neonates with bilateral choanal atresia with minimal complications. In this paper, with a follow-up time of 2 years, 52 neonates

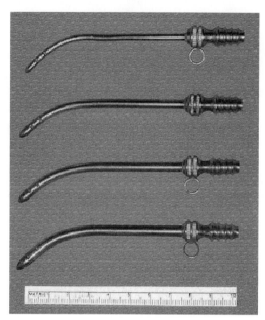

Fig. 2. Fearon dilators.

with bilateral choanal atresia were dilated. Stents were placed for an average of 12 weeks. In this series, only three of 52 infants required sequential dilation, and only two of 52 required subsequent revision surgery, via a transpalatal route, for persistent unilateral stenosis.

Samadi and colleagues[8] used a transnasal approach in 62 children, and had a "success rate" determined by being asymptomatic at 1-year follow-up of 100%. The group of children included mixed uni- and bilateral atresia, and were stented for a median duration of 41 days. The re-operation rate of the transnasal treatment was not stated explicitly because they were analyzed in a larger group of 78 children undergoing a mixture of procedures, but 70 of 78 required more than one procedure. Many procedures were simply removal of stents under anesthetic. However, a median of 2.7 procedures for unilateral and 4.9 for bilateral cases was required. Only 24% of the cases were endoscopically assisted.

Hengerer[11] reported a series of 73 patients, 18 of which had a transnasal puncture and stenting. Nine of the 18 patients required a total of 24 revisions. Hengerer concluded that there was a higher recurrence rate in transnasal procedures compared to an additional endoscopic resection.

Transpalatal Resection

Transpalatal surgery was the first surgical repair that permitted good exposure of the choanal abnormality and correction of the atresia. It was the main technique alongside simple dilation until the advent of endoscopic techniques.

A U-shaped flap in the palate is made, with care to preserve the greater palatine artery and nerve. The anterior palatine bone, vomer and atretic plate are removed under direct vision. This technique allows correction of all of the anatomical abnormalities, including the medialization of the lateral wall at the anterior pterygoid plates; the technique has a success rate of more than 80%, with few cases requiring re-operation.[40]

Complications are unusual but include blood loss requiring transfusion, palatal flap breakdown, or fistula. More significant, however, is the high rate of crossbite abnormalities, high arched palate, and subsequent orthodontic treatment. Freng[41] examined 55 children with choanal atresia of whom 35 underwent a transpalatal repair, and compared them with a group of 265 children without choanal atresia. He observed that there were narrow maxillary dental arches in the operated group compared to the unoperated choanal atresia group and the control group, and an increased cross bite abnormality in 52% of the operated group, compared with 4% in the control group.

A recent study with long-term follow-up examined 26 children who were treated with the transpalatal approach. Eighteen patients treated with the transpalatal approach had some degree of high arched palate deformity, and 12 developed a crossbite requiring orthodontic treatment. This trend was not seen in patients who received treatment with the transnasal and endoscopic techniques.[11] Both studies showed a higher rate of palatal abnormalities in younger children, consistent with a growth spurt of the palate in younger children, although growth continues until adulthood.[42]

Endoscopic Resection

In part because of dissatisfaction with the long-term complications of the transpalatal repair, transnasal microscopic techniques were developed.[43] Initially using the operating microscope, it has now become truly an endoscopic transnasal repair. The use of the endoscope was promoted by Stankiewicz,[44] who reported four cases. Subsequent to his report, many papers on variations of the endoscopic technique have been published (**Table 2**).

The technique is straight-forward to perform, although it may be more difficult to perform in a neonate's nose or—especially—if there is a very narrow or anatomically abnormal nose. The nose is decongested and a 2.8- or 4-mm endoscope is used to visualize the atretic plate. The plate is perforated either under direct vision through the nose, or more commonly, using dilators observed via the postnasal space with mirror or 120° endoscope. After a passage is made into the postnasal space, the opening is enlarged, typically by removing the posterior part of the septum with back-biting through-cutters, microdebrider or guarded drill. It is important to avoid injury to the turbinates, which may result in intranasal synechiae, and to protect the alar and columellar cartilages as instruments are passed into the nose. Most authors agree that it is essential to make a generous opening through the posterior nose, as there is a tendency for it to close over time. It may be difficult to pass instruments through a neonatal nose; however, small diameter endoscopes and pediatric ESS equipment makes this possible in most cases. Some surgeons recommend elevating mucosal flaps; a variety of flaps have been described, but this approach is difficult in the neonatal nose and it is not proven that preserving flaps of mucosa prevents restenosis.[45–47] However, it is a good surgical principle that minimizing the healing reaction will reduce subsequent scarring and cicatrisation.

As shown in **Table 2**, there are a number of small series of endoscopic choanal atresia repairs. The success rates are generally high, with a low revision rate. It is often necessary to subsequently reduce or remove granulation tissue around the choanae. Many of these children receive two or more procedures. The mortality is low, although large series often report a small mortality related to associated medical conditions, especially in syndromic children, usually from subsequent cardiac death.

Table 2
Endoscopic atresia repairs

Study	Year	Patients	Number Not Stented	Stenting Period	Follow-Up (Months)	Revision Rate (%)
Stankiewicz[44]	1990	4	0	2–3 week	5–24	25
Lazar and Younis[65]	1995	10	0	?	18–24	30
Panwar and Martin[66]	1996	5	5	—	3–15	0
Anderhuber and Stammberger[67]	1997	7	0	3–4 week	36	14
Sadek[68]	1998	8	8	0	1–18	12.5
Josephson and colleagues[69]	1998	15	0	?	?	13
Wiatrak[70]	1998	11	1	6 week	3–89	9
Saetti and colleagues[71]	1998	31	4	?	?	25
Fong and colleagues[72]	1999	8	6	?	1–27	38
Tzifa and Skinner[73]	2001	3	3	—	12–48	0
Ku and colleagues[74]	2001	6	0	1–2 week	14–18	33
Uri and Greenberg[75]	2001	7	0	8–12 week	12–96	14
Khafagy[76]	2002	9	0	5–8 week	12–18	22
Van Den Abbeele and colleagues[54]	2002	40	?	24–48 h	?–18	15
Pasquini and colleagues[77]	2003	14	12	72 h–3 week	2–64	7
Rombaux and colleagues[78]	2003	7	0	—	12–36	14
Kubba and colleagues[30]	2004	46	10	6 weeks	3–25	?
Schoem[55]	2004	13	0	—	12	0
Cedin and colleagues[79]	2006	10	0	—	6–36	0
Yaniv and colleagues[80]	2007	17	17	6 week	10–60	12
Durmaz and colleagues[38]	2008	13	12	6 week	12–60	8
Teissier and colleagues[9]	2008	80	0	24 h	Mean 43, range not stated	8

Initially, the endoscopic techniques were used mainly in older children with unilateral choanal atresia, but as surgeons' confidence in the endoscopic technique, aligned with improvements in equipment, has increased, a number of groups have published on endoscopic repair in neonates who have had procedures within a few days of birth.[9,30,48] It is clear that surgery for bilateral atresia, especially in the first 10 days of life, has a higher recurrence rate of stenosis,[9,30] and in this group it is not clear that extensive endoscopic surgery has much to offer over simple dilation and stenting.[39]

AIDS TO SURGERY
Mitomycin C

Mitomycin C is an antiproliferative agent that inhibits fibroblast growth and proliferation. Its use to prevent scar tissue and granulation formation in ophthalmic surgery and its increasing use in otolaryngology for glottic and subglottic stenosis have stimulated surgeons to try it to prevent the cicatrisation and scarring after choanal atresia surgery.[49,50] It is usually applied at a concentration of 0.4 mg/ml on a cotton pledget for 2 to 4 minutes. After initial enthusiasm, several case series has shown no convincing effect of mitomycin on the long-term success rates, although a randomized trial has not been performed.[9,30,51] Furthermore, there are long-term concerns about the application of a potentially oncogenic medication in a child who has a benign condition,[52] so at this time there is not enough evidence to support the routine use of mitomycin C.

Stents

Stenting of the opened choanae is a traditional part of the postoperative management of choanal atresia. Park and colleagues[53] reported in 2000 that only three of 95 members of the American Society of Pediatric Otolaryngology did not routinely use stents. Since then, there has been a steady trickle of papers suggesting that stents are not always necessary after endoscopic surgery.[54–56] Even in centers that customarily use stents, there is no clear-cut evidence that stents prevent stenosis after removal,[9,30] and some series show adverse effects of stenting in children with unilateral stenosis.[57] Nevertheless, it is probably advisable to place stents in children who have a higher risk of failure; this would include neonates and bilateral choanal stenosis.

It is important when placing stents to avoid injury to the alar and septal cartilages or palate due to necrosis or infection. As a guiding principle, the maximum size dilator should not exceed the size of the anterior nares. In neonates, this size is most commonly a 3.0 or 3.5 mm inner diameter endotracheal tube. The tube is folded and a posterior fenestration is created. The fenestrated, folded end straddles the vomer and a mirror exam of the nasopharynx assures precise positioning of the stent. The stent is fixed in position with two independent 4 - 0 prolene sutures: one for each side of the nose. Each separate suture is placed around the alveolar ridge for extra tissue support, thus maintaining an inferior force on the stent minimizing any alar or septal pressure ulceration and/or necrosis (**Fig. 3**). Cleaning consists of saline irrigation and suctioning as required. Occasionally, the instillation of hydrogen peroxide is required to clear crusts that may develop within the stents. Patients should be discharged home only after their caregivers have completed a CPR course and have

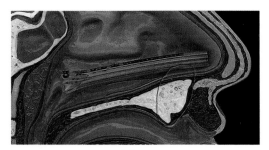

Fig. 3. Circumalveoalar suture to secure nasal stent.

demonstrated proficiency in the suctioning and care of the stents. Furthermore, a home suction machine and adequate nursing support should be available.

Computer-Assisted Surgery

There is increasing use of CT-navigation systems in ESS, especially for skull base cases. Although most cases of choanal atresia can be safely managed simply with good quality pre-operative CT images, in difficult cases with other skull base abnormalities there may be a role for CT-navigation.[58,59]

Laser Assisted Surgery

Lasers allow accurate dissection of tissue and may minimize bleeding, but they carry with them additional risks. A number of papers have examined the use of a variety of lasers to open the posterior choanae.[60–62] However, several deaths have occurred after nasal use of Nd-YAG lasers from air embolism, and there is probably little advantage over conventional instruments.[63,64]

SUMMARY

Regrettably, no randomized controlled trials of treatment for choanal atresia exist, so evidence for best practice is based on case series and personal experience. An increasing literature demonstrates the safety and efficacy of endonasal treatment with either puncture and stenting or with endoscopic opening of the posterior choanae. However, the value of additional treatments, such as mitomycin and laser-assisted techniques, is not proven. Further research should be directed to the avoidance of morbidity in two areas: firstly, the high rates of multiple revision surgeries in children with bilateral atresia, and secondly, to determine the value of prolonged nasal stenting after adequate endoscopic surgical resection.

REFERENCES

1. Flake CG, Ferguson CF. Congenital choanal atresia in infants and children. Ann Otol Rhino Laryngol 1961;70:1095–110.
2. Fraser JS. Congenital atresia of the choanae. Br Med J 1910;2:1968–71.
3. Brown OE, Pownell P, Manning SC. Choanal atresia: a new anatomic classification and clinical management applications. Laryngoscope 1996;106(1 Pt 1):97–101.
4. Shirkhoda A, Biggers WP. Choanal atresia: a case report illustrating the use of computed tomography. Radiology 1982;142(1):93–4.
5. Hasegawa M, Oku T, Tanaka H, et al. Evaluation of CT in the diagnosis of congenital choanal atresia. J Laryngol Otol 1983;97(11):1013–5.
6. Tadmor R, Ravid M, Millet D, et al. Computed tomographic demonstration of choanal atresia. AJNR Am J Neuroradiol 1984;5(6):743–5.
7. Stankiewicz JA. Pediatric endoscopic nasal and sinus surgery. Otolaryngol Head Neck Surg 1995;113(3):204–10.
8. Samadi DS, Shah UK, Handler SD. Choanal atresia: a twenty-year review of medical comorbidities and surgical outcomes. Laryngoscope 2003;113(2):254–8.
9. Teissier N, Kaguelidou F, Couloigner V, et al. Predictive factors for success after transnasal endoscopic treatment of choanal atresia. Arch Otolaryngol Head Neck Surg 2008;134(1):57–61.
10. Keller JL, Kacker A. Choanal atresia, CHARGE association, and congenital nasal stenosis. Otolaryngol Clin North Am 2000;33(6):1343–51, viii.

11. Hengerer AS, Brickman TM, Jeyakumar A. Choanal atresia: embryologic analysis and evolution of treatment, a 30-year experience. Laryngoscope 2008;118(5): 862–6.
12. Dupe V, Matt N, Garnier JM, et al. A newborn lethal defect due to inactivation of retinaldehyde dehydrogenase type 3 is prevented by maternal retinoic acid treatment. Proc Natl Acad Sci U S A 2003;100(24):14036–41.
13. Hehr U, Muenke M. Craniosynostosis syndromes: from genes to premature fusion of skull bones. Mol Genet Metab 1999;68(2):139–51.
14. Greenberg F. Choanal atresia and athelia: methimazole teratogenicity or a new syndrome? Am J Med Genet 1987;28(4):931–4.
15. Wilson LC, Kerr BA, Wilkinson R, et al. Choanal atresia and hypothelia following methimazole exposure in utero: a second report. Am J Med Genet 1998;75(2): 220–2.
16. Barbero P, Ricagni C, Mercado G, et al. Choanal atresia associated with prenatal methimazole exposure: three new patients. Am J Med Genet A 2004;129A(1): 83–6.
17. Foulds N, Walpole I, Elmslie F, et al. Carbimazole embryopathy: an emerging phenotype. Am J Med Genet A 2005;132A(2):130–5.
18. Barbero P, Valdez R, Rodriguez H, et al. Choanal atresia associated with maternal hyperthyroidism treated with methimazole: a case-control study. Am J Med Genet A 2008;146A(18):2390–5.
19. Cocks HC, Thompson S, Turner FE, et al. Role and regulation of the fibroblast growth factor axis in human thyroid follicular cells. Am J Physiol Endocrinol Metab 2003;285(3):E460–9.
20. Ramsden JD, Cocks HC, Shams M, et al. Tie-2 is expressed on thyroid follicular cells, is increased in goiter, and is regulated by thyrotropin through cyclic adenosine 3′,5′-monophosphate. J Clin Endocrinol Metab 2001;86(6): 2709–16.
21. Hall BD. Choanal atresia and associated multiple anomalies. J Pediatr 1979; 95(3):395–8.
22. Hittner HM, Hirsch NJ, Kreh GM, et al. Colobomatous microphthalmia, heart disease, hearing loss, and mental retardation–a syndrome. J Pediatr Ophthalmol Strabismus 1979;16(2):122–8.
23. Graham JM Jr. A recognizable syndrome within CHARGE association: Hall-Hittner syndrome. Am J Med Genet 2001;99(2):120–3.
24. Pagon RA, Graham JM Jr, Zonana J, et al. Coloboma, congenital heart disease, and choanal atresia with multiple anomalies: CHARGE association. J Pediatr 1981;99(2):223–7.
25. Blake KD, Prasad C. CHARGE syndrome. Orphanet J Rare Dis 2006;1:34.
26. Leclerc JE, Fearon B. Choanal atresia and associated anomalies. Int J Pediatr Otorhinolaryngol 1987;13(3):265–72.
27. Jongmans MC, Admiraal RJ, van der Donk KP, et al. CHARGE syndrome: the phenotypic spectrum of mutations in the CHD7 gene. J Med Genet 2006;43(4): 306–14.
28. Sanlaville D, Verloes A. CHARGE syndrome: an update. Eur J Hum Genet 2007; 15(4):389–99.
29. Miller MJ, Martin RJ, Carlo WA, et al. Oral breathing in newborn infants. J Pediatr 1985;107(3):465–9.
30. Kubba H, Bennett A, Bailey CM. An update on choanal atresia surgery at Great Ormond Street Hospital for Children: preliminary results with Mitomycin C and the KTP laser. Int J Pediatr Otorhinolaryngol 2004;68(7):939–45.

31. Muzumdar D, Ventureyra EC. Inadvertent intracranial insertion of a soft rubber tube in a patient with Treacher-Collins syndrome: case report and review of literature. Childs Nerv Syst 2008;24(5):609–13.

32. Nathoo N, Nadvi SS. Intracranial malposition of a nasogastric tube following repair of choanal atresia. Br J Neurosurg 1999;13(4):409–10.

33. Freng A. Congenital choanal atresia. Etiology, morphology and diagnosis in 82 cases. Scand J Plast Reconstr Surg 1978;12(3):261–5.

34. Effat KG. Use of the automatic tympanometer as a screening tool for congenital choanal atresia. J Laryngol Otol 2005;119(2):125–8.

35. Slovis TL, Renfro B, Watts FB, et al. Choanal atresia: precise CT evaluation. Radiology 1985;155(2):345–8.

36. Otto AW, Lehrbach DER. Pathologischen Anatomic des Menschenund der Thiere. Berlin: Recker 1830;1:181–3 [German].

37. Emmert C. Stenochorie und Atresie der Choannen. Lehrbach der Speciellen Chirurgie 1854;2:535–8.

38. Durmaz A, Tosun F, Yldrm N, et al. Transnasal endoscopic repair of choanal atresia: results of 13 cases and meta-analysis. J Craniofac Surg 2008;19(5): 1270–4.

39. Gujrathi CS, Daniel SJ, James AL, et al. Management of bilateral choanal atresia in the neonate: an institutional review. Int J Pediatr Otorhinolaryngol 2004;68(4): 399–407.

40. Ferguson JL, Neel HB 3rd. Choanal atresia: treatment trends in 47 patients over 33 years. Ann Otol Rhinol Laryngol 1989;98(2):110–2.

41. Freng A. Growth in width of the dental arches after partial extirpation of the mid-palatal suture in man. Scand J Plast Reconstr Surg 1978;12(3):267–72.

42. Lang J, Baumeister R. [Postnatal growth of the nasal cavity]. Gegenbaurs Morphol Jahrb 1982;128(3):354–93.

43. Fearon B, Dickson J. Bilateral choanal atresia in the newborn: plan of action. Laryngoscope 1968;78(9):1487–99.

44. Stankiewicz JA. The endoscopic repair of choanal atresia. Otolaryngol Head Neck Surg 1990;103(6):931–7.

45. Dedo HH. Transnasal mucosal flap rotation technique for repair of posterior choanal atresia. Otolaryngol Head Neck Surg 2001;124(6):674–82.

46. Nour YA, Foad H. Swinging door flap technique for endoscopic transeptal repair of bilateral choanal atresia. Eur Arch Otorhinolaryngol 2008;265(11):1341–7.

47. Stamm AC, Pignatari SS. Nasal septal cross-over flap technique: a choanal atresia micro-endoscopic surgical repair. Am J Rhinol 2001;15(2):143–8.

48. Lapointe A, Giguere CM, Forest VI, et al. Treatment of bilateral choanal atresia in the premature infant. Int J Pediatr Otorhinolaryngol 2008;72(5):715–8.

49. Holland BW, McGuirt WF Jr. Surgical management of choanal atresia: improved outcome using mitomycin. Arch Otolaryngol Head Neck Surg 2001;127(11): 1375–80.

50. Prasad M, Ward RF, April MM, et al. Topical mitomycin as an adjunct to choanal atresia repair. Arch Otolaryngol Head Neck Surg 2002;128(4):398–400.

51. Al-Ammar AY. Effect of use of mitomycin C on the outcome of choanal atresia repair. Saudi Med J 2007;28(10):1537–40.

52. Agrawal N, Morrison GA. Laryngeal cancer after topical mitomycin C application. J Laryngol Otol 2006;120(12):1075–6.

53. Park AH, Brockenbrough J, Stankiewicz J. Endoscopic versus traditional approaches to choanal atresia. Otolaryngol Clin North Am 2000;33(1):77–90.

54. Van Den Abbeele T, Francois M, Narcy P. Transnasal endoscopic treatment of choanal atresia without prolonged stenting. Arch Otolaryngol Head Neck Surg 2002;128(8):936–40.
55. Schoem SR. Transnasal endoscopic repair of choanal atresia: why stent? Otolaryngol Head Neck Surg 2004;131(4):362–6.
56. Cedin AC, Peixoto Rocha JF Jr, Deppermann MB, et al. Transnasal endoscopic surgery of choanal atresia without the use of stents. Laryngoscope 2002; 112(4):750–2.
57. Al-Ammar AY. The use of nasal stent for choanal atresia. Saudi Med J 2008;29(3): 437–40.
58. Westendorff C, Dammann F, Reinert S, et al. Computer-aided surgical treatment of bilateral choanal atresia. J Craniofac Surg 2007;18(3):654–60.
59. Postec F, Bossard D, Disant F, et al. Computer-assisted navigation system in pediatric intranasal surgery. Arch Otolaryngol Head Neck Surg 2002;128(7): 797–800.
60. Furuta S, Itoh K, Shima T, et al. Laser beam in treating congenital choanal atresia in three patients. Acta Otolaryngol Suppl 1994;517:33–5.
61. Pototschnig C, Volklein C, Appenroth E, et al. Transnasal treatment of congenital choanal atresia with the KTP laser. Ann Otol Rhinol Laryngol 2001;110(4):335–9.
62. D'Eredita R, Lens MB. Contact-diode laser repair of bony choanal atresia: a preliminary report. Int J Pediatr Otorhinolaryngol 2008;72(5):625–8.
63. Yuan HB, Poon KS, Chan KH, et al. Fatal gas embolism as a complication of Nd-YAG laser surgery during treatment of bilateral choanal stenosis. Int J Pediatr Otorhinolaryngol 1993;27(2):193–9.
64. Aqil M, Ulhaq A, Arafat A, et al. Venous air embolism during the use of a Nd YAG laser. Anaesthesia 2008;63(9):1006–9.
65. Lazar RH, Younis RT. Transnasal repair of choanal atresia using telescopes. Arch Otolaryngol Head Neck Surg 1995;121(5):517–20.
66. Panwar SS, Martin FW. Trans-nasal endoscopic holmium: YAG laser correction of choanal atresia. J Laryngol Otol 1996;110(5):429–31.
67. Anderhuber W, Stammberger H. Endoscopic surgery of uni- and bilateral choanal atresia. Auris Nasus Larynx 1997;24(1):13–9.
68. Sadek SA. Congenital bilateral choanal atresia. Int J Pediatr Otorhinolaryngol 1998;42(3):247–56.
69. Josephson GD, Vickery CL, Giles WC, et al. Transnasal endoscopic repair of congenital choanal atresia: long-term results. Arch Otolaryngol Head Neck Surg 1998;124(5):537–40.
70. Wiatrak BJ. Unilateral choanal atresia: initial presentation and endoscopic repair. Int J Pediatr Otorhinolaryngol 1998;46(1–2):27–35.
71. Saetti R, Emanuelli E, Cutrone C, et al. [The treatment of choanal atresia]. Acta Otorhinolaryngol Ital 1998;18(5):307–12.
72. Fong M, Clarke K, Cron C. Clinical applications of the holmium: YAG laser in disorders of the paediatric airway. J Otolaryngol 1999;28(6):337–43.
73. Tzifa KT, Skinner DW. Endoscopic repair of unilateral choanal atresia with the KTP laser: a one stage procedure. J Laryngol Otol 2001;115(4):286–8.
74. Ku PK, Tong MC, Tsang SS, et al. Acquired posterior choanal stenosis and atresia: management of this unusual complication after radiotherapy for nasopharyngeal carcinoma. Am J Otolaryngol 2001;22(4):225–9.
75. Uri N, Greenberg E. Endoscopic repair of choanal atresia: practical operative technique. Am J Otolaryngol 2001;22(5):321–3.

76. Khafagy YW. Endoscopic repair of bilateral congenital choanal atresia. Laryngo-scope 2002;112(2):316–9.
77. Pasquini E, Sciarretta V, Saggese D, et al. Endoscopic treatment of congenital choanal atresia. Int J Pediatr Otorhinolaryngol 2003;67(3):271–6.
78. Rombaux P, de Toeuf C, Hamoir M, et al. Transnasal repair of unilateral choanal atresia. Rhinology 2003;41(1):31–6.
79. Cedin AC, Fujita R, Cruz OL. Endoscopic transeptal surgery for choanal atresia with a stentless folded-over-flap technique. Otolaryngol Head Neck Surg 2006; 135(5):693–8.
80. Yaniv E, Hadar T, Shvero J, et al. Endoscopic transnasal repair of choanal atresia. Int J Pediatr Otorhinolaryngol 2007;71(3):457–62.

Surgical Management of Benign Sinonasal Masses

Richard J. Harvey, MD[a],*, Patrick O. Sheahan, MD[b],
Rodney J. Schlosser, MD[b]

KEYWORDS

- Endoscopic • Skull base • Tumor • Sinonasal
- Angiofibroma • Juvenile nasopharyngeal angiofibroma
- Inverted papilloma • Osteoma

Benign sinonasal tumors encompass a collection of pathologic findings that include neoplastic masses and fibro-osseous lesions. These conditions are common, with radiologic evidence of osteoma present in up to 1% of all radiographs[1] and up to 3% of all CT scans.[2] This represents an incidence of 10 to 80 per 100,000 annually. Most are not symptomatic, however, and often present only when functional impairment of the paranasal sinus system occurs with significant growth. Although the classic order of incidence for tumor frequency is osteoma occurring more frequently than hemangioma and hemangioma occurring more frequently than papilloma, it is the papillomas that dominate the clinical presentation. Subsequently, inverted papilloma (IP) is the archetypical case example by which the management of benign sinonasal masses is defined.

PHILOSOPHY OF MANAGEMENT

The management of benign sinonasal masses should follow a balanced algorithm of the need for resection weighed against the adverse effects of surgical removal. Lateral rhinotomy and subtotal maxillectomy for such conditions as IP, osteoma, or fibrous dysplasia (FD) may result in greater morbidity than observation alone, particularly if such lesions are asymptomatic. Conversely, surgical removal of benign sinonasal masses should be contemplated when they are causing symptoms or pending complications or when the suspicion of malignancy exists (**Box 1**).

[a] Rhinology and Skull Base Surgery, Department of Otolaryngology/Skull Base Surgery, St. Vincent's Hospital, 354 Victoria Street, Darlinghurst, Sydney, NSW 2010, Australia
[b] Rhinology and Skull Base Surgery, Department of Otolaryngology/Head and Neck Surgery, Medical University of South Carolina, 135 Rutledge Avenue, Charleston, SC 29425, USA
* Corresponding author.
E-mail address: richard@sydneyentclinic.com (R. Harvey).

Otolaryngol Clin N Am 42 (2009) 353–375
doi:10.1016/j.otc.2009.01.006
0030-6665/09/$ – see front matter © 2009 Elsevier Inc. All rights reserved.

> **Box 1**
> **Indications for nasal surgery**
>
> *Indications for surgery of benign sinonasal masses*
>
> Symptoms directly related to pathologic findings (ie, obstructive sinusitis)
>
> Pending complications
>
> Suspicion or potential for malignancy

Complete tumor removal is always the desired treatment end point. Unlike malignancy, however, total en bloc excision with significant normal tissue removal can be excessive for some of these lesions and can result in unacceptable cosmesis, functional impairment, dental disruption, epiphora, orbital displacement, and nerve injury. These adverse effects may be acceptable for the management of malignant disease when the consequences of persistent local, regional, or distant disease are significant, but for benign disease, subtotal resection for the purposes of relieving the current symptomatology may be better practice when the potential for morbidity is high. When the suspicion for malignancy or potential malignant change is high (eg, IP), this morbidity needs to be balanced.

Common sites of tumor involvement for which this morbidity must be weighed are the dura and periorbita. There are many well described techniques for reconstructing these areas that are highly reliable,[3] but resection of the dura or periorbita removes a natural barrier to tumor spread. Removal of soft tissues tumors from bone is significantly easier than direct dural or periorbital removal, and observation of residual benign tumor around the dura, periorbita, or carotid may be more prudent than a partial disruptive attempt at removal. Aggressive attempts to remove tumor from these soft tissue barriers are unlikely to result in wide negative margins, and a small breech may result in intracranial or orbital recurrence of benign disease that can subsequently require radical treatment with significant morbidity. In contrast to the surgical philosophy for sinonasal malignancies, the authors' approach to confirmed benign disease involving these areas is more conservative to ensure that the surgical "cure" is not worse than the disease. A staged second resection may be more prudent.

Surgeons have always been cognizant of the need to keep morbidity low for benign conditions. The surgical management of benign conditions has commonly proceeded through limited approaches (eg, early intranasal procedures for IP with high recurrence rates), however. Limited approaches have often resulted in incomplete removal of disease at common sites (**Box 2**). Lack of vision, heavy reliance on angled instruments, and "scraping" dissection techniques all increase the risk for recurrence at these

> **Box 2**
> **Common sites of residual disease**
>
> Dental roots
>
> Frontal sinus and recess
>
> Lateral sphenoid
>
> Anterior maxillary wall
>
> Nasolacrimal duct
>
> Infratemporal fossa extension (including pterygopalatine fossa [PPF] and infra-orbital fissure [IOF])

areas. The authors typically approach these lesions with an en bloc resection philosophy but with strict attention to sites of tumor attachment even if tumors need to be debulked to visualize margins properly.

This article describes an aggressive surgical approach to these lesions while maintaining respect for their benign nature and the importance of preserving natural barriers to growth (spread), such as the dura and periorbita.

SYMPTOMS

The growth of many benign masses within the paranasal sinuses is slow, and the clinical presentation is tempered by adaptation on the part of patients. Adaptation describes the phenomenon of decreased symptom awareness secondary to gradual impairment of function over time. Nasal obstruction is the most common presentation despite adaptation. Most patients (58%–76%) have unilateral nasal obstruction.[4,5] The symptom duration may be misleadingly short, because many patients complain of a short symptom course with a concurrent viral upper respiratory tract infection. Although the patient history may be brief, the pathologic condition may have been present in considerable size for many months with adaptation to the functional component.

Epistaxis is also common for benign lesions (17%–21%).[4,5] Initially, this symptom may seem to be more strongly associated with malignant disease. Benign lesions often cause disruption to nasal airflow, however, with subsequent turbulence, crusting, and small areas of mucositis and mucosal excoriation. Patients often blow the affected side of their nose with greater force to relieve symptoms, and self-digitalization is commonly performed to help clear crusting. These all increase the chance of nasal bleeding in benign disease.

Pain is commonly perceived in up to 18% of cases.[5] The pain experienced is rarely severe, sharp, or debilitating. Subtle pressure and facial ache are more frequently encountered. This may be the result of ostial obstruction with changes in luminal pressure or inflammatory dysfunction of the sinuses. Additionally, it can be generated by dural or periorbital compression or contact. The ability of benign masses to cause persistent pain without evidence of sinus dysfunction is still debated. Many rhinologic surgeons have encountered patients, without surrounding sinus changes or dural or periorbital contact, with pain as their presenting feature. This situation is not uncommonly encountered, because many of these patients with headache of alternative origin have had a CT scan or other radiologic imaging and the subsequent finding of what might be an incidental lesion. After exclusion of other headaches causes, and especially in the presence of localization of pain, many of these patients have received benefit from tumor removal. The nature of pain generation may be based on periosteal reaction or localized osteitis.

Persistent sensation of postnasal drainage (PND) and bilateral nasal obstruction can occur in 12% and 14% of patients, respectively. PND is likely to be the result of mucociliary dysfunction, air turbulence, and subsequent changes in mucus rheology. Bilateral obstruction usually results from secondary septal deformity compromising the contralateral nasal cavity. Acute sinusitis is uncommon (9%). Mucociliary function is often retained until late in tumor growth, and bacterial infection of a compromised sinus is not common. The presentation of a nasal mass and epiphora also appears later in the disease progression.[5] Olfactory loss is rare, because contralateral function usually prevents clinical syraptoms. Eye symptoms can occur from growth into the orbit with proptosis, and then diplopia, as common orbital symptoms. Visual loss is extremely rare.

PATHOLOGIC FINDINGS ENCOUNTERED

IPs, juvenile nasopharyngeal angiofibromas (JNAs), hemangiomas, and fibro-osseous masses dominate the published literature. This does not necessarily reflect incidence but, as a result of clinical impact, challenges in management and difficulties in surgical removal. **Table 1** presents a comprehensive but not necessarily complete list of benign neoplasms encountered in the nasal cavity and paranasal sinuses. Although it is important to have a structured comprehensive list (see **Table 1**) when unusual masses are encountered or for examination purposes, a common and practical grouping for these conditions is often structured as five simple groups: fibro-osseous (FD, chondroma, and osteoma), IP, neural-related (schwannoma, neuroma, and meningioma), vascular (JNA, hemangioma, and pyogenic granuloma), and odontogenic.

Inverted Papilloma

This is the most common epithelial tumor of the sinonasal tract. The incidence of IP has been documented at 0.2 to 0.6 cases per 100,000 people anually.[6,7] It is

Table 1
Sinonasal lesions or pathologic findings

Tissue of Origin	Benign Tumor
Epithelial	
Epidermoid or squamous	Papilloma
Nonepidermoid	Adenoma Monomorphic Pleomorphic Oncocytoma
Neuroectodermal	Meningioma Neurofibroma Glioma Ectopic pituitary adenoma
Odontogenic	Ameloblastoma
Mesenchymal	
Vascular	Hemangioma Capillary Cavernous Angiofibroma Angiomyolipoma Paraganglioma
Muscular	Leiomyoma Rhabdomyoma
Cartilaginous	Chondroma Chondroblastoma
Osseous	Osteoma Osteoblastoma
Lymphoreticular	Plasmacytoma (EMP)
Notochord	Chordoma
Tissue eosinophil	LCH or eosinophilic granuloma
Other	Fibroma Lipoma Myxoma

Abbreviation: EMP, extramedullary plasmacytoma.

synonymous with inverting papilloma, epithelial papilloma, papillary sinusitis, schneiderian papilloma, inverted schneiderian papilloma, soft papilloma, transitional cell papilloma, polyp with inverting metaplasia, and benign transitional cell growth. Although these names have been used interchangeably to describe this condition, its current description should be IP. Sinonasal papilloma was first described by Ward[8] in 1854, but it was Hyams[9] who helped to define the pathoclinical understanding of the condition. The subdivisions of inverted, septal (fungiform), and oncocytic (cylindric) are still widely accepted today.[10] These lesions are the most common benign epithelial tumors of the nose. They comprise less than 5% of all tumors of the nose,[11] but IP is frequently encountered in the clinical environment because of its potential for growth, malignant change, and high recurrence rate. IP occurs in the fifth to eight decade of life and is generally more common in men than in women. An association of IP with inflammatory polyps is well described, but most are isolated lesions. Only 4.9% of patients present with bilateral or multifocal disease.[12] A human papilloma virus (HPV) origin has been widely investigated. The septal type is most commonly associated with HPV 6 and 11, but even with in situ hybridization techniques, HPV DNA has only been demonstrated in less than 50% of cases.[10,13,14] The overall evidence for a causal link is not strong but may explain uncommon multifocal disease.

The classic clinical findings are of a nodular, papillomatous, unilateral mass (**Fig. 1**). An endophytic or "inverted" growth pattern characterizes these tumors. There is a thickened squamous epithelial proliferation and a mixed chronic inflammatory infiltrate. A downward growth pattern into a fibromyxoid stroma is classic. There are two classic surgical features of IP. The presence of osteitis within the mass can often identify the site of attachment.[15–17] Bony changes at the attachment site also lead to a rough base, and histologic examination has demonstrated tumor pseudopods extending into the bone, thus requiring bony resection at the attachment.[17]

Atypia, dysplasia, carcinoma in situ, and squamous cell carcinoma can all occur in papilloma. Malignant change within the inverted type of papilloma has been well

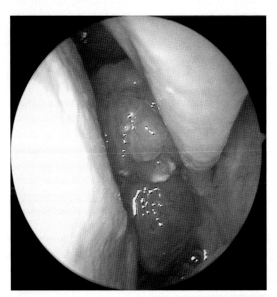

Fig. 1. The classic appearance of IP arising in the left sphenoethmoidal recess.

documented.[18] Krouse[12] originally described a 9.1% rate of squamous cell carcinoma in his cohort. This has been supported by a recent meta-analysis of published case series that reported a synchronous carcinoma rate of 7.1% and a metachronous rate of 11%.[19] It was widely speculated that the atypical and dysplastic changes were precancerous,[12] but this is not supported by the literature. Degree of atypia, the mitotic index, and recurrence seem to have little correlation with carcinoma transformation.[20,21] Carcinoma in situ should be closely followed, because these cases may represent precancerous change or undetected carcinoma from sampling errors.[19]

Lateral rhinotomy for surgical removal was the standard of care until the past 2 decades. This was based on Weissler's recurrence rates of 71% for the intranasal approaches, 56% for the limited Caldwell-Luc or external ethmoid approaches, and 29% for the lateral rhinotomy.[21] The intranasal approaches were little more than a polypectomy in the pre-endoscopic era, however. Subsequent studies by Tufano and colleagues[5] and Woodworth and colleagues[22] and a literature meta-analysis have demonstrated a significant advantage to endoscopic resection. A collation of the literature reports recurrence rates of 12.8% for endoscopic resection, 17.0% for lateral rhinotomy, and 34.2% for other limited resections.[19] Selection bias may exist for some of the published reports, but the Krouse staging system is well accepted in the literature to provide a comparison basis (**Table 2**).

Juvenile Nasopharyngeal Angiofibroma

JNA is an uncommon tumor (<1%) of the sinonasal system,[23] but it has a disproportionately high representation in the literature because of its clinical impact, potential for morbidity, and difficulties in surgical resection. It is a misnomer, with the site of origin accepted as an area in the lateral nasal wall near the sphenopalatine foramen. The lesions occur almost exclusively in men and during the second and third decades of life. There is some debate about the potential for JNA to represent a vascular malformation rather than a tumor.[24] Spontaneous regression has been reported. There is a familial predisposition to JNA, with the lesion being encountered 25 times more frequently in those carrying the familial adenomatous polyposis gene.[25,26]

The tumor appears as a purple-gray pedunculated mass centered on the sphenopalatine foramen (**Fig. 2**). Histologically, there is a vascular component of thin-walled vessels of varying sizes. They lack elastic fibers and usually have a partial or incomplete smooth muscle layer.[27] A fibrous stroma extends throughout the lesion. Androgen receptors have been detected within the stroma.[10] The classic radiologic feature of JNA is anterior bowing of the posterior maxillary sinus wall, the Holman-Miller sign.[28] Intracranial extension of JNA may occur, with tumor spreading through

Table 2	
Krouse staging for inverted papilloma	
Stage	
T1	Tumor isolated to one area of the nasal cavity without extension to the paranasal sinuses
T2	Tumor involves medial wall of the maxillary sinus, ethmoid sinuses, or osteomeatal complex
T3	Tumor involves the superior, inferior, posterior, anterior, or lateral wall of the maxillary sinus, frontal sinus, or sphenoid sinus
T4	Tumor with extrasinonasal extent or malignancy

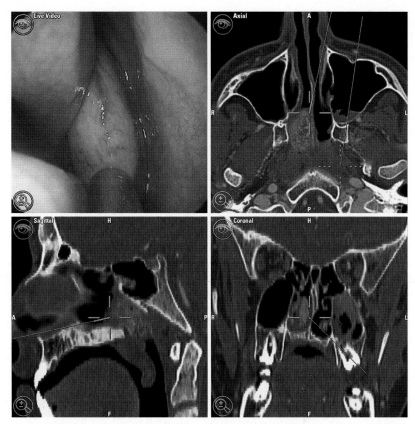

Fig. 2. The pale mucosal covering of a JNA occupying the posterior right nasal cavity. The contrasted CT images demonstrate its typical origin near the sphenopalatine foramen. The vascularity of the tumor, which is well shown in the CT images, is not immediately apparent on examination. An injudicious biopsy can result in heavy epistaxis.

well described routes to the skull base.[29] This spread is dominated by an extradural pattern.[29,30] The Andrew's classification is currently used for staging (**Table 3**).[31]

The endoscopic route has become widely accepted for managing most tumors.[32] Even large tumors involving the middle cranial fossa can be successfully removed endoscopically (**Fig. 3**). The midface degloving approach is occasionally used for extensive intracranial involvement.[33,34] A careful devascularization of the tumor before removal is the key to successful endoscopic surgical management. This can be achieved by lateral ligation of the feeding arteries (see **Fig. 2**) or by preoperative embolization. Radiotherapy and hormonal therapy have little role in modern management.

Hemangioma

Lobular capillary hemangioma (LCH) dominates the vascular neoplastic masses in the nose and paranasal sinuses. LCH is synonymous with pyogenic granuloma and vascular pregnancy tumor. Pyogenic granuloma is a poor name, however, because the condition is neither an infectious process nor a granulomatous one. These lesions are common throughout life but are uncommon in persons younger than 16 years of age.[10] LCH presents as a red-purple, lobulated, smooth mass (**Fig. 4**). It classically

Table 3
Andrew's (modified Fisch) classification for juvenile nasopharyngeal angiofibroma

Type	Tumor Extent
I	Limited to the nasopharynx and nasal cavity, bone destruction negligible or limited to the sphenopalatine foramen
II	Invades the pterygopalatine fossa or the maxillary, ethmoid, or sphenoid sinus with bone destruction
IIIa	Invades the infratemporal fossa or the orbital region without intracranial involvement
IIIb	Invades the infratemporal fossa or orbit with intracranial extradural (parasellar) involvement
IVa	Intracranial intradural tumor without infiltration of the cavernous sinus, pituitary fossa, or optic chiasm
IVb	Intracranial intradural tumor with infiltration of the cavernous sinus, pituitary fossa, or optic chiasm

arises from the septum, but it also arises from the head of the inferior turbinate. Histologically, LCH is characterized by lobules of central capillaries in the submucosal space. There are surrounding feeding vessels. There is a prominent endothelial lining with tufting and mitoses. Atypical mitoses may be associated, but there is little evidence of transformation to angiosarcoma.[10] Cavernous hemangiomas are much less common in the sinonasal tract than LCH. They are more frequently located in the middle turbinates (**Fig. 5**), in the lateral nasal wall, and within bony structures.

Osteoma and Fibro-Osseous Lesions

Osteoma is perhaps the most common benign tumor of the sinonasal system.[4] It is present in 1% of all radiographs[1] and in an even higher number of CT scans (**Fig. 6**).[2] Presenting in the third to fourth decade of life, osteomas have a preponderance to occur in men (1.5–2:1 ratio). They arise most commonly in the frontal and ethmoid sinuses and less commonly from the maxillary and sphenoid sinuses.[2,35,36] Endoscopically, they appear as a simple, smooth, mucosal-covered mass. Their

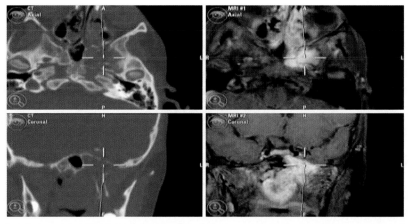

Fig. 3. Intracranial extension of a JNA often follows classic pathways. This lesion has developed through the pterygopalatine fossa, involving the foramen rotundum and the middle cranial fossa floor.

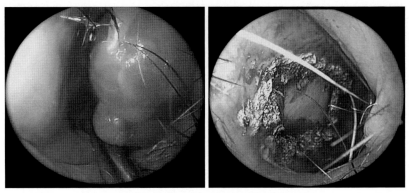

Fig. 4. (*Left*) Large (1.5 cm) left anterior septal LCH. (*Right*) Excision is a simple zone 1 approach with low recurrence.

histology is defined by dense, predominately mature, lamellar bone. A variable amount of interosseus space with hematopoietic elements is present. Two subtypes are recognized, ivory and mature (osteoma spongiosum).[37] Ivory osteomas have hard dense bone with few fibrous components. Mature variants have cancellous bone and interosseous spaces. Surgically, this is important, because the ivory subtype requires extensive drilling. Their growth rate is slow and estimated to be approximately 1.61 mm/y (range: 0.44–6.0 mm/y).[38] There are developmental, traumatic, and infectious theories regarding their etiology, all with limited evidence.[2] Extensive osteoma, especially with anterior frontal or anterior orbital attachment, may still provide an indication for open approaches: osteoplastic flap or Lynch procedures (**Fig. 7**). The complications, such as frontal stenosis, need to be weighed carefully against ease of access secondary to removing the lateral wall of the frontal recess in the external approach, however.[39–41]

FD is also common within the bones of the skull base. It is usually mono-ostotic and can present as a nasal mass. The classic radiologic features of a ground-glass appearance make this condition easier to confirm without surgical intervention

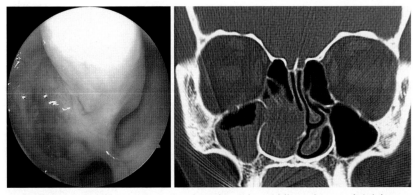

Fig. 5. (*Left*) Cavernous hemangioma involves the right middle turbinate. (*Right*) Intraosseous component is common. (*Left*) Synechiae are a secondary phenomenon. Multiple nasal packing was performed before formal postepistaxis evaluation finally identified the pathologic condition.

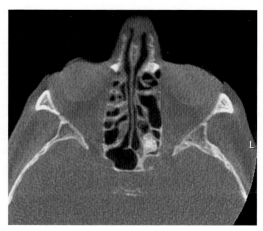

Fig. 6. The most common benign neoplasm of the nose. A small osteoma of the left posterior ethmoid is an incidental finding in this patient. Up to 3% of CT scans show such pathologic findings.

(**Fig. 8**). Management is generally conservative,[42] because many of these lesions have slow growth rates and often slow or regress after puberty.

Odontogenic Masses

Odontogenic pathologic conditions are mentioned here to provide the endoscopic surgeon a framework with which to classify the numerous pathologic findings encountered. Infective masses include periapical or radicular cysts (**Fig. 9**). Developmental conditions are dominated by dentigerous cysts (an ectopic or unerupted tooth) and odontogenic keratocysts (OKCs). An OKC is a benign but locally aggressive developmental odontogenic cyst. It is thought to arise from the dental lamina. The dental lamina is a band of epithelial tissue seen in histologic sections of a developing tooth. Additionally, ameloblastoma and calcifying epithelial tumor contribute to the majority of neoplastic odontogenic lesions.

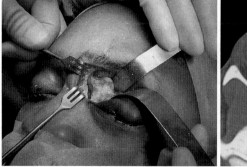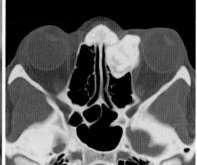

Fig. 7. Open approaches, such as a Lynch procedure (*left*), may still be suitable for bony tumors with anterior and orbital involvement (*right*).

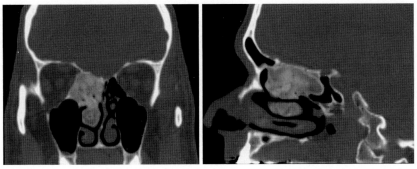

Fig. 8. Mono-ostotic FD of the right ethmoid. The ground-glass appearance, intact cortical lamina, and confinement to a single bony site are classic features of this condition.

Syndromes

There are some well-defined clinical syndromes that are associated with some of the previously mentioned benign lesions. The most commonly encountered are the following:

Osteoma: Gardner's syndrome has a classic triad of colorectal polyps, skeletal abnormalities, and supranumerary teeth.[43] It is an autosomal-dominant constellation of osteomas, fibromas, lipomas, and intestinal polyps. Malignant degeneration of the intestinal polyps is common in affected patients.[44]

OKC: Gorlin's syndrome (nevoid basal cell carcinoma [BCC] syndrome) is an autosomal-dominant syndrome with multiple BCCs, skeletal abnormalities (mainly bifid rib), OKCs, cranial calcifications, and medulloblastoma.[45]

FD: McCune-Albright syndrome demonstrates the association of polyostotic FD, café-au-lait spots, and endocrine abnormalities with precocious puberty in female and male patients, thyroid disease, acromegaly, and Cushing's syndrome.[46]

PREOPERATIVE ASSESSMENT
Radiologic Evaluation

The purpose of radiologic evaluation is several-fold. Primarily, it is to determine the extent of disease. Clinical evaluation may reveal a small soft tissue mass in the middle

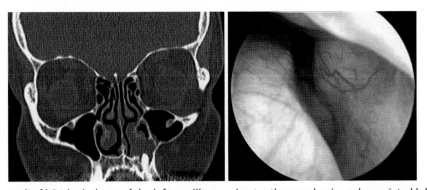

Fig. 9. (*Left*) Periapical cyst of the left maxillary canine tooth caused pain and associated left maxillary sinusitis. (*Right*) Only careful examination of the left nasal floor near the inferior meatus demonstrates the mass.

meatus, but extensive involvement of the frontal sinus with dural exposure may be present. Similarly, a nasal cavity filled with tumor may only be arising from the lateral nasal wall with little or no sinus involvement. Determining the site of attachment and involvement of the frontal sinus, evaluation of areas at risk from surgery (medial orbital wall, skull base, and lateral sphenoid wall), and evaluation of areas for surgical planning are important in the presurgical evaluation.

CT

CT is the cornerstone of radiologic assessment. Classically, soft tissue changes fill the paranasal sinuses, and the delineation of obstructive changes with mucus-filled sinuses cannot easily be separated from the soft tissue component of the tumor. The "bony erosion" is commonly used to describe the surrounding anatomy to the tumor mass. This usually represents pressure-induced remodeling (expansion and atrophy) of the bone (primarily) rather than the aggressive bone destruction that occurs in malignant disease (see **Fig. 3**).

MRI

At the authors' institutions, MRI is indicated when there is skull base or orbital erosion, possible frontal extension, or extrasinus disease. It is important to define the adjacent soft tissue changes to an area of erosion. CT opacity may represent tumor, mucocele, encephalocele, or intracranial extension. This is also true for sphenoid opacity or erosion on CT. The surgical plan to remove disease from critical structures should be anticipated in advance so that wide exposure to these areas can be created during surgery to allow for safe drilling around the orbital apex or carotid (**Fig. 10**).

Frontal sinus involvement is a common indication for the use of MRI. Determination of frontal sinus tumor extension allows an appropriate surgical plan that may encompass a combined endoscopic and trephine or osteoplastic flap approach. This decision should be one that is anticipated before surgery and discussed with the patient rather than one that arises during surgery after inability to complete tumor resection from an entirely endoscopic route.

Embolization

The vascularity of JNA is important in the planning of surgical resection.[47,48] Blood supply is determined by the size and extension of the tumor. In the initial stages, there is a consistent vascular supply from the distal branches of the external carotid artery by way of the internal maxillary artery. In the advanced stages, the tumor may receive important vessels from the internal carotid artery (ICA), especially from collateral branches of the ophthalmic artery.[49,50] Preoperative carotid angiography greatly assists in determining the vascular contributions to the tumor and in identifying significant arteriovenous shunts.[48–50] Even with high-resolution angiography, only blood vessels with diameters exceeding 200 μm can be visualized.[48] Arteriovenous shunts of smaller caliber may not be identified with angiography and may present a potential risk during embolization.[48,49] JNA can have a high incidence of arteriovenous shunts and larger particles of polyvinyl alcohol ($\geq$140 μm in caliber) are recommend for preoperative embolization.[51] Some researchers argue for the need to perform direct intratumoral embolization in addition to preoperative embolization in cases of JNA with significant vascular contribution from the ICA.[49] At the authors' institutions, if there is good access laterally to feeding tumor vessels (see **Fig. 2**), embolization is not essential; however, for large tumors in which a structured approach to vascular control is not available, embolization is used.

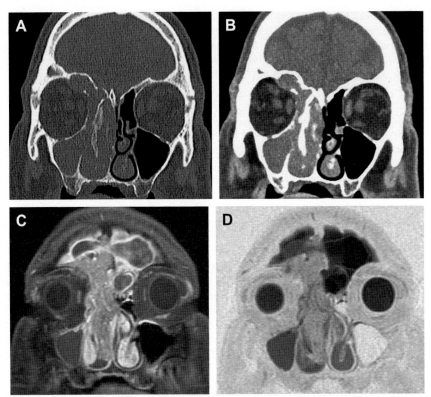

Fig. 10. IP evaluation. CT scans of bone (*A*) and soft tissue (*B*) demonstrate the site of attachment with an osteitic right middle turbinate. T1-weighted MRI with contrast (*C*) and inverse T2-weighted MRI (*D*) demonstrate tumor extent and delineate obstructive changes.

Image Guidance

Although not an absolute necessity, image guidance surgery (IGS) is useful for many tumor cases. It is important to note that it is not a replacement for sound knowledge of skull base and paranasal anatomy and proper equipment to perform such procedures.[52] IGS is valuable for identifying surgical landmarks when there is extensive disease. It can ensure that the frontal recess has been widened to the maximal limits allowed by the patient's anatomy. IGS is an excellent education tool for the surgeon, residents, and students when in the operating room (OR). Perhaps most importantly, there is a learning curve for the use of IGS, registration, and OR setup. If IGS is never used until a situation arises for which its use is critical, staff, the surgeon, and the radiology department are unfamiliar and unprepared to use it. Most IGS-related cost represents an initial capital expense, with most current models incurring small ongoing per case costs.

Medical Presurgical Treatment

Anecdotally, the authors have found that large tumors predispose to obstructive inflammatory sinus changes. These changes result in a moderate degree of edema in the mucosal lining of areas not directly involved by tumor. Obtaining sound anatomic landmarks for the safe progression of endoscopic removal is important, and the authors pretreat many patients who have extensive pathologic findings with antibiotics and oral steroids. This affords better operative conditions and earlier recovery of regenerating mucosa. Comorbidities allowing, the authors start oral prednisone and antibiotics 7 days before surgery. This decision is based on endoscopic and radiologic assessment and not on clinical symptoms.

OPERATIVE TECHNIQUE

The focus is on endoscopic resection of the sinonasal masses. There are a variety of open approaches that can be applied and have been well described;[21,34] however, they have a limited role in the management of benign disease at the authors' institutions. The midface degloving approach with a large osteoplastic flap is perhaps one open approach that is still rarely used for managing lesions in which an endoscopic approach may not suffice. The coronal incision and osteoplastic flap, along with the frontal trephine, are two important open adjuncts that are used to manage frontal sinus extension. Transfacial incisions are rarely used.

Importantly, the philosophy of complete resection should be retained without the need for traditional en bloc surgery. The limits of the area to be removed and drilled should be defined before resection begins; in fact, the authors attempt to define their surgical margins before surgery. This ensures that a surgical plan is adhered to and enhances total removal. The authors believe that there needs to be shift away from the pathoetiologic focus of traditional teachings and emphasize the need to resect anatomic zones or regions. This is not pathology-specific surgery but site-specific surgery. The foundations of this approach are to gain good visualization and access to the anatomic region of origin and interest.

Multiple staging systems, although well described for prognostication in the management of malignant disease, are becoming more frequent for benign conditions. Examples by Cannady and colleagues,[53] Jameson and Kountakis,[54] Krouse,[12] and Woodworth and colleagues[22] all touch on important aspects in the groupings of their patients. Nevertheless, it is fundamentally the completeness of surgical resection of the tumor that dictates the final outcome for benign disease. Synchronous and metachronous malignant disease may occur, but the impact of these events on outcome is unlikely to be reflected in any of the proposed staging systems.

The authors predefine the regions or zones that require endoscopic access and resection (**Table 4**). Easy disorientation can occur during open or endoscopic surgery within the complex anatomy of the skull base. The limits of tissue removal may too easily align with surgeon comfort rather than with anatomic boundaries defined by the presurgical clinical and radiologic examinations. Open craniofacial surgery and the principles of en bloc resection from its oncologic foundations in managing malignant disease are often followed, by some surgeons, to ensure that the appropriate margins have been reached. With careful planning and preoperative radiologic evaluation, it is possible to define the zone of resection likely to be required. **Table 4** outlines the authors' current surgical approach to endoscopic resection. This approach is defined from practical surgical experience and is based on current limitations of the transnasal route. These zones were developed and are used at the Medical University of South Carolina (MUSC) Rhinology and Skull Base and St. Vincent's Rhinology and Skull Base Divisions when planning surgical access in endoscopic tumor removal (**Fig. 11**A). They are defined as follows. In zone 1, the tumor is limited to the septum; turbinates; middle meatus; ethmoid, frontal, and sphenoid sinuses; and medial orbital wall. Surgery may include turbinectomies; septectomy; middle meatal antrostomy (MMA); and frontal, sphenoid, and ethmoid surgery. Basic endoscopic sinus surgery

Table 4
Surgical resection zones

MUSC Zone	Anatomic Region	Surgery Techniques	Instrumentation
Zone 1	Tumor limited to septum; turbinates; middle meatus; ethmoid, frontal, or sphenoid sinuses; and medial orbital wall (IP, hemangioma, chondroma)	Surgery includes turbinectomies and septectomy	Basic ESS instrumentation
Zone 2	Tumor extends to involve maxillary sinus medial to ION, limited posterior wall, or maxillary floor (IP, JNA)	MMA, frontal recess surgery (Draf 1–3, trephine, or osteoplastic), sphenoid surgery, ethmoid surgery Some sinus surgery to include SPA management or modified EMM needed for tumor surveillance	Angled instrumentation and bipolar diathermy or endoscopic clip applicators Maxillary trephination may be used Rongeurs or chisel required for bone removal
Zone 3	Tumor involves NLD, medial buttress, or maxilla lateral to ION and up to zygomatic recess (IP, JNA)	Requires DCR, possible transseptal approach, possible endoscopic Denker's maxillotomy, or open approach (sublabial Caldwell-Luc type approach)	Angled instrumentation has limitations in access Standard ESS instruments by means of transseptal approach or maxillary trephine may be required
Zone 4	Tumor involves anterior maxillary wall with minimal extension into premaxillary soft tissue	Surgery requires transseptal approach, endoscopic Denker's maxillotomy, or premaxillary ESS approach Sublabial open type approach Open lateral rhinotomy or midface degloving	ESS instruments by means of transseptal approach or maxillary trephine may be required Angled ipsilateral endoscopic instruments are of little utility
Zone 5	Tumor involves premaxillary tissue or skin	Surgery requires open approach	Open surgical instrumentation

Abbreviations: DCR, Dacryocystorhinostomy; ESS, Endoscopic sinus surgery; ION, Inferior orbital nerve; MMA, Middle meatal antrostomy; MUSC, Medical University of South Carolina; NLD, Nasolacrimal duct; SPA, Sphenopalatine artery.

instrumentation is required (**Fig. 11**B). In zone 2, the tumor extends to involve the maxillary sinus medial to the inferior orbital nerve (ION), limited posterior wall, or maxillary floor. MMA or modified endoscopic medial maxillectomy (MMM) is needed for tumor surveillance. Sinus surgery to include MMA with or without MMM, sphenopalatine artery management, and some angled instrumentation is needed (**Fig. 11**C). In zone 3, the tumor involves the maxilla lateral to the ION and up to the zygomatic recess. The nasolacrimal duct (NLD) or medial buttress may need resection. Surgery may require dacryocystorhinostomy (DCR), a possible transseptal approach,

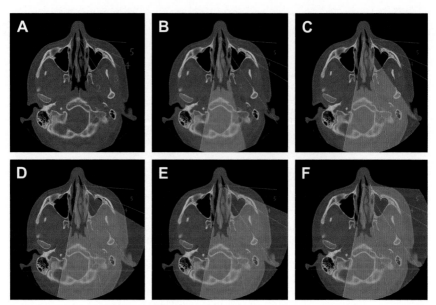

Fig. 11. (*A*) MUSC endoscopic resection zones. (*B–F*) Zones 1 through 5 demonstrate increasing anterior and lateral disease. The details of the zones are outlined in **Table 4**.

a possible sublabial maxillotomy,[55] or medial buttress removal. Traditional open approaches are described for tumors in this location (sublabial Caldwell-Luc type approach, open lateral rhinotomy, and midface degloving). Angled instrumentation is mandatory for ipsilateral surgery (**Fig. 11**D). In zone 4, the tumor involves the anterior maxillary wall without extension into premaxillary soft tissue. Surgery requires transseptal dissection with direct drilling to the anterior maxillary wall (mucosal side) or one of the previously described external approaches (**Fig. 11**E). In zone 5, the tumor involves premaxillary tissue or skin. Surgery requires an open approach (**Fig. 11**F).

Vascular Control

This is arguably the most common reason for incomplete resection, and not just for endoscopic cases. Poor hemostasis can lead to increased difficulty in recognizing the most important anatomic landmarks and identifying the sinus outflow pathways. It enhances the risks for intraoperative complications and postoperative scarring. Most importantly, it leads to an incomplete operation.

Frontal Recess

Disease of the frontal sinus, lateral to the plane of the lamina papyracea, is often not accessible for total resection by means of a transnasal-only approach,[22] even when a Draf 3 procedure has been performed. Other adjunctive procedures may be necessary. The frontal trephine[56] and osteoplastic flap form the basis for achieving additional access. Understanding the need for these in the preoperative assessment is key. They are easy to perform, but the need for them should be defined before surgery and not discovered as unexpectedly necessary during surgery. Use of MRI and CT can help in this assessment (see **Fig. 10**).

Access is not the only concern. Reconstruction of the frontal recess may be necessary if the pathologic finding(s) has been removed from within the frontal sinus. A combination of maximal widening of the frontal recess (Draf 2a, 2b, or 3 procedure), mucosal preservation, and possible silastic sheet stenting for 5 to 7 days after surgery may be appropriate in this circumstance. Additionally, inadvertent frontal recess obstruction may occur if surgery is performed adjacent to the frontal recess. A Draf 2a procedure is routinely performed for most endoscopic resections. This ensures correct localization of the frontal recess and posterior table and aids in postoperative care. A simple classification system is used (**Table 5**) that mirrors cerebrospinal fluid defect repair previously proposed by Woodworth and colleagues.[57] This helps to aid assessment before surgery.

Nasolacrimal Duct

The lower NLD should simply be removed and reconstructed when disease is adjacent or involves this area. Working around this structure simply decreases visualization and increases the risk for positive margins. High patency rates are reported for primary and revision DCR performed for disease involving the NLD.[58–60] The authors have found little morbidity from resection and reconstruction of the nasolacrimal system during endoscopic surgery. The current technique used at the authors' institutions does not necessarily require full sac exposure. Marsupialization of a 6- to 8-mm segment of the distal membranous duct suffices in most cases.

Medial Buttress and Anterior Maxillary Wall Involvement

When the medial buttress (medial rim of the piriform aperture) and bony anterior wall are involved, the area often needs to be drilled. Ipsilateral access often does not allow full access to these areas. The options include an endoscopic version of Denker's medial maxillotomy or a transseptal approach. A medial maxillotomy carries the risk for alar retraction, although not as commonly as when performed by means of a lateral rhinotomy, because lateral alar ligamentous support is less disrupted. The anterior superior alveolar nerve is usually damaged in this approach and can carry the morbidities of dental pain and paraesthesia. The transseptal approach may provide superior access to this area.[61]

Table 5		
Frontal sinus evaluation algorithm		
Degree of Frontal Extension	**Area Involved**	**Ancillary Procedure Required**
Frontal sinus	Lateral lamina papyracea Medial to lamina papyracea	Trephine or osteoplastic flap likely Draf 2b/3 or trephine
Frontal recess	Nasofrontal beak, intersinus septum, or frontal recess proper	Draf 2b or 3 as a minimum Reconstruction and short-term silastic stenting required if extensive bone exposure
Adjacent to frontal recess	Anterior ethmoid, middle turbinate, or medial orbital wall	Draf 2a for identification to ensure whether resection, reconstruction, or packing is going to interfere with the frontal recess

Premaxillary Soft Tissue

If premaxillary tissue is involved, an open sublabial or midface degloving approach is likely to be more suitable. An endoscopic premaxillary dissection plane can be created, but access is superior and soft tissue margins are better obtained by means of an open route.

Supraorbital Ethmoid Cell

The supraorbital ethmoid (SOE) cell presents a unique surgical problem for the treating rhinologist. With any anterior approach (open or endoscopic), there is great difficultly in removing disease from the increasingly narrow cleft of the SOE, formed between the orbit and anterior cranial fossa, as dissection proceeds posteriorly. Instrumentation may simply not fit into this cleft. Even with removal of orbital bone (the medial wall and roof) and the ethmoid roof, the cleft of the dura and periorbita is still restrictive (**Fig. 12**). Only a subcranial or frontal craniotomy approach allows one to elevate the anterior cranial fossa dura, remove the superior bone, and then address the disease in this cleft. Identification of disease in this area before surgery is important to balance the approach-related morbidity and need for completeness of resection.

Dental Roots

The adult maxillary sinus pneumatizes under the nasal floor in most adults. The bone between the dental roots and sinus mucosa is, on average, only 2 mm for the second premolar tooth. Significant morbidity can arise from aggressive drilling in this area. Identifying the maxillary dental relation is important for preoperative counseling (**Fig. 13**).

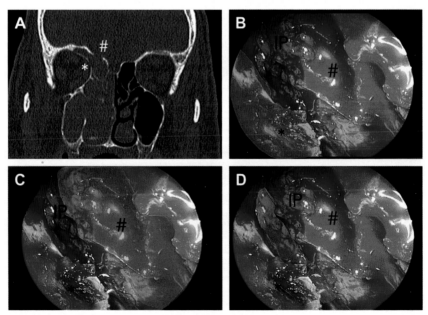

Fig. 12. The SOE problem in tumor resection. The SOE forms a narrow cleft between the orbit (*) and anterior cranial fossa (#). The IP can be seen in this cleft. (A) CT scan is for reference. The orbital wall (B), anterior cranial fossa (C), and SOE (D) arrangement make resection, and especially drilling, challenging in these cases.

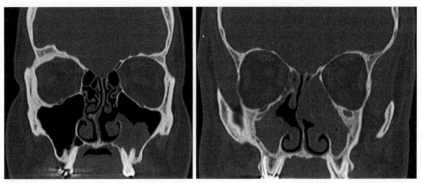

Fig. 13. (*Left*) Dental root damage is likely if there is overly aggressive drilling in the left maxillary sinus floor of a patient who has an IP. (*Right*) Maxillary sinus development affords a much greater safety margin for bone removal.

Dura and Periorbita

The facial layers of the dura and periorbita represent specialized periosteal layers that form a natural barrier to prevent the spread of benign disease. For the orbit, extensive removal of the lamina papyracea can be performed with minimal impact on the mechanics of the extraocular muscles. As removal extends to involve the orbital floor (medial to the infraorbital nerve), the incidence of transient diplopia increases. With the periorbita intact, however, this is rarely a long-term problem. Loss of integrity of the dura or periorbita, although easily reconstructed, increases the risk for intraorbital or intracranial spread. This can be a significant source of morbidity and potential mortality. An IP in the anterior cranial fossa invariably results in some loss of pial or parenchymal frontal lobe tissue in an attempt at complete removal, because the dissection plane has been lost.

POSTOPERATIVE CARE

Packing has a limited role. Extensive tight ribbon gauze is generally not necessary and is uncomfortable for the patient. Silastic sheeting is used routinely to cover the anterior septum, particularly for transseptal approaches.[61] Prolonged endoscopic surgery is associated with significant excoriation and mucosal abrasion to the anterior septum even with careful technique. Heavy fibrinous exudate can occur and cause nasal obstruction, adhesion, and discomfort if not managed. Silastic sheeting (0.4 mm) secured with through-and through Prolene suture assists with this problem. Exposed bone is generally covered with Gelfoam (Pfizer, New York, New York). A gloved Merocel dressing (Medtronic, Mystic, Connecticut) is placed as a middle meatal spacer or in the new cavity created. This is less for hemostasis and more for preventing extensive crusting. It is secured with transseptal Prolene suture. High-volume irrigations start on the first postoperative day. The authors find that this improves patient comfort and breathing and, counterintuitively, reduces bleeding. Antibiotics are given for 14 days after surgery, because there is exposed bone and foreign material in the cavity. The gloved Merocel spacer is removed on day 7. This generally provides a moist environment with soft clot that can easily be suctioned in the outpatient clinic. Pain management has evolved over the past few years in the authors' experience. Combination acetaminophen and opiates are used initially. With extensive bone exposure, however, a secondary pain phenomenon is perceived around postoperative day 5 to 7. This may be similar to the pain experienced by patients who have had a tonsillectomy and are undergoing secondary healing. Nonsteroidal anti-inflammatory drugs greatly help to reduce this phenomenon.

SUMMARY

Benign sinonasal masses are common and can be the cause of significant morbidity. A sound approach is required to balance carefully the need for removal with the impact of surgery on the patient's life. Surgery is indicated when control of symptoms directly related to pathologic findings is required, when there are pending complications, or when the potential or suspicion of malignancy exists. Surgery should not be subtotal. Complete removal of these lesions is curative. Maximal endoscopic exposure, aggressive bone removal, and reconstruction of the functional components of the sinonasal system should be paramount. The morbidity of surgery around the dental roots, dura, periorbita, or exposed critical structures (eg, ICA) should influence the aggressiveness of surgical resection, however. Re-exploration and removal of focal disease recurrence, if required, may be more prudent. Endoscopic surgical resection has replaced transfacial approaches at many institutions. The patient experience has been greatly enhanced by endoscopic surgery. Pain, recovery, hospital stay, and disfigurement can all be reduced with an aggressive endoscopic approach. The potential for complications differs little from the days of open surgery, however.

REFERENCES

1. Mehta BS, Grewal GS. Osteoma of the paranasal sinuses along with a case report of an orbito-ethmoidal osteoma. J Laryngol Otol 1963;77:601–10.
2. Eller R, Sillers M. Common fibro-osseous lesions of the paranasal sinuses. Otolaryngol Clin North Am 2006;39(3):585–600.
3. Hegazy HM, Carrau RL, Snyderman CH, et al. Transnasal endoscopic repair of cerebrospinal fluid rhinorrhea: a meta-analysis. Laryngoscope 2000;110(7): 1166–72.
4. Melroy CT, Senior BA. Benign sinonasal neoplasms: a focus on inverting papilloma. Otolaryngol Clin North Am 2006;39(3):601–17.
5. Tufano RP, Thaler ER, Lanza DC, et al. Endoscopic management of sinonasal inverted papilloma. Am J Rhinol 1999;13(6):423–6.
6. Buchwald C, Nielsen LH, Nielsen PL, et al. Inverted papilloma: a follow-up study including primarily unacknowledged cases. Am J Otol 1989;10(4):273–81.
7. Verner JL, Maguda TA, Young JM. Epithelial papillomas of the nasal cavity and sinuses. AMA Arch Otolaryngol 1959;70:574–8.
8. Ward N. A mirror of the practice of medicine and surgery in the hospitals of London. London Hospital Lancet 1854;2:480–2.
9. Hyams VJ. Papillomas of the nasal cavity and paranasal sinuses. A clinicopathological study of 315 cases. Ann Otol Rhinol Laryngol 1971;80(2):192–206.
10. Wenig BM. Atlas of head and neck pathology. 2nd edition. Philadelphia/London: Elsevier Saunders; 2008.
11. Vrabec DP. The inverted Schneiderian papilloma: a 25-year study. Laryngoscope 1994;104(5 Pt 1):582–605.
12. Krouse JH. Endoscopic treatment of inverted papilloma: safety and efficacy. Am J Otol 2001;22(2):87–99.
13. Respler DS, Jahn A, Pater A, et al. Isolation and characterization of papillomavirus DNA from nasal inverting (Schneiderian) papillomas. Ann Otol Rhinol Laryngol 1987;96(2 Pt 1):170–3.

14. Weber RS, Shillitoe EJ, Robbins KT, et al. Prevalence of human papillomavirus in inverted nasal papillomas. Arch Otolaryngol Head Neck Surg 1988;114(1):23–6.
15. Lee DK, Chung SK, Dhong HJ, et al. Focal hyperostosis on CT of sinonasal inverted papilloma as a predictor of tumor origin. AJNR Am J Neuroradiol 2007; 28(4):618–21.
16. Yousuf K, Wright ED. Site of attachment of inverted papilloma predicted by CT findings of osteitis. Am J Rhinol 2007;21(1):32–6.
17. Chiu AG, Jackman AH, Antunes MB, et al. Radiographic and histologic analysis of the bone underlying inverted papillomas. Laryngoscope 2006;116(9): 1617–20.
18. Snyder RN, Perzin KH. Papillomatosis of nasal cavity and paranasal sinuses (inverted papilloma, squamous papilloma). A clinicopathologic study. Cancer 1972;30(3):668–90.
19. Mirza S, Bradley PJ, Acharya A, et al. Sinonasal inverted papillomas: recurrence, and synchronous and metachronous malignancy. J Laryngol Otol 2007;121(9):857–64.
20. Christensen WN, Smith RR. Schneiderian papillomas: a clinicopathologic study of 67 cases. Hum Pathol 1986;17(4):393–400.
21. Weissler MC, Montgomery WW, Turner PA, et al. Inverted papilloma. Ann Otol Rhinol Laryngol 1986;95(3 Pt 1):215–21.
22. Woodworth BA, Bhargave GA, Palmer JN, et al. Clinical outcomes of endoscopic and endoscopic-assisted resection of inverted papillomas: a 15-year experience. Am J Rhinol 2007;21(5):591–600 [erratum appears in Am J Rhinol 2008 Jan-Feb;22(1):97].
23. Mann WJ, Jecker P, Amedee RG. Juvenile angiofibromas: changing surgical concept over the last 20 years. Laryngoscope 2004;114(2):291–3.
24. Beham A, Beham-Schmid C, Regauer S, et al. Nasopharyngeal angiofibroma: true neoplasm or vascular malformation? Adv Anat Pathol 2000;7(1):36–46.
25. Guertl B, Beham A, Zechner R, et al. Nasopharyngeal angiofibroma: an APC-gene-associated tumor? [see comment]. Hum Pathol 2000;31(11):1411–3.
26. Valanzano R, Curia MC, Aceto G, et al. Genetic evidence that juvenile nasopharyngeal angiofibroma is an integral FAP tumour. Gut 2005;54(7):1046–7.
27. Beham A, Fletcher CD, Kainz J, et al. Nasopharyngeal angiofibroma: an immunohistochemical study of 32 cases. Virchows Arch A Pathol Anat Histopathol 1993; 423(4):281–5.
28. Sessions RB, Wills PI, Alford BR, et al. Juvenile nasopharyngeal angiofibroma: radiographic aspects. Laryngoscope 1976;86(1):2–18.
29. Radkowski D, McGill T, Healy GB, et al. Angiofibroma. Changes in staging and treatment. Arch Otolaryngol Head Neck Surg 1996;122(2):122–9.
30. Bales C, Kotapka M, Loevner LA, et al. Craniofacial resection of advanced juvenile nasopharyngeal angiofibroma. Arch Otolaryngol Head Neck Surg 2002; 128(9):1071–8.
31. Andrews JC, Fisch U, Valavanis A, et al. The surgical management of extensive nasopharyngeal angiofibromas with the infratemporal fossa approach. Laryngoscope 1989;99(4):429–37.
32. Douglas R, Wormald PJ, Douglas R, et al. Endoscopic surgery for juvenile nasopharyngeal angiofibroma: where are the limits? Current 2006;14(1):1–5.
33. Cansiz H, Guvenc MG, Sekerciolu N, et al. Surgical approaches to juvenile nasopharyngeal angiofibroma. J Craniomaxillofac Surg 2006;34(1):3–8.
34. Danesi G, Panciera DT, Harvey RJ, et al. Juvenile nasopharyngeal angiofibroma: evaluation and surgical management of advanced disease. Otolaryngol Head Neck Surg 2008;138(5):581–6.

35. Atallah N, Jay MM. Osteomas of the paranasal sinuses. J Laryngol Otol 1981; 95(3):291–304.
36. Boysen M. Osteomas of the paranasal sinuses. J Otolaryngol 1978;7(4):366–70.
37. Fu YS, Perzin KH. Non-epithelial tumors of the nasal cavity, paranasal sinuses, and nasopharynx. A clinicopathologic study. II. Osseous and fibro-osseous lesions, including osteoma, fibrous dysplasia, ossifying fibroma, osteoblastoma, giant cell tumor, and osteosarcoma. Cancer 1974;33(5):1289–305.
38. Koivunen P, Lopponen H, Fors AP, et al. The growth rate of osteomas of the paranasal sinuses. Clin Otolaryngol Allied Sci 1997;22(2):111–4.
39. Dedo HH, Broberg TG, Murr AH. Frontoethmoidectomy with Sewall-Boyden reconstruction: alive and well, a 25-year experience. Am J Rhinol 1998;12(3):191–8.
40. Neel HB 3rd, McDonald TJ, Facer GW. Modified Lynch procedure for chronic frontal sinus diseases: rationale, technique, and long-term results. Laryngoscope 1987;97(11):1274–9.
41. Schenck NL. Frontal sinus disease. III. Experimental and clinical factors in failure of the frontal osteoplastic operation. Laryngoscope 1975;85(1):76–92.
42. London SD, Schlosser RJ, Gross CW. Endoscopic management of benign sinonasal tumors: a decade of experience. Am J Rhinol 2002;16(4):221–7.
43. Buch B, Noffke C, de Kock S. Gardner's syndrome—the importance of early diagnosis: a case report and a review. SADJ 2001;56(5):242–5.
44. Senior BA, Lanza DC. Benign lesions of the frontal sinus. Otolaryngol Clin North Am 2001;34(1):253–67.
45. Palacios E, Serou M, Restrepo S, et al. Odontogenic keratocysts in nevoid basal cell carcinoma (Gorlin's) syndrome: CT and MRI evaluation. Ear Nose Throat J 2004;83(1):40–2.
46. Zacharin M. The spectrum of McCune Albright syndrome. Pediatr Endocrinol Rev 2007;4(Suppl 4):412–8.
47. Laurent A, Wassef M, Chapot R, et al. Partition of calibrated tris-acryl gelatin microspheres in the arterial vasculature of embolized nasopharyngeal angiofibromas and paragangliomas. J Vasc Interv Radiol 2005;16(4):507–13.
48. Petruson K, Rodriguez-Catarino M, Petruson B, et al. Juvenile nasopharyngeal angiofibroma: long-term results in preoperative embolized and non-embolized patients. Acta Otolaryngol 2002;122(1):96–100.
49. Lefkowitz M, Giannotta SL, Hieshima G, et al. Embolization of neurosurgical lesions involving the ophthalmic artery. Neurosurgery 1998;43(6):1298–303.
50. Casasco A, Houdart E, Biondi A, et al. Major complications of percutaneous embolization of skull-base tumors. AJNR Am J Neuroradiol 1999;20(1):179–81.
51. Schroth G, Haldemann AR, Mariani L, et al. Preoperative embolization of paragangliomas and angiofibromas. Measurement of intratumoral arteriovenous shunts. Arch Otolaryngol Head Neck Surg 1996;122(12):1320–5.
52. Fried MP, Parikh SR, Sadoughi B. Image-guidance for endoscopic sinus surgery. Laryngoscope 2008;118(7):1287–92.
53. Cannady SB, Batra PS, Sautter NB, et al. New staging system for sinonasal inverted papilloma in the endoscopic era. Laryngoscope 2007;117(7):1283–7.
54. Jameson MJ, Kountakis SE. Endoscopic management of extensive inverted papilloma. Am J Rhinol 2005;19(5):446–51.
55. James D, Crockard HA. Surgical access to the base of skull and upper cervical spine by extended maxillotomy. Neurosurgery 1991;29(3):411–6.
56. Zacharek MA, Fong KJ, Hwang PH. Image-guided frontal trephination: a minimally invasive approach for hard-to-reach frontal sinus disease. Otolaryngol Head Neck Surg 2006;135(4):518–22.

57. Woodworth BA, Schlosser RJ, Palmer JN. Endoscopic repair of frontal sinus cerebrospinal fluid leaks. J Laryngol Otol 2005;119(9):709–13.

58. Ben Simon GJ, Joseph J, Lee S, et al. External versus endoscopic dacryocystorhinostomy for acquired nasolacrimal duct obstruction in a tertiary referral center. Ophthalmology 2005;112(8):1463–8.

59. Cokkeser Y, Evereklioglu C, Er H, et al. Comparative external versus endoscopic dacryocystorhinostomy: results in 115 patients (130 eyes). Otolaryngol Head Neck Surg 2000;123(4):488–91.

60. Dolman PJ, Dolman PJ. Comparison of external dacryocystorhinostomy with nonlaser endonasal dacryocystorhinostomy. Ophthalmology 2003;110(1):78–84.

61. Harvey RJ, Sheahan PO, Debanth NI, et al. Trans-septal approach for extended endoscopic resections of the maxilla and infra-temporal fossa. Amer J Rhinol 2009, in press.

Surgical Management of Polyps in the Treatment of Nasal Airway Obstruction

Samuel S. Becker, MD

KEYWORDS
- FESS • Nasal polyps • Sinonasal polyps • Polyp treatment
- Nasal obstruction

In addition to their role in chronic rhinosinusitis and nasal congestion, sinonasal polyps are associated with significant nasal obstruction. Via a purely mechanical effect (ie, obstruction at its simplest level), polyps alter and otherwise block the normal flow of air through the nose. Similarly, by blocking the drainage pathways of the paranasal sinuses, sinus inflammation and its associated symptom of congestion occur. Because the pathway that leads to the formation of sinonasal polyps has not been completely elucidated, effective long-term treatments remain difficult to pinpoint.

Management of these polyps, therefore, is a difficult challenge for the contemporary otolaryngologist. Some of the more common medical treatment options include: topical and oral steroids; macrolide antibiotics; diuretic nasal washes; and intrapolyp steroid injection. Surgical options include polypectomy and functional endoscopic sinus surgery (FESS). In addition, novel treatments for polyps are introduced with some frequency. This article presents an overview of management options for sinonasal polyps, focusing on the indications, efficacy, and complications of the more common interventions.

DIAGNOSIS AND PREVALENCE OF SINONASAL POLYPS

Diagnosis of sinonasal polyps relies primarily on nasal endoscopy, with computed tomography (CT) to evaluate the extent of disease. Although unilateral polyposis often requires adjunctive studies such as magnetic resonance (MR) imaging for further evaluation, endoscopy and CT are usually sufficient to evaluate bilateral, symmetric polyposis.

In the attempt to create valid, reproducible rhinoscopic methods to characterize bilateral sinonasal polyps, multiple staging systems have been proposed.[1,2]

Becker Nose and Sinus Center, 2301 Evesham Road, Suite 404, Voorhees, NJ 08043, USA
E-mail address: sam.s.becker@gmail.com

Otolaryngol Clin N Am 42 (2009) 377–385
doi:10.1016/j.otc.2009.01.002
0030-6665/09/$ – see front matter © 2009 Elsevier Inc. All rights reserved.

Examination of five of these scoring systems found reproducibility in three of the systems. Interestingly, the same study also found that polyp size (and score) correlated more directly to symptoms of nasal congestion than to nasal blockage.[3] This distinction between nasal blockage and nasal congestion is often overlooked but is important.

Work continues on the creation of a reproducible, easy to perform endoscopic scoring system. CT scans are helpful in attempts to quantify the extent of polyp disease and they are essential before any surgical intervention. CT characterization of sinonasal polyps has been well-elucidated by a variety of studies and includes infundibulum enlargement, bony attenuation of the ethmoid trabecula, and the presence of nonenhancing soft tissue formations of a mucoid matrix density, among other traits.[4,5] As polyps are expansile and, in some cases, may expand and erode the skull base,[6] CT is essential for gathering data on the state of the skull base in these patients.

The prevalence of sinonasal polyps is a matter of continued debate. Although most authors cite a prevalence of 1% to 4%,[7] some studies report rates as high as 32%.[8] One study noted a 4.2% prevalence of polyps in a group of patients followed for asthma and rhinitis,[9] while a separate, population based questionnaire sent out by researchers in Finland demonstrated a prevalence of 4.3%.[10] In neither of these studies, however, did respondents undergo nasal endoscopy, which is the gold standard for diagnosis of nasal polyposis. When nasal endoscopy was performed by Johansson and colleagues on a random sample of 1387 Swedish citizens, polyps were identified in 2.7% of the subjects. In their study from 2004, Larsen and Tos[8] identified polyps in 32% of nasal endoscopies performed during 69 consecutive autopsies. Of patients who had polyps, however, 72% of the polyps were smaller than 5 mm in greatest diameter and were not likely to be clinically relevant. The conclusion that small polyps may lead to few symptoms is supported by a 2002 study by Larsen and Tos, which demonstrated that only a small subset of those patients with nasal polyps develop sinonasal complaints.[11]

The prevalence of both symptomatic and asymptomatic nasal polyposis is increased in certain subsets of the population. Patients who have cystic fibrosis, asthma, age greater than 60 years, Churg-Strauss syndrome, or sarcoidosis, or who are male, have been shown to suffer from increased rates of nasal polyposis.[12–15]

PHYSIOLOGY OF SINONASAL POLYPS

Debate continues about the exact pathophysiology of sinonasal polyps, despite much research in this area. Several studies support the idea of the development of polyps as a byproduct of sinonasal inflammation. Although the source of inflammation may be variable (eg, mechanical trauma, bacteria, viruses, fungi, and environmental allergens have all been suggested), researchers theorize that these inciting events lead to disruption of the epithelial lining and initiate a resultant inflammatory cascade. If this inflammation does not subside in its normal timely fashion, stromal edema consolidates and may result in polyp formation.[16]

It has been suggested that an ineffective local Th1-based immune response in these patients is associated with increased Th2-based activity, which contributes to a chronic infection as well as to an increased presence of eosinophils, which then lead to further polyp formation.[17] It has been further proposed that the weakened Th1-response in these patients may be secondary to the down-regulation of some specific toll-like receptors involved in the innate immune response.[18,19] Sinonasal polyps are highly associated with the presence of tissue eosinophilia.

As mentioned, the source of this eosinophilia continues to be investigated. Some authors have focused on a decreased rate of local eosinophilic apoptosis and have postulated the elevated expression of surviving, an inhibitor of protein apoptosis, as the source of this reduced eosinophilic apoptosis.[20,21] Others have documented the increased expression of the chemokines eotaxin and Regulated on Activation Normal T Expressed and Secreted (RANTES) as having a major role in the increased eosinophilic inflammation.[22,23] Others have focused on increased levels of such pro-inflammatory cytokines as tumor necrosis factor, interferon, granulocyte-macrophage colony-stimulating factor (GM-CSF), and interleukin (IL)-5 as a source of the increased inflammatory cells in polyps.[24,25]

The failure of lymphangiogenesis in sinonasal mucosa has also been suggested as a contributing factor to the persistence of stromal edema and eventual polyp formation.[26] Anatomic factors may also play a role in initiation of this inflammatory cascade, as polyps have been noted to appear predominately in structurally tight areas of the sinonasal pathway. Abnormalities in nitrous oxide metabolism, superantigen production, and elevated levels of metalloproteinases are just a few of the other abnormalities found in association with sinonasal polyps.[27–29] Although much has been learned in the past few years concerning the development of sinonasal polyps, much more remains to be elucidated.

MEDICAL TREATMENT OF POLYPS

Patients who have nasal polyposis often experience severe nasal airway obstruction, and have been shown to carry a significantly greater health burden than patients who have chronic rhinosinusitis but no polyp disease.[30] Treatment options vary and they include topical and oral steroids, intrapolyp steroid injection, office polypectomy, and surgery (most commonly FESS). Lesser known and less widely accepted treatments include the use of macrolides,[31] intranasal capsaicin,[32–34] intranasal furosemide,[35] Amphotericin B nasal spray,[36] intranasal lysine-acetylsalicylic acid,[37] UV phototherapy, and anti-leukotriene medications.

Despite this lengthy list of treatment options for nasal polyps, the mainstay of contemporary medical management continues to be intranasal and oral systemic corticosteroids.[38] Steroids likely act on polyps by decreasing the concentration of eosinophils and IgE via the up-regulation of anti-inflammatory genes.[39,40] Some authors have demonstrated increased apoptosis of inflammatory cells and fibroblasts in nasal polyps after steroid administration.[41–43] Through gene array techniques, other researchers have shown the impact of steroids on gene expression.[44] Several studies have demonstrated the clinical efficacy of topical steroids in patients with nasal polyps,[45,46] while other studies have demonstrated on a histologic level a decrease of inflammatory cells after use of topical steroids.[47,48] Fillici and colleagues[49] demonstrated in a randomized, double-blind placebo-controlled study the efficacy of intranasal steroid sprays. In their study, 157 patients with bilateral nasal polyposis were randomized to receive nasal steroid spray or placebo. Patients who received steroids showed statistically and clinically significant improvement in nasal symptoms and polyp size when compared with those who received placebo. Although topical steroids are usually applied via nasal spray, one paper has demonstrated efficacy of manual application directly into the frontal sinus; many other rhinologists have begun to advocate the off-label use of stronger steroids such as Pulmicort for use in nasal washes or applied directly as nasal drops.[50] Systemic steroids are more potent, and have been shown to be more effective at decreasing polyp eosinophilia when compared with steroid sprays.[51]

A recent Cochrane database review of the effectiveness of oral steroids on sino-nasal polyps demonstrated that, although there exists a need for well-designed prospective randomized controlled trials, existing studies do support efficacy of oral steroids as treatment for polyposis.[52] One such study did document the clinically significant improvement in symptoms in patients with sinonasal polyps after a 2-week course of prednisolone.[53] Any consideration of systemic steroids must, of course, include screening patients for relative contraindications (diabetes, emotional instability, hypertension, glaucoma, history of tuberculosis), as well as informing patients of potential systemic side effects.

STEROID INJECTION OF POLYPS

Intranasal steroid injection has been used as a means to deliver a high concentration of steroids directly into inflammatory lesions, such as polyps, without the systemic side effects normally associated with steroids. There is, unfortunately, no level I evidence in support of steroid injections for sinonasal polyposis. Most studies are small, anecdotal, or retrospective. Of particular concern is the associated risk of ocular complication with intranasal steroid injection.

Specifically, there have been sporadic reports of temporary and permanent visual loss after intranasal steroid injection most likely caused by retinal artery embolization and vasospasm. Retrograde embolization may occur when the small steroid particle flows in reverse though the anterior or posterior ethmoid arteries to the ophthalmic artery and then into the central retinal artery where it causes a vaso-occlusive event. Although it is unusual for this to occur, it has been suggested that the risk of compli-cation may be decreased further by following some specific guidelines. These guide-lines include: recommendation for the choice of a steroid with a small particle size such as Triamcinolone acetonide; drawing up this steroid with a small gauge needle; and pre-procedure use of a topical vasoconstrictor to reduce nasal vascular conges-tion. The use of Triamcinolone acetonide has the added advantage of being a steroid suspension of small particles whose local effects continue for several weeks. Recom-mendations have also been made against intra-operative injection. It remains the case that more is unknown about the benefits and risks of steroid injection for sinonasal polyps than is known. Although steroid injection appears to be an effective nonsurgical modality for treating polyps, it is unclear how it compares to topical and oral steroids in regards to efficacy and systemic absorption. There is a small but real risk associated with steroid injection. The risks and benefits should be discussed with the patient. Informed consent should be obtained before administration of a steroid injection.

SURGICAL TREATMENT OF POLYPS

It has been suggested that up to 50% of patients who have sinonasal polyps may eventually require surgical intervention.[54] Although office polypectomy is performed less frequently today than in the past, it continues to be a useful tool for use by the contemporary otolaryngologist. In traditional office polypectomy, polyps are removed with a surgical tonsil snare after appropriate topical anesthesia and vasoconstriction. The principles for office polypectomy remain essentially unchanged from their description by Hippocrates in 400 BC in which he secured polyps through the loop end of a tin curette tied to a string, and avulsed them through the mouth by pulling on the string.[55] In more recent times, authors have described polypectomy in the clinic setting using powered endonasal instrumentation as more precise and less traumatic than traditional office snare polypectomy.[56,57] Although it is largely impractical to perform polypectomy in the clinic setting on patients who have a large polyp burden, it remains a viable option for patients who have a small volume of polyps, or patients who have had a few recalcitrant polyps grow back after surgery, despite aggressive medical therapy.

It has been demonstrated that, in patients who have a high burden of sinonasal polyps, sinus surgery can result in a marked reduction of polyps with a consequent improvement in nasal obstruction and quality of life.[58] Although patients who have sinonasal polyps often have associated anatomic abnormalities and thinning of their skull base, which places them at increased intraoperative risk, advances in endoscopic and computer navigation technology, powered instrumentation, and increasingly effective anesthesia have all combined to make surgery in these patients relatively safe. In the few polyp patients who do suffer anterior skull base trauma, the more common site is the anterior aspect of the ethmoid roof just posterior to the frontal recess, and not the lateral lamella of the cribriform plate as may be commonly expected.[59]

Several studies have documented the efficacy of endoscopic sinus surgery for sinonasal polyposis. One study by Batra and colleagues[60] recorded marked improvement in sinonasal symptomotology in patients with nasal polyps and asthma who underwent FESS. Another paper with a mean follow-up period of 5 years found improved functional outcomes in polyp patients who underwent sinus surgery with improvement in nasal obstruction, rhinorrhea, facial pain, and anosmia.[61] Multiple other studies have been published with similar findings supportive of the efficacy of endoscopic sinus surgery as an effective means for the treatment of symptoms secondary to sinonasal polyposis.[62,63]

Most sinus surgery for nasal polyposis involves standard, as well as powered endonasal instrumentation, for polyp removal and "nasalization" of the sinuses. Over the years, several "novel" tools have been applied to the removal of sinonasal polyps. One such tool, the KTP laser, was reported to be very effective in the surgical management of recurrent nasal polyps.[64] Other clinicians have also focused on the role of KTP laser in the management of recurrent polyps. Dr. Howard Levine reported an 81% success rate in a series of 52 patients treated with KTP laser in the face of recurrent polyposis.[65] Others have reported success with the Nd:YAG laser for the treatment of small polyps. Described advantages of laser use in the surgical management of sinus and nasal polyps include improved hemostasis capabilities and flexible operating modes. Although this technology seems appealing, there is currently no compelling data to support its use for polyp management.

Other tools have also been suggested as a means to surgically remove polyps with improved hemostasis. Coblation surgery in particular has been described as "associated with a statistically significant lower estimated blood loss and blood loss per minute when compared with traditional microdebridement technique."[66] These results are preliminary and will require future studies for validation. Balloon technology has been introduced as a minimally invasive means for the treatment of sinonasal disease. It should be noted that because the balloon does not remove tissue or bone but rather enlarges existing ostia, it has not been deemed an effective tool for the treatment of sinonasal polyps.

COMBINED TREATMENT OF POLYPS

Although multiple studies have shown the utility of sinus surgery for patients who have nasal polyposis, it should not be thought of as a panacea but rather as a method to start to manage patients with an excessive polyp burden because the surgically excised polyps will inevitably recur without aggressive medical management. Deal and Kountakis[30] demonstrated an association between the presence of nasal polyposis and an increased need for revision surgery. Wynn and Har-El[67] also showed significantly higher rates of recurrent surgery in patients with nasal polyposis than those without polyps. Despite the increased rates of revision, it has been documented that patients with polyps may achieve similar improvement after sinus surgery as non-polyp patients.[68] To diminish the need for and frequency of revision surgery, patients with sinonasal polyps must be treated with an aggressive medical regimen before and after surgery. There is evidence that administration of systemic steroids in the postoperative period for patients who have polyps may have a significant impact on their postoperative course.[69] Surgery for patients who have polyps should be viewed as the first step in management of a chronic disease process that will require careful monitoring and treatment with topical and oral medications.

SUMMARY

The contemporary otolaryngologist has a variety of means to treat nasal obstruction that results from polyposis. Although the goal is create a favorable local sinonasal environment in which medical therapy can successfully keep polyps from reforming, many patients – especially those with a large polyp burden – require surgery to help them achieve this favorable environment. Fortunately, advances in the understanding of sinus anatomy and changes with polyposis, along with many available technological advancements, combine to make surgery safer, more efficient, and more complete than in the past.

REFERENCES

1. Lildholt T, Rundcrantz H, Bende M, et al. Glucocorticoid treatment for nasal polyps. The use of topical budesonide, intramuscular betamethasone, and surgical treatment. Arch Otolaryngol Head Neck Surg 1997;123:595–600.
2. Lund VJ, Mackay IS. Staging in rhinosinusitis. Rhinology 1993;31:183–4.
3. Johansson L, Akerlund A, Holmberg K, et al. Evaluation of methods for endoscopic staging of nasal polyposis. Acta Otolaryngol 2000;120:72–6.
4. Drutman J, Harnsberger H, Babbel R, et al. Sinonasal polyposis: investigation by direct coronal CT. Neuroradiology 1994;36(6):469–72.
5. Som P, Sacher M, Lawson W, et al. CT appearance distinguishing benign nasal polyps from malignancies. J Comput Assist Tomogr 1987;11(1):129–33.
6. Yazbak PA, Phillips JM, Ball PA, et al. Benign nasal polyposis presenting as an intracranial mass: case report. Surg Neurol 1991;36:380–3.
7. Bateman N, Fahy C, Woolford T. Nasal polyps: still more questions than answers. J Laryngol Otol 2003;117:1–9.
8. Larsen P, Tos M. Origin of nasal polyps: an endoscopic autopsy study. Laryngoscope 2004;114(4):710–9.
9. Settipane GA, Chafee FH. Nasal polyps in asthma and thinits: a review of 6037 patients. J Allergy Clin Immunol 1977;59:17–21.
10. Heman J, Kapiro J, Poussa T, et al. Prevalence of asthma, aspirin intolerance, nasal polyposis and chronic obstructive pulmonary disease in a population-based study. Int J Epidemiol 1999;28:717–22.
11. Larsen K, Tos M. The estimated incidence of symptomatic nasal polyps. Acta Otolaryngol 2002;122:179–82.
12. Olsen KD, Neel HB 3rd, Deremee RA, et al. Nasal manifestations of allergic granulomatosis and angiitis (Churg-Strauss syndrome). Otolaryngol Head Neck Surg 1980;88:85–9.

13. Settipane GA. Epidemiology of nasal polyps. Allergy Asthma Proc 1996;17: 231–6.
14. Rugina M, Serrano E, Klossek J, et al. Rpidemiological and clinical aspects of nasal polyposisin France; the ORLI group experience. Rhinology 2002;40(2):75–9.
15. Hadfield PJ, Rowe-Jones JM, Mackay IS. The prevalence of nasal polyps in adults with cystic fibrosis. Clin Otolaryngol 2000;25:19–22.
16. Norlander T, Westrin K, Fukami M, et al. Experimentally induced polyps in the sinus mucosa: a structural analysis of the initial stages. Laryngoscope 1996; 106(2):196–203.
17. Ramanathan M, Lee W, Spannhake E, et al. Th2 cytokines associated with chronic rhinosinusitis with polyps down-regulate the antimicrobial immune function of human sinonasal epithelial cells. Am J Rhinol 2008;22(2):115–21.
18. Ramanathan M, Lee W, Dubin M, et al. Sinonasal epithelial cell expression of toll-like receptor 9 is decreased in chronic rhinosinusitis with polyps. Am J Rhinol 2007;21(1):110–6.
19. Lane A, Truong-Tran Q, Schleimer R. Altered expression of genes associated with innate immunity and inflammation in recalcitrant rhinosinusitis with polyps. Am J Rhinol 2006;20:138–44.
20. Qiu Z, Han D, Zhang L, et al. Expression of survivin and enhanced polypogenesis in nasal polyps. Am J Rhinol 2008;22(2):106–10.
21. Kowalski M, Grzegorczyk J, Pawliczak R, et al. Decreased apoptosis and distinct profile of infiltrating cells in the nasal polyps of patients with aspirin hypersensitivity. Allergy 2002;57:493–500.
22. Meyer JE, Bartels J, Gorogh T, et al. The role of RANTES in nasal polyposis. Am J Rhinol 2005;19:15–20.
23. Olze H, Forster U, Zuberbier T, et al. Eosinophilic nasal polyps are a rich source of eotaxin, eotaxin-2 and eotaxin-3. Rhinology 2006;44:145–50.
24. Ohori J, Ushikai M, Sun D, et al. TNF-alpha upregulates VCAM-1 and NF-kappa B in fibroblasts from nasal polyps. Auris Nasus Larynx 2007;34:177–83.
25. Rudack C, Stoll W, Bachert C. Cytokines in nasal polyposis, acute and chronic sinusitis. Am J Rhinol 1998;12(6):383–8.
26. Kim T, Lee S, Lee H, et al. D2-40 immunohistochemical assessment of lymphangiogenesis in normal an dedemetous sinus mucosa and nasal polyp. Laryngoscope 2007;117:442–6.
27. Bernstein J, Kansal R. Superantigen hypothesis for the early development of chronic hyperplastic sinusitis with massive nasal polyposis. Curr Opin Otolaryngol Head Neck Surg 2005;13:39–44.
28. Cannady S, Batra P, Leahy R, et al. Signal transduction and oxidative processes in sinonasal polyposis. J Allergy Clin Immunol 2007;120(6):1346–53.
29. Lechapat-Zalcman E, Coste A, D'Ortho M, et al. Increased expression of matrix metalloproteinase-9 in nasal polyps. J Pathol 2001;193:233–41.
30. Deal T, Kountakis S. Significance of nasal polyps in chronic rhinosinusitis: symptoms and surgical outcomes. Laryngoscope 2004;114(11):1932–5.
31. Ichimura K, Shimazaki Y, Ishibashi T, et al. Effect of new macrolide roxithromycin upon nasal polyps associated with chronic sinusitis. Auris Nasus Larynx 1996;23: 48–56.
32. Baudoin T, Kalogjera L, Hat J. Capsaicin significantly reduces sinonasal polyps. Acta Otolaryngol 2000;120(2):307–11.
33. Zheng C, Wang Z, Lacroix J. Effect of intranasal treatment with capsaicin on the recurrence of polyps after polypectomy and ethmoidectomy. Acta Oto-Laryngologica 2000;120(1):62–6.

34. Zheng C, Wang Z, Lacroix J. Effect of intranasal treatment with capsaicin on polyp recurrence after polypectomy and ethmoidectomy. Lin Chuang Er Bi Yan Hou Ke Za Zhi 2000;14(8):344–6 [Chinese].
35. Passali D, Mezzedimi C, Passali G, et al. Treatment of recurrent chronic hyperplastic sinusitis with nasal polyposis. Arch Otolaryngol Head Neck Surg 2003; 129(6):656–9.
36. Helbling A, Baumann A, Hanni C, et al. Amphotericn B nasal spray has no effect on nasal polyps. J Laryngol Otol 2006;120:1023–5.
37. Nucera E, Schiavino D, Milani S, et al. Effects of lysine-acetylsalicylate (LAS) treatment in nasal polyposis: two controlled long term prospective follow up studies. Thorax 2000;55(Suppl 2):S75–8.
38. Nores J, Avan P, Bonfils P. Medical management of nasal polyposis: a study in a series of 152 consecutive patients. Rhinology 2003;41(2):97–102.
39. Tao Z, Kong Y, Xiao B, et al. Effects of corticosteroid on eosinophils and expression of transforming growth factor beta 1 in nasal polyps. J Clin Otorhinolaryngol 2003;17(8):474–5.
40. Benson M. Pathophysiological effects of glucocorticoids on nasal polyps: an update. Curr Opin Allergy Clin Immunol 2005;5(1):31–5.
41. Meagher LC, Cousin JM, Seckl JR, et al. Opposing effects of glucocorticoids on the rate of apoptosis in neutrophilic and eosinophilic granulocytes. J Immunol 1996;156(11):4422–8.
42. Saunders MW, Wheatley AH, George SJ, et al. Do corticosteroids induce apoptosis in nasal polyp inflammatory cells? In vivo and in vitro studies. Laryngoscope 1999;109(5):785–90.
43. Sumiko H, Kazuhito A, Mayumi N, et al. Induction of apoptosis in nasal polyp fibroblasts by glucocorticoids in vitro. Acta Otolaryngol 2003;123:1075–9.
44. Bolger W, Joshi A, Spear S, et al. Gene expression analysis in sinonasal polyposis before and after oral corticosteroids: a preliminary investigation. Otolaryngol Head Neck Surg 2007;137:27–33.
45. Jankowski R, Schrewelius C, Bonfils P, et al. Efficacy and tolerability of budenoside aqueous nasal spray treatment in patients with nasal polyps. Arch Otolaryngol Head Neck Surg 2001;127:447–52.
46. Penttila M, Poulsen P, Hollingworth K, et al. Dose-related efficacy and tolerability of fluticasone propionate nasal drops 400 mg once daily and twice daily in the treatment of bilateral nasal polyposis: a placebo-controlled randomised study in adult patients. Clin Exp Allergy 2000;30:94–102.
47. Kanai N, Denburg J, Jordana M, et al. Nasal polyp inflammation: effect of topical nasal steroid. Am J Respir Crit Care Med 1994;150(4):1094–100.
48. Hamilos DL, Thawley SE, Kramper MA, et al. Effect of intranasal fluticasone on cellular infiltration, endothelial adhesion molecule expression, and proinflammatory cytokine mRNA in nasal polyp disease. J Allergy Clin Immunol 1999;103: 79–87.
49. Fillici F, Passali D, Puxeddo R, et al. A randomized controlled trial showing efficacy of once daily intranasal budenoside in nasal polyposis. Rhinology 2000; 38(4):185–90.
50. Citardi M, Kuhn F. Endoscopically guided frontal sinus beclomethasone instillation for refractory fronal sinus/recess mucosal edema and polyposis. Am J Rhinol 1998;12(3):179–82.
51. Jankowski R, et al. Clinical factors influencing the eosinophil infiltration of nasal polyps. Rhinology 2002;40(4):173–8.

52. Patiar S, Reece P. Cochrane database review of oral steroids for nasal polyps. The Cochrane Collection 2007;3:1–17.
53. Hissaria P, Smith W, Wormald P, et al. Short course of systemic corticosteroids in sinonasal polyposis: a double blind randomized placebo-controleed trial with evaluate of outcome measures. J Allergy Clin Immunol 2006;118:128–33.
54. Bonfils P. Medical treatment of naso-sinus polyposis: a prospective study of 181 patients. Ann Otol Rhinol Laryngol 1998;115:202–14.
55. Lascaratos JG, Segas JV, Assimakopoulos DA. Treatment of nasal polyposis in Byzantine times. Ann Otol Rhinol Laryngol 2000;109:871–6.
56. Hawke WM, McCombe AW. How I do it: nasal polypectomy with an arthroscopic bone shaver: the Stryker "Hummer". J Otolaryngol 1995;24(1):57–9.
57. Krouse JH, Christmas DA. Powered nasal polypectomy in the office setting. Ear Nose Throat J 1996;75(9):608–10.
58. Chiu AG, Kennedy DW. Surgical management of chronic rhinosinusitis and nasal polyposis: a review of the evidence. Curr Allergy Asthma Rep 2004;4(6):486–9.
59. Grevers G. Anterior skull base trauma during endoscopic sinus surgery for nasal polyposis preferred sites for iatrogenic injuries. Rhinology 2001;39:1–4.
60. Batra P, et al. Outcome analysis of endoscopic sinus surgery in patients with nasal polyps and asthma. Laryngoscope 2003;113(10):1703–6.
61. Garrel R, Gardiner Q, Khudjadze M, et al. Endoscopic surgical treatment of sino-nasal polyposis-medium term outcomes. Rhinology 2003;41:91–6.
62. Poetker D, Mendolia-Loffredo S, Smith T. Outcomes of endoscopic sinus surgery for chronic rhinosinusitis associated with sinonasal polyposis. Am J Rhinol 2007; 21(1):84–8.
63. Toros S, Bolukbasr S, Naiboglu B, et al. Comparative outcomes of endoscopic sinus surgery in patients with chronic sinusitis and nasal polyps. Eur Arch Otorhinolaryngol 2007;264:1003–8.
64. Wang H, Wang P, Tsai Y, et al. Endoscope-assisted KTP laser sinus clear-out procedure for recurrent ethmoid polyposis. J Clin Laser Med Surg 2003;21(2): 93–8.
65. Levine H. Lasers and Nasal and Sinus Surgery: KTP/532 Laser and Nasal and Sinus Surgery. In: Levine H, Clemente M, editors. Sinus Surgery. New York: Thieme Medical Publishers; 2004.
66. Eloy J, Walker T, Casiano R, et al. Effect of Coblation Polypectomy on Estimated Blood Loss in Endoscopic Sinus Surgery: A Pilot Study. Presentation at American Rhinologic Society Fall Meeting. Chicago. September 20, 2008.
67. Wynn R, Har-El G. Recurrence rates after endoscopic sinus surgery for massive sinus polyposis. Laryngoscope 2004;114:811–3.
68. Bhattacharyya N. Influence of polyps on outcomes after endoscopic sinus surgery. Laryngoscope 2007;117:1834–8.
69. Wright E, Agrawal S. Impact of perioperative systemic steroids on surgical outcomes in patients with chronic rhinosinusitis with polyposis: evaluation with novel perioperative sinus endoscopy (POSE) scoring system. Laryngoscope 2007;117S:1–27.

Case Studies in the Surgical Management of Pediatric Nasal Airway Obstruction

Larry H. Kalish, MBBS (Hons I), MS, MMed(Clin Epi), FRACS[a], Joao F. Nogueira, MD[b],
Aldo C. Stamm, MD, PhD[b],*

KEYWORDS

- Pediatric nasal obstruction • Bacterial meningitis
- Nasal bleeding • Gradual-onset nasal obstruction
- Nasal obstruction case studies

A blocked or "stuffy" nose represents one of the most common patient complaints. The list of possible diagnoses is long. The problem can be self-limited or constant, a stand-alone concern or part of an array of symptoms. Children begin life as obligate nasal breathers and nasal obstruction in neonates can present as a dramatic airway insult. As the child ages, nasal blockage is a symptom commonly attributed to simple rhinitis or adenoid hypertrophy with little consideration given to the possibility of a significant underlying problem. This article presents two cases that highlight the consequences of a delayed diagnosis and the complexities of managing obstructed lesions in children.

CASE REPORT 1: 21-MONTH-OLD FEMALE WITH BACTERIAL MENINGITIS

A 21-month-old female patient presented to a community hospital with a bacterial meningitis. She had mild hypertelorism and a stuffy nose attributed to a cleft soft palate. After appropriate medical intervention, the patient was discharged home without further assessment of her nasal stuffiness. She was then readmitted within a few weeks with a recurrence of her meningitis. After resolution of the second episode, a CT scan was performed that demonstrated a skull-base defect in the region of the planum sphenoidale. An MRI was performed and showed an encephalocele originating from the third ventricle protruding through the skull base into the posterior nasal space abutting the back of the septum (**Fig. 1**). The patient was then transferred to Edmundo Vasconcelos Hospital in Brazil for definitive management.

[a] Department of Otorhinolaryngology, Concord Hospital, Sydney, NSW Australia
[b] Department of Otorhinolaryngology, Edmundo Vasconcelos Hospital, Sao Paulo ENT Center, Rua Afonso Braz 525 Cj 13 045-11011 São Paulo SP, Brazil
* Corresponding author.
E-mail address: cof@centrodeorl.com.br (A.C. Stamm).

Otolaryngol Clin N Am 42 (2009) 387–398
doi:10.1016/j.otc.2009.01.007
0030-6665/09/$ – see front matter © 2009 Elsevier Inc. All rights reserved.

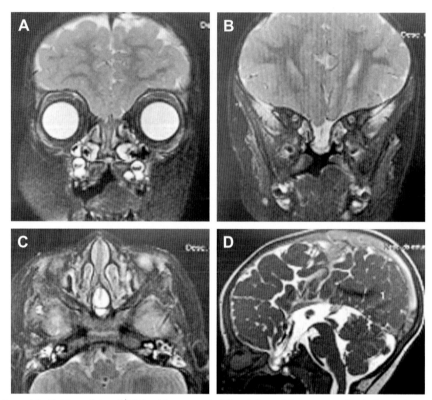

Fig. 1. (A, B) T2-weighted MRI with coronal, (C) axial, and (D) parasagittal views demonstrating the meningoencephalocele originating from the third ventricle protruding through the skull base into the posterior nasal space abutting the back of the septum.

Preoperative Considerations

The presentation of a child with a midline defect, such as a cleft palate and hypertelorism, should alert the clinician to the possibility of other midline defects[1] and prompt the investigation of "trivial" complaints, such as a stuffy or blocked nose. Aberrant embryogenesis leads to three main types of anomalies: nasal dermoid, anterior encephalocele, and a nasal glioma. Each may present in a similar manner, including with nasal obstruction. The optimal timing for surgical repair of congenital skull-base defects has not been definitively determined with consideration given to the risks and benefits for each patient. In the case of an encephalocele, intact mucosal membrane and dura separating the intracranial contents from the nasal cavity may not always be adequate to prevent meningitis, although the risk for meningitis in the absence of a cerebrospinal fluid (CSF) leak has been reported as low for the first 5 years of life and it may be safe to delay definitive surgical repair until the child is of sufficient size to make endoscopic repair feasible (typically age 2–3 years).[2,3] Actively leaking defects should be repaired earlier if possible, because the risk of meningitis in the presence of dural and mucosal defects is probably higher. The presentation in this case, with recurrent meningitis and the associated midline defects, prompted us to choose a more definitive surgical approach. It has also been suggested that a child with a sincipital or basal defect and mild hypertelorism should have the encephalocele treated in early childhood to allow the facial skeleton to remodel with growth.[4]

However, in this case, the encephalocele was situated in a posterior and completely intranasal position, the hypertelorism was not likely related directly to the intranasal mass, and the encephalocele was unlikely to affect facial growth.

The position and size of the mass need to be considered preoperatively. In this case, although the mass was relatively small, it was in a nonfavorable position, arising from the ethmoid roof in the midline with an intact non-displaced septum and inferior turbinates. Often, large intranasal masses displace the septum and turbinates, making access easier. Basal encephaloceles may harbor vital herniated structures. This makes it important to consult with a neurologist/neurosurgeon before surgery to make every effort to preserve tissue during repair. Any element of hydrocephalus should be dealt with first, followed by an elective single-stage endoscopic repair.[5]

Surgical Technique

The surgery was performed under general anesthesia, with the patient positioned with 30° head elevation. An image-guidance system was set up and used during the surgery. The nose was prepared with topical vasoconstriction using 1:1000 adrenalin-soaked neuropatties for 10 minutes and then the anterior part of the nasal septum was infiltrated with xylocaine and adrenaline (1:100,000). A traditional 4-mm, 0° nasal endoscope was used for the majority of the procedure to optimize the visual fields. Smaller 2.7-mm endoscopes are avoided unless anatomic constraints prevent use of the wider endoscopes. Access was gained through a hemi-transfixion incision on the right side of the nasal septum and the mucosa was raised along a subperichondrial and subperiosteal plane to the back of the septum. Superior and inferior parallel releasing incisions were then made along the maxillary crest and superior septum toward the posterior choanae and sphenoid ostium respectively, creating a long vascularized mucosal flap pedicled on the sphenopalatine artery. A similar flap was created on the left side, although this was not extended as far anteriorly, thus preserving the mucosa over the caudal septum. To maximize access and working space, the middle turbinate on the right side was resected. The mucosa was preserved in case additional free mucosal grafts were required to close any skull-base defects. Nasal septal cartilage was removed, preserving an appropriate caudal strut for tip support, and saved for possible use in the reconstruction of the skull-base defect.

To make use of all possible avenues, we passed a nasoendoscope through the cleft palate as an alternative way of visualizing the mass in the posterior nasal cavity as the lesion was situated at the posterior part of the nasal septum. We used special pediatric instruments, such as pediatric dissectors, aspirators, sickle knifes, and small Kerrison punches.

The meningoencephalocele was identified and resected from the nasal floor up to the skull base using bipolar cautery (**Fig. 2**). The abnormal herniation of the meninges and brain was carefully repositioned.

The bony skull base had a V- or funnel-shaped defect (**Fig. 3**). This did not support a cartilage graft to hold the meningoencephalocele. So, instead we used fascia lata for an intracranial support and the two sphenopalatine artery septal vascularized flaps were laid over the defect (**Fig. 4**). Fibrin glue was placed principally around the edges of the flap (**Fig. 5**) and then Gelfoam was placed over the reconstruction, completely covering it to prevent the dressing or catheter from accidentally pulling on the graft when removed. A Foley catheter was inserted and inflated to keep the nasal packing in place. A lumbar drainage catheter was inserted at the start of the procedure and kept in situ postoperatively.

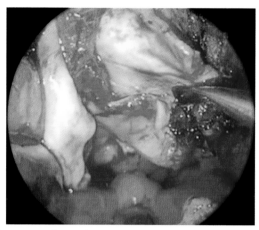

Fig. 2. Bipolar diathermy, used to reduce the meningocele, exposed the edges of the defect (covered by neuropathies). The meningocele is clearly demonstrated at the end of the suction tube.

After the procedure, the child was sedated for 2 days to facilitate the use of the nasal packing. Antibiotics were given to the patient before the procedure and for 10 days after the surgery.

On the third postoperative day, the Foley catheter was removed and all sedation ceased. There were no signs of a CSF leak. The child was discharged from the hospital with no signs of CSF leak or infection on the sixth postoperative day.

One minor complication postoperatively was a representation with nasal obstruction. Again a broad differential needs to be considered, including such postoperative complications as bleeding with resulting clot, crusting, recurrence of the encephalocele, septal hematoma or collection, mucosal congestion, and synechiae. In this case, nasal obstruction was due to the Gelfoam, which slipped back into the nasal cavity, obstructing airflow but not causing respiratory distress. This was removed under vision in the clinic and no other problems were encountered.

During follow-up each week, the nasal area was examined and suctioned in the clinic. These nasal toilets were performed with great care to avoid causing any undue stress to the patient. Imaging studies were performed 30 days after the procedure.

There was no evidence of recurrence, any complications, or CSF leaks.

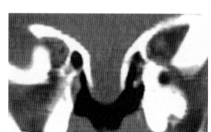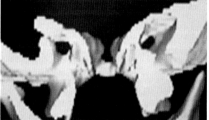

Fig. 3. Coronal CT scan and three-dimensional reconstruction demonstrating the funnel-shaped skull-base defect.

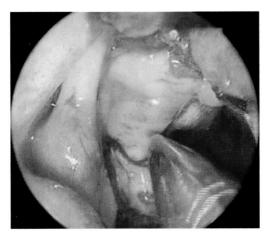

Fig. 4. Vascularized flap seen rotated over the previously demonstrated defect.

Discussion

Transnasal endoscopic techniques can now be performed relatively safely in fairly young children for the treatment of complex pathology, such as choanal atresia, orbital cellulitis, and meningoencephaloceles.[2,6–8] However, pediatric patients require meticulous preparation, specialized instrumentation, and specialized staff involved in their perioperative care. The two main challenges in this case were access and closure. For access, we used a binostril technique and made use of the septal cleft to maximize exposure. To ensure adequate skull-base closure, we used nasal septum flaps pedicled at the sphenopalatine artery. These vascularized flaps receive direct blood supply from the sphenopalatine artery, making them much more robust as grafts than alternative graft sources in the closure of skull-base defects. In adults, the use of these flaps is almost routine in skull-base surgeries performed at many medical centers;[9,10] however, their use has not been well described in pediatric patients. The creation of the flaps bilaterally not only allowed for plenty of tissue to cover the skull-base defect but also facilitated access.

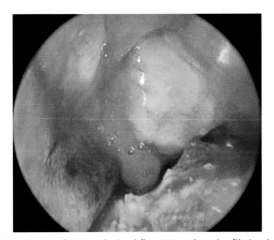

Fig. 5. Fibrin glue is seen over the vascularized flap. Note that the fibrin glue is concentrated around the edges of the flap with minimal glue over the center of the flap.

Potential flap complications include mucoceles, synechia, infection, and failure, such as failure stemming from retraction of the graft over time, especially in anterior-based defects.

Another point to consider is the nasal packing. There are few nasal packs specially designed for pediatric patients. We try to minimize the use of packing. We used Gelfoam soaked in antibiotics in the nasal cavity to protect the graft from additional packing and offer some support. Although this is generally a safe and reliable option, the displacement of the packing postoperatively demonstrates a potential complication, such as the nasal obstruction seen in this case. Rarely it can pose a greater risk, such as aspiration of the packing material. Part of the reason a Foley catheter was inserted was not only to support the grafts, but also to prevent the displacement of the packing into the nasopharynx. Specific to this patient was the cleft soft palate, which allowed for improved access during the case. However, postoperatively the cleft palate did not provide any support for the packing, which probably made displacement more likely.

There is no consensus in the literature for the length of time nasal packing should remain in place. A balance between needing to keep the patient sedated to tolerate the packs and removing the packs too soon needs to be considered. We removed the Foley catheter balloon 2 days after the surgery, but the absorbable material was left in place to be resorbed or washed out.

A multidisciplinary team is also fundamental to a good outcome. The team managing this patient was made up of a pediatrician, a pediatric anesthesiologist, an otolaryngologist, a neurosurgeon, an intensive care pediatrician, and a radiologist, who were all instrumental in the success.

CASE 2: 14-YEAR-OLD MALE WITH NASAL BLEEDING AND ONSET NASAL OBSTRUCTION

A 14-year-old male presented with repetitive episodes of minor nasal bleeding and a gradual onset nasal obstruction over 3 years. Initially, the nasal obstruction was intermittent and fluctuated from side to side, but then the nasal obstruction became more persistent on the left side. The bleeding was considered minor and he underwent chemical cauterization with trichloroacetic acid 70% on several occasions. He also had a number of left middle-ear infections over the last year. Eventually he presented with poor nasal airflow interfering with his sporting activity. An endoscopy was performed, which demonstrated a purplish nasal mass occluding the posterior nasal cavity (**Fig. 6**). There were no orbital or visual changes, cranial nerve function was normal, and the only positive finding on examination was in the left middle-ear.

In a younger child, such as the child discussed in case 1, the top differential diagnoses include a glioma, dermoid, encephalocele, or a dacryocystocele. In an older child, especially a male, then a juvenile nasopharyngeal angiofibroma (JNA) must feature high on the differential list. There are other possible diagnoses. If the mass exhibits rapid growth or malignant potential, possible diagnoses include hemangioma, a lymphoma, craniopharyngioma, and rhabdomyosarcoma. If the mass arises from the posterior nasopharynx, then possible diagnoses include a Rathke's pouch or Thornwaldt's cyst. See **Box 1** for summary.

A CT scan and an MRI scan were performed demonstrating a posterior nasal mass with some sphenopalatine fossa widening and extension into the sphenoid, confirming a clinical diagnosis of a JNA (**Figs. 7–9**). This diagnosis should always be clinical as biopsy of the lesion can have catastrophic outcomes and should never even be contemplated if a JNA is in the differential diagnosis.

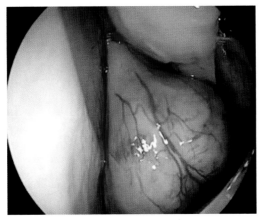

Fig. 6. The polypoid mass in the left posterior nasal passage is only evident with an endoscope. Note how the mass can be easily mistaken for an inflammatory mass or even normal anatomy.

Preoperative Considerations

We elected to resect the JNA endoscopically after an embolization had been performed. Increasing evidence shows that, with improvements in endoscopic techniques and perioperative care, the endoscopic approach, assisted by preoperative embolization, leads to less intraoperative blood loss, a shorter surgical procedure, a shorter length of hospital stay, and fewer complications, compared with the conventional techniques.[11–14] There is also a suggestion of potentially lower recurrence rate with the

---

Box 1
Differential diagnosis for mass causing pediatric nasal obstruction

Young child (∼2–8 years)

    Glioma

    Dermoid

    Encephalocele

    Dacryocystocele

Older child, especially if male (∼10 years through early teens)

    JNA[a][1]

    Hemangioma

    Lymphoma

    Craniopharyngioma

    Rhabdomyosarcoma

    Rathke's pouch

    Thornwaldt's cyst

[1] Confirm diagnosis with CT or MRI
[a] Do not biopsy if JNA is in the differential diagnosis. Outcome can be catastrophic.

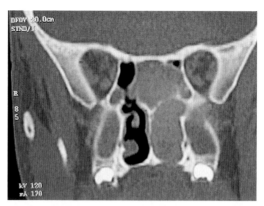

Fig. 7. Coronal bony window CT scan demonstrating the mass completely obstructing the left posterior nasal cavity with erosion through the floor of the sphenoid.

endoscopic procedure even after accounting for selection biases in studies. This lower rate is attributed to meticulous removal of the angiofibroma infiltrating the pterygoid canal and basisphenoid, which is better attained with endoscopic approaches.[15] Preoperative embolization has been shown to reduce intraoperative blood loss[16] but can have rare but potentially devastating side effects, such as thromboembolic events,[17] and needs to be performed within 72 hours of the surgery. Studies have reported comparable outcomes without embolization. No randomized trials have been performed examining the issue of whether the decision to use embolization is linked to preferences among surgeons or institutions, rather than diagnostic findings.[18–20] Embolization may fail for many reasons, such as if the contralateral external carotid or either internal carotid systems supplies blood to the tumor. It is our experience that, in cases where the embolization was performed no more than 48 hours before the resection, surgical conditions are optimal if preoperative angiography demonstrates greater than 90% to 95% devascularization of the tumor.

Surgical Technique

As in case study 1, the surgery was performed under general anesthesia, with the patient positioned supine, with 30° head elevation. The nose was prepared with

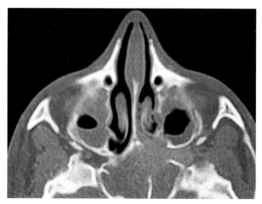

Fig. 8. Axial bony window CT scan demonstrating widening of the sphenopalatine fossa and extension into the sphenoid.

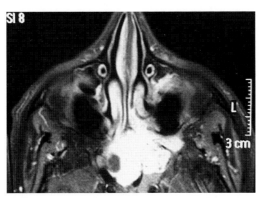

Fig. 9. T1-weighted MRI with gadolinium demonstrating the vascularized mass extending into the pterygopalatine fossa.

topical vasoconstriction using 1:1000 adrenalin-soaked neuropatties for 10 minutes. Then the anterior part of the nasal septum was infiltrated with xylocaine and adrenaline (1:100,000).

The initial approach involved a complete left uncinectomy and wide maxillary antrostomy, exposing the entire posterior wall of the maxillary sinus. This was followed by an anterior and posterior ethmoidectomy and opening of the sphenoid sinus with removal of the ipsilateral middle turbinate to maximize tumor exposure. The posterior wall of the maxillary sinus was then removed using a Kerrison punch and high-speed diamond drill, exposing the maxillary artery, which was coagulated and clipped at this point. The tumor was dissected by entering a submucosal subperiosteal plane and lifted away from the underlying bony margins. Minor bleeding was controlled with bipolar and monopolar diathermy and bony bleeding with a diamond drill. The infraorbital nerve was identified and preserved and the tumor completely isolated (**Fig. 10**). The most difficult part of the tumor removal was its nasopharyngeal attachment, which was removed with suction dissectors and monopolar diathermy. After complete tumor dissection, the mass was too large to be removed via the nostril, so it was delivered into the oral cavity and removed through the mouth. Hemostasis was achieved and the septum was left intact throughout the case. The operative site was covered with Spongostan and a Merocel pack was left in situ for 48 hours. After removal of the pack, nasal airflow was excellent and no further bleeding occurred. The patient made an unremarkable recovery with minimal complaints other than some minor nasal obstruction secondary to nasal crusting. This resolved by the second week postoperatively. There were no other concerns and the patient remains recurrence-free.

Discussion

The prevalence of nasal obstruction in children is high. Allergic rhinitis, one of the most common causes of nasal obstruction, is prevalent in around 29% of children age 13 to 14 years, giving some indication of how common a blocked and stuffy nose can be.[21] Many doctors can be complacent in the face of a "stuffy" nose, but vigilance and a thorough nasal examination is required whenever there is asymmetry, pain, unilateral discharge, epistaxis, diploplia, a unilateral middle-ear effusion, or just progression in the absence of other symptoms. Any unilateral polypoid mass should be regarded as highly suspicious and the next step is always imaging to assess the vascularity of the mass, its origin, communication with the brain or orbit, and any feature that

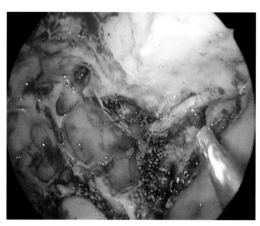

Fig. 10. Clinical photograph taken at the end of the case demonstrating the infraorbital nerve (at the end of the suction tube) and the wide surgical field postexcision.

may suggest malignancy. The classical features for a JNA include a highly vascular mass arising at the sphenopalatine fossa. This mass usually—but not always—results in widening of the fossa. There may be anterior displacement if the posterior maxillary wall, often referred to as the Holman Miller sign, and widening of the pterygomaxillary and the superior orbital fissures may be evident. There is no role for in office biopsy even if the diagnosis is uncertain and the mass has the appearance of an inflammatory polyp. There are various staging systems for JNA. The Radkowski classification accurately describes the clinical behavior and can be easily correlated with various surgical approaches.[22]

As discussed, the surgical treatment for JNA can be open or endoscopic with current evidence suggesting lower morbidity, reduced cost, and improved outcomes with endoscopic approaches.[11–14] Angiofibromas in the nasal cavity, with extension into the sinuses, extension into pterygopalatine fossa, and limited extension into the infratemporal fossa, can be removed endoscopically with a good success rate.[23] Even with larger tumors, which may extend laterally into the infratemporal fossa, surgeons have adapted novel endoscopic approaches to permit safe removal. A two-surgeon technique with a transeptal approach for better leverage of the tumor has facilitated the removal of more laterally displaced tumors.[24] Similarly, endoscopic removal of angiofibromas with early intracranial or intracavernous infiltration has been described in an increasing number of case reports and case series.[13,23,25,26] Large tumors can be delivered through the mouth, as in our case, or reduced in size in situ using a laser or a harmonic scalpel.[27,28]

REFERENCES

1. Giffoni SD, Cendes F, Valente M, et al. Midline facial defects with hypertelorism and low-grade astrocytoma: a previously undescribed association. Cleft Palate Craniofac J 2006;43:748–51.
2. Woodworth BA, Schlosser RJ, Faust RA, et al. Evolutions in the management of congenital intranasal skull base defects. Arch Otolaryngol Head Neck Surg 2004;130:1283–8.
3. Hoving EW, Vermeij-Keers C. Frontoethmoidal encephaloceles, a study of their pathogenesis. Pediatr Neurosurg 1997;27:246–56.

4. Macfarlane R, Rutka JT, Armstrong D, et al. Encephaloceles of the anterior cranial fossa. Pediatr Neurosurg 1995;23:148–58.
5. Hoving EW. Nasal encephaloceles. Childs Nerv Syst 2000;16:702–6.
6. Lanza DC, O'Brien DA, Kennedy DW. Endoscopic repair of cerebrospinal fluid fistulae and encephaloceles. Laryngoscope 1996;106:1119–25.
7. Marshall AH, Jones NS, Robertson IJ. Endoscopic management of basal encephaloceles. J Laryngol Otol 2001;115:545–7.
8. Kanowitz SJ, Bernstein JM. Pediatric meningoencephaloceles and nasal obstruction: a case for endoscopic repair. Int J Pediatr Otorhinolaryngol 2006;70:2087–92.
9. Hadad G, Bassagasteguy L, Carrau RL, et al. A novel reconstructive technique after endoscopic expanded endonasal approaches: vascular pedicle nasoseptal flap. Laryngoscope 2006;116:1882–6.
10. Stamm AC, Pignatari S, Vellutini E, et al. A novel approach allowing binostril work to the sphenoid sinus. Otolaryngol Head Neck Surg 2008;138:531–2.
11. Yiotakis I, Eleftheriadou A, Davilis D, et al. Juvenile nasopharyngeal angiofibroma stages I and II: a comparative study of surgical approaches. Int J Pediatr Otorhinolaryngol 2008;72:793–800.
12. Hofmann T, Bernal-Sprekelsen M, Koele W, et al. Endoscopic resection of juvenile angiofibromas—long term results. Rhinology 2005;43:282–9.
13. Onerci TM, Yucel OT, Ogretmenoglu O. Endoscopic surgery in treatment of juvenile nasopharyngeal angiofibroma. Int J Pediatr Otorhinolaryngol 2003;67:1219–25.
14. Pryor SG, Moore EJ, Kasperbauer JL. Endoscopic versus traditional approaches for excision of juvenile nasopharyngeal angiofibroma. Laryngoscope 2005;115:1201–7.
15. Howard DJ, Lloyd G, Lund V. Recurrence and its avoidance in juvenile angiofibroma. Laryngoscope 2001;111:1509–11.
16. Glad H, Vainer B, Buchwald C, et al. Juvenile nasopharyngeal angiofibromas in Denmark 1981–2003: diagnosis, incidence, and treatment. Acta Otolaryngol 2007;127:292–9.
17. Onerci M, Gumus K, Cil B, et al. A rare complication of embolization in juvenile nasopharyngeal angiofibroma. Int J Pediatr Otorhinolaryngol 2005;69:423–8.
18. Fonseca AS, Vinhaes E, Boaventura V, et al. Surgical treatment of non-embolized patients with nasoangiofibroma. Braz J Otorhinolaryngol 2008;74:583–7.
19. Borghei P, Baradaranfar MH, Borghei SH, et al. Transnasal endoscopic resection of juvenile nasopharyngeal angiofibroma without preoperative embolization. Ear Nose Throat J 2006;85:740–3, 746.
20. Andrade NA, Pinto JA, Nobrega Mde O, et al. Exclusively endoscopic surgery for juvenile nasopharyngeal angiofibroma. Otolaryngol Head Neck Surg 2007;137:492–6.
21. Asher MI, Montefort S, Bjorksten B, et al. Worldwide time trends in the prevalence of symptoms of asthma, allergic rhinoconjunctivitis, and eczema in childhood: ISAAC Phases One and Three Repeat Multicountry Cross-sectional Surveys. Lancet 2006;368:733–43.
22. Radkowski D, McGill T, Healy GB, et al. Changes in staging and treatment. Arch Otolaryngol Head Neck Surg 1996;122:122–9.
23. Wormald PJ, Van Hasselt A. Endoscopic removal of juvenile angiofibromas. Otolaryngol Head Neck Surg 2003;129:684–91.
24. Robinson S, Patel N, Wormald PJ. Endoscopic management of benign tumors extending into the infratemporal fossa: a two-surgeon transnasal approach. Laryngoscope 2005;115:1818–22.

25. Nicolai P, Berlucchi M, Tomenzoli D, et al. Endoscopic surgery for juvenile angiofibroma: when and how. Laryngoscope 2003;113:775–82.

26. Roger G, Tran Ba Huy P, Froehlich P, et al. Exclusively endoscopic removal of juvenile nasopharyngeal angiofibroma: trends and limits. Arch Otolaryngol Head Neck Surg 2002;128:928–35.

27. Mair EA, Battiata A, Casler JD. Endoscopic laser-assisted excision of juvenile nasopharyngeal angiofibromas. Arch Otolaryngol Head Neck Surg 2003;129: 454–9.

28. Chen MK, Tsai YL, Lee KW, et al. Strictly endoscopic and harmonic scalpel–assisted surgery of nasopharyngeal angiofibromas: eligible for advanced stage tumors. Acta Otolaryngol 2006;126:1321–5.

Case Studies in the Surgical Management of Nasal Airway Obstruction

Adam M. Becker, MD, Stilianos E. Kountakis, MD, PhD, FACS*

KEYWORDS

- Nasal • Nasal obstruction • Encephalocele
- Pleomorphic adenoma • Epistaxis • Nasal mass

Nasal obstruction is one of the most common complaints evaluated by the otolaryngologist. In addition to being an important risk factor for obstructive sleep apnea, nasal obstruction is associated with such extranasal symptoms as headache, fatigue, sleep disturbance, and daytime somnolence, and contributes to overall diminished health and quality of life.[1–3] The differential diagnosis is extensive, ranging from anatomic malformation to unusual but life-threatening disease states. Patients often suffer from a combination of etiologies, further confounding the clinician's ability to establish a diagnosis. Treatment planning therefore depends on careful history-taking; detailed physical examination, including nasal endoscopy; and the appropriate use of sinonasal imaging. Medical therapy focuses on treatment of the underlying mucosal disease, whereas surgical intervention is directed towards the areas of anatomic obstruction. In this discussion, we present two unusual cases of nasal obstruction.

CASE 1: 31-YEAR-OLD WITH NASAL OBSTRUCTION AND EPISTAXIS

A 31-year-old female presented with a 2-month history of nasal obstruction, swelling along the right nasal dorsum, and intermittent, self-limited epistaxis. Her sense of smell was unaltered, and there was no associated discomfort.

On physical examination, the patient was found to have fullness along the right nasal dorsum and a submucosal mass obstructing the right nasal cavity and displacing the nasal septum to the left.

Rigid nasal endoscopy was performed, demonstrating a mass originating from the right nasal septum and abutting the right lateral nasal wall with no overt invasion.

Department of Otolaryngology–Head and Neck Surgery, Medical College of Georgia, 1120 Fifteenth Street, Augusta, GA 30912-4060, USA
* Corresponding author.
E-mail address: skountakis@mcg.edu (S.E. Kountakis).

Otolaryngol Clin N Am 42 (2009) 399–404
doi:10.1016/j.otc.2009.01.003
0030-6665/09/$ – see front matter © 2009 Elsevier Inc. All rights reserved.

oto.theclinics.com

MRI revealed a well-circumscribed soft tissue mass measuring 1.0 × 0.7 cm (**Fig. 1**). The mass originated from the right nasal septum and extended to the right lateral nasal wall with remodeling of the nasal process of the maxilla. No bone erosion was seen and the septum appeared intact.

A biopsy was obtained and it was consistent with a pleomorphic adenoma. The patient underwent an endoscopic wide local excision of the mass with resection of septal perichondrium as the deep margin. Final pathology showed that all margins were negative and the patient is without evidence of disease at 12-month follow-up (**Fig. 2**).

Although the majority of pleomorphic adenomas are found in the major salivary glands, many examples of intranasal benign mixed tumors have been documented and described. One of the largest series to date was an analysis of more than 10,000 salivary gland tumors by Compango and Wong.[4] In their review, 40 patients with nasal pleomorphic adenoma were identified. The vast majority of tumors (90%) originated from the nasal septum. Other sites included the lateral nasal wall and nasopharynx. The majority of tumors were noted in the third to sixth decades of life and, although these investigators did not find a disparity between male and female patients, others have reported a female predilection.[5] Nasal obstruction and epistaxis are the most common presenting symptoms. However, nasal swelling, nasal mass, epiphora, and mucopurulent rhinorrhea may also be seen. Rhinoscopy generally shows a submucosal polypoid mass, which may bleed easily.[5] CT often demonstrates a well-circumscribed mass with bony remodeling, whereas MRI typically exhibits a mass with low to intermediate signal intensity on T1-weighted images and high signal intensity on T2-weighted images.[6] In contrast to those tumors that originate within major salivary glands, intranasal pleomorphic adenomas histologically exhibit increased myoepithelial cellularity with little stromal component. Recurrence rates have been reported from 2.4% to 7.5%.

CASE 2: 44-YEAR-OLD WITH UNILATERAL NASAL OBSTRUCTION

A 44-year-old female presented with unilateral nasal obstruction without significant rhinorrhea. A detailed history revealed that she recently recovered from meningitis and had experienced a previous episode of meningitis several years before. There was no prior history of head and neck surgery or trauma. Her other medical history was significant for hypertension and seizures.

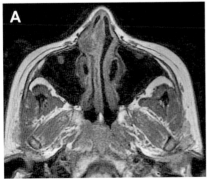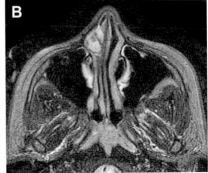

Fig. 1. MRI revealing a mass in the anterior nasal cavity arising from the septum. (A) T1 axial image. (B) T2 axial image.

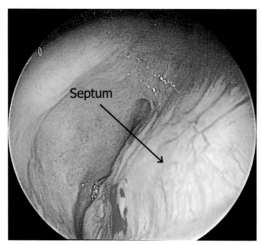

Fig. 2. Endoscopic picture 12 months postoperatively without evidence of persistent or recurrent tumor.

Physical examination demonstrated a large nasal mass lateral to the left middle turbinate extending outside the middle meatus, filling the nasal cavity (**Fig. 3**). There was no evidence of clear rhinorrhea and the mass was not pulsatile.

An MRI showed a right lateral lamella cribriform encephalocele measuring 1 × 3 cm (**Fig. 4**). CT evaluation showed a skull-base defect in continuation with the nasal mass (**Fig. 5**).

The encephalocele was approached endoscopically for resection and skull-base reconstruction. The middle turbinate was medialized and the area of the frontal recess was serially dilated with Afrin-soaked neurosurgical pledgets.

Once adequate exposure was obtained, the stalk of the encephalocele was amputated with bipolar electrocautery at the level of the skull base. Several dural veins were identified entering the meningocele and cauterized with bipolar electrocautery.

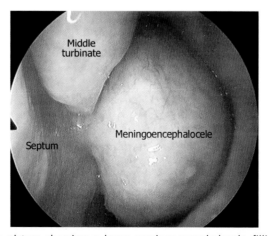

Fig. 3. Endoscopic picture showing a large meningoencephalocele filling the left nasal cavity.

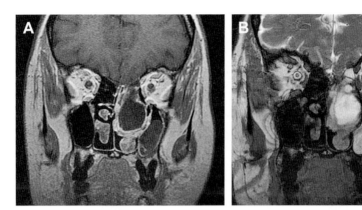

Fig. 4. MRI showing a large meningoencephalocele filling the left nasal cavity. (*A*) T1 coronal image. (*B*) T2 coronal image.

The encephalocele was then removed en bloc for pathologic evaluation. At this point, the brain was noted to be herniating through a 1-cm defect in the lateral lamella of the cribiform plate. The defect was sequentially fulgurated along its inferior aspect with bipolar electrocautery to reduce the herniation into the anterior cranial fossa. Following this, the skull base surrounding the defect was denuded in preparation for grafting.

A mucosal graft was harvested from the right middle turbinate, and the mucosal surface marked with ink to ensure proper positioning over the defect. Anterior ethmoid bone was harvested, shaped, and carefully placed into position in an underlay fashion. The mucosal graft was then placed (**Fig. 6**) and held in position with Gelfoam (Pfizer Inc., New York, New York) soaked in tissue sealant. Bioresorbable dressing was then placed to allow for additional support of the graft.

The patient did well and was discharged on the third postoperative day. As of her 2-year follow-up appointment, she has been free of recurrence or cerebrospinal fluid (CSF) leak (**Fig. 7**).

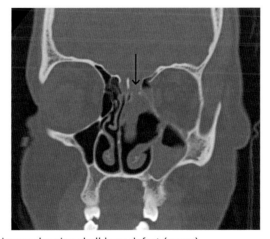

Fig. 5. CT coronal image showing skull-base defect (*arrow*).

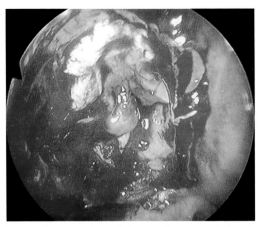

Fig. 6. Endoscopic picture after resection of the meningoencephalocele. The mucosal graft covers the skull-base defect.

Endonasal endoscopic treatment of encephaloceles is well documented. Intranasal encephaloceles are present in only 3% to 12% of patients with CSF rhinorrhea.[7-9] The etiologies are varied and include congenital, traumatic (including iatrogenic), and idiopathic causes. Congenital encephaloceles usually present early in life, although some may present in adulthood.[10] Those discovered beyond childhood are usually traumatic or spontaneous. Spontaneous intranasal encephaloceles are postulated to result from elevated CSF pressures that exert hydrostatic forces on anatomically fragile areas of the skull base and may be associated with such conditions as benign intracranial hypertension and empty sella syndrome.[8] The majority of encephaloceles occur in the lateral sphenoid sinus or the lateral cribriform plate.[7,8,11]

Serious complications of untreated symptomatic encephaloceles include meningitis and pneumocephalus. The risk of meningitis from CSF rhinorrhea is reported to be up to 40% in long-term follow-up.[7] Debate continues on how best to manage asymptomatic encephaloceles and decisions to treat are based on patient factors and surgeon preference.

Over the past 15 years, endoscopic techniques have revolutionized the management of encephaloceles and have nearly eliminated the intracranial complications

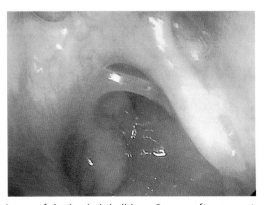

Fig. 7. Endoscopic picture of the healed skull base 2 years after reconstruction.

associated with transcranial procedures. A reduction in intracranial morbidity reduces both financial costs and the length of hospitalization. The primary complications associated with endoscopic excision of encephaloceles are those inherent to standard endoscopic sinus surgery. Excision of encephaloceles within the sphenoid sinus cavity presents the additional risk of injury to the optic nerve, the cavernous sinus, and the internal carotid artery. The transpterygoid approach to the lateral sphenoid sinus exposes the sphenopalatine ganglion to injury and subsequent xerophthalmia.[12]

SUMMARY

Nasal obstruction is a common presenting complaint to the otolaryngologist head and neck surgeon. The causes are diverse and the accurate diagnosis depends on careful history and physical examination. The management is targeted towards medical therapy to treat reversible etiologies or surgery to correct anatomic obstruction. The endonasal endoscopic approach has been used successfully for the last 15 years in the resection of nasal masses. This approach has the distinct advantage of panoramic visualization while performing surgery via a natural orifice. If needed, this approach can be combined with an external approach to increase exposure or provide access to otherwise unreachable areas, such as the frontal sinus or anterior cranial fossa.

REFERENCES

1. Udaka T, Susuki H, Fujimura T, et al. Chronic nasal obstruction causes daytime sleepiness and decreased quality of life even in the absence of snoring. Am J Rhinol 2007;21(5):564–9.
2. Udaka T, Suzuki H, Fujimura T, et al. Relationships between nasal obstruction, observed apnea, and daytime sleepiness. Otolaryngol Head Neck Surg 2007; 137(4):669–73.
3. Rhee JS, Book DT, Burzynski M, et al. Quality of life assessment in nasal airway obstruction. Laryngoscope 2003;113(7):1118–22.
4. Compagno J, Wong RT. Intranasal mixed tumors (pleomorphic adenomas): a clinicopathologic study of 40 cases. Am J Clin Pathol 1977;68(2):213–8.
5. Jackson LE, Rosenberg SI. Pleomorphic adenoma of the lateral nasal wall. Otolaryngol Head Neck Surg 2002;127(5):474–6.
6. Yiotakis I, Dinopoulou D, Ferekidis E, et al. Pleomorphic adenoma of the nose. Rhinology 2001;39(1):55–7.
7. McMains KC, Gross CW, Kountakis SE. Endoscopic management of cerebrospinal fluid rhinorrhea. Laryngoscope 2004;114(10):1833–7.
8. Schlosser RJ, Bolger WE. Management of multiple spontaneous nasal meningoencephaloceles. Laryngoscope 2002;112(6):980–5.
9. Lai SY, Kennedy DW, Bolger WE. Sphenoid encephaloceles: disease management and identification of lesions within the lateral recess of the sphenoid sinus. Laryngoscope 2002;112(10):1800–5.
10. Nishizawa S, Ohta S, Yamaguchi M. Encephalocele in the ethmoid sinus presenting as a massive intracerebral hemorrhage after a "polypectomy:" a case report. Am J Otolaryngol 2005;26(1):67–70.
11. Lanza DC, O'Brien DA, Kennedy DW. Endoscopic repair of cerebrospinal fluid fistulae and encephaloceles. Laryngoscope 1996;106(9):1119–25.
12. Bolger WE. Endoscopic transpterygoid approach to the lateral sphenoid recess: surgical approach and clinical experience. Otolaryngol Head Neck Surg 2005; 133(1):20–6.

Case Studies in the Surgical Management of Nasal Airway Obstruction

Kristin A. Seiberling, MD, Peter-John Wormald, MD, FRACS, FCS (SA)*

KEYWORDS

- Nasal airway obstruction • Septal deviation
- Meningoencephalocele • Endoscopic septoplasty
- Benign nasal tumor • Skull-base defects

This article focuses on the workup and treatment of two distinct cases of nasal obstruction. The first case has to do with a 24-year old male who presented with a brief seizure. Review of systems was positive only for longstanding right nasal obstruction. Imaging studies were consistent with a meningoencephalocele. The patient was taken to surgery for excision of the nasal mass and repair of the skull-base defect. Case two involves the treatment of a male with chronic nasal obstruction due to an S-shaped septal deviation and turbinate hypertrophy. The case illustrates the role of endoscopic septoplasty and shows how the endoscopic septoplasty technique is applied. The article also discusses the management of the enlarged turbinates.

CASE ONE: 23-YEAR-OLD MALE WITH SEIZURE

A 23-year-old previously healthy male presented to the emergency room after experiencing a brief seizure. At the time, he had no headache, photophobia, fevers, chills, or neck stiffness. Review of systems was positive only for longstanding right-sided nasal obstruction. He denied a history of sinusitis, allergies, postnasal drip, epistaxis, or congestion. Facial pain, numbness, and swelling were absent. His remaining medical history was negative. On examination, nasal endoscopy revealed a large right-sided nasal mass. The mass was purplish and appeared smooth. The septum was bowed to the opposite side without any evidence of erosion.

Preoperative Evaluation

This patient presented with a nasal mass of unclear etiology. The first step in the work-up of any nasal mass is imaging. It is imperative to obtain imaging before

Department of Otolaryngology Head and Neck Surgery, The Queen Elizabeth Hospital, 28 Woodville Road, Woodville South 5011, South Australia, Australia
* Corresponding author.
E-mail address: peter.wormald@adelaide.edu.au (P-J. Wormald).

Otolaryngol Clin N Am 42 (2009) 405–417
doi:10.1016/j.otc.2009.01.011
0030-6665/09/$ – see front matter. Crown Copyright © 2009 Published by Elsevier Inc. All rights reserved.

performing a biopsy to avoid the potential downfall of biopsying a mass that contains brain tissue or meninges. If there is concern for intracranial extension or communication, both CT and MRI are necessary and complementary imaging modalities because a CT scan of the sinuses will demonstrate any bony defects in the skull base while the MRI will more clearly define the intracranial component and cerebrospinal fluid (CSF) signal. In this patient, the CT of sinuses demonstrated a large nasal mass extending from the skull base into the right nasal cavity. On sagittal views, a skull-base defect was apparent along the right fovea (**Fig. 1**). The MRI scan demonstrated herniation of meninges through the skull-base defect into the nasal cavity (**Fig. 2**). The nasal mass was determined to be a meningocele. The patient was subsequently taken to the operating theater for endoscopic repair of the meningocele.

Preoperative Considerations

The surgeon should be prepared to repair either a small or large skull-base defect, depending on intraoperative findings. Preoperative imaging often underestimates the size of the skull-base defect. Surgical repair varies with the size of the defect. A larger skull-base defect needs a stronger repair consisting of fascia and mucosal free grafts. A smaller defect may be repaired with a fat plug and mucosal graft. Although pedicled septal mucosal flaps are not routinely used to repair these lesions, the surgeon should be prepared to use them if the defect is large enough. In addition, preoperative scans may not be able to accurately differentiate between a meningocele and meningoencephalocele. It is ultimately up to the surgeon to correctly identify during the case whether the mass contains meninges only (meningocele) or meninges with brain tissue (meningoencephalocele). This identification is critical as it may alter the choice of surgical repair of the skull-base defect as discussed below. A lumbar drain is not recommended in the case of large skull-base defects because the drain, rather than helping to seal the defect, creates a greater potential for air to be sucked intracranially. Lastly, image guidance should be available and used if necessary.

Surgical Technique

The patient was positioned in the supine position with the head of bed elevated at 30°. The nasal cavity was infiltrated with local anesthetic. Neuropatties saturated with topical cocaine (10%) mixed with normal saline and adrenaline were placed in the

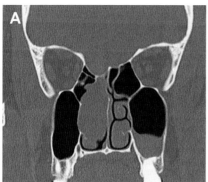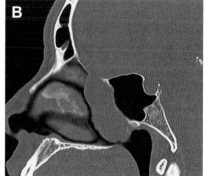

Fig. 1. (*A*) Coronal CT scan shows a large right nasal mass extending from the skull base and filling the right nasal cavity. (*B*) Sagittal scan demonstrates a defect in the skull base with extension of the mass into the nasal cavity.

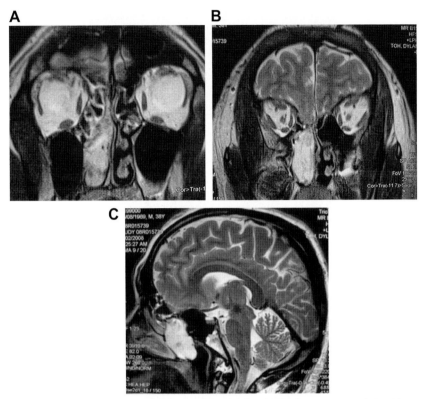

Fig. 2. (*A* and *B*) Coronal contrast-enhanced T1-weighted MRI demonstrates right-side nasal mass with intracranial communication. (*C*) Sagittal T2-weighted MRI.

nasal cavity bilaterally. The uncinate process was removed using the swinging-door technique. Next, the natural ostium of the maxillary sinus was identified and widened. This was followed by an anterior and posterior ethmoidectomy. When the sphenoethmoidal recess was entered, care was taken not to enter into the sac of the meningocele. The sac was seen extending from the skull base into the nasal cavity adjacent to the septum and middle/superior turbinate in the sphenoethmoidal recess (**Fig. 3**). The natural ostium of the sphenoid sinus was identified medial to the superior turbinate and widened in a medial and inferior direction. The anterior wall of the sphenoid sinus was removed to the level of the skull base. The remaining posterior ethmoids were opened to improve access and exposure of the skull base. The middle turbinate was removed flush with the neck of the meningocele sac at its exit from the skull base. The mucosa of the middle turbinate was saved to be used as a free mucosal graft later in the repair. The entire sac was visualized and incised to reveal its contents. When the sac was incised, both brain and meninges herniated through the opening. Half of the sac appeared to contain nonfunctional brain tissue. The sac and protruding contents were carefully debrided with a shaver until the extent of the skull-base defect could be visualized. When using the shaver, the tissue should be handled gently and every attempt should be made to identify and cauterize any vessels before debriding the tissue. This may be accomplished by using the suction in the shaver to capture the tissue before oscillating the blade. The surgeon should look at the tissue in the mouth

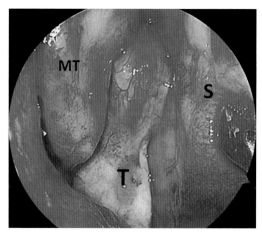

Fig. 3. The meningoencephalocele (T) can be seen extending from the skull base between the septum (S) and middle turbinate (MT).

of the blade and stop to cauterize vessels if visualized. Without this careful dissection, traumatized vessels could potentially retract intracranially and bleed. During this procedure, the surgeon should stop using the shaver as the sac gets smaller and as the shaver gets close to the skull base. At this time, the dissection should be performed meticulously with bipolar cautery. The bipolar cautery was used to effectively shrink the prolapsing brain tissue and meninges until it was flush with the skull-base defect. The mucosa around the defect was removed and the edges of the skull-base defect were freshened using a blunt probe and a sickle knife. Care was taken not to enlarge the skull-base defect while creating the ledge for the graft to be placed under. Proper closure and, ultimately, the success of the repair rely on the creation of a plane between the edges of the skull-base defect and surrounding dura. In the case of a meningoencephalocele, the prolapsed brain tissue is often found to contact the skull-base defect and to adhere to the dura around the defect. When this occurs, repair with a fat plug is not suitable because there is insufficient space intracranially to place the plug. The fat plug can be used in defects up to 1.5 cm if there is sufficient space intracranially in which to place the fat. Where there is prolapse of brain through the skull-base defect, the repair should be performed with two pieces of fascia lata covered either by a pedicled vascularized mucosal flap or free mucosal graft. Prior to placing the fascia, a malleable suction Freer elevator may be used to gently mobilize the brain tissue from the dural edges around the defect to create sufficient space to place the graft intracranially. In this case, the defect was filled with prolapsed brain tissue, so two pieces of fascia lata were harvested from the lateral thigh. The skull-base defect was measured using the tip of a 3-mm curette. A piece of fascia lata just slightly larger (by 5 mm on all sides) than the defect was fashioned. The first layer of fascia was then placed in an underlay manner between the skull-base defect and dura. The edges of the graft were smoothed out to eliminate any folds. Folds in the graft indicate that the graft is too large and may not seal the leak. A second piece of fascia was placed in an overlay fashion and finished with the free middle turbinate mucosal graft (**Fig. 4**). The layers were sealed with synthetic tissue glue and two pieces of Gelfoam. The nasal cavity was packed with gauze soaked in bismuth iodoform paraffin paste. The placement of two large layers of Gelfoam before the nasal packing helps prevent the gauze from sticking to the grafts during removal. The

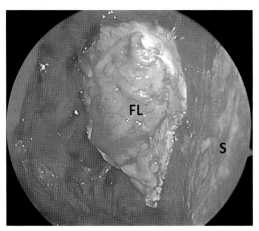

Fig. 4. The second fascia lata (FL) graft has been placed in an overlay fashion over the first fascia lata graft. S, septum.

packing was removed on postoperative day 1 and the patient was discharged from the hospital on postoperative day 2. Discharge medications included a 7-day course of broad-spectrum antibiotics and pain medication. The patient was instructed to refrain for 2 weeks from blowing his nose, lifting over 20 lb, or participating in strenuous exercise. The patient has made a full recovery without evidence of any further CSF leak.

Discussion

Intranasal meningoencephaloceles are rare with an estimated incidence of 1 per 40,000 live births.[1,2] They are characterized by a protrusion of meninges and glial tissue through a skull-base defect into the nasal cavity. They may be categorized as spontaneous (congenital or acquired) or traumatic in origin. The majority are congenital anomalies thought to arise from the failure of closure of the neural tube. Thus, most are diagnosed early in the pediatric population as either an isolated malformation or as part of a congenital anomaly. There have been few reports of intranasal meningoencephaloceles presenting in the adult population. Most adult cases are diagnosed after recurrent episodes of meningitis or in association with a CSF leak. The diagnosis is made by imaging and not biopsy. A CT scan can delineate the skull-base defect, while the MRI may demonstrate CSF within the sac, the presence of brain tissue extending into the nasal cavity, and flow voids associated with vasculature. As discussed, the preoperative images may be misleading and fail to distinguish between a meningocele and a meningoencephalocele with a 100% certainty. Neurosurgery should be consulted to advise on the safety of brain resection in the case of a meningoencephalocele. Once the diagnosis has been made, surgical planning should begin. Endoscopic repair has been successful in most cases.[3–6] The key to successful surgery is clear identification of the skull-base defect and secure placement of the graft. To provide improved access and allow for two surgeons to work simultaneously, a septal window may be created (**Fig. 5**). This facilitates the dissection and removal of larger tumors in which retraction is performed by one surgeon while the other one dissects.

As discussed previously, defects larger than 15 mm or smaller defects with brain prolapse should be repaired with two layers of fascia lata rather than the bath-plug technique. We have recently started using the Hadad pedicled mucosal flap and feel that this adds solidity to the repair. We now routinely use this flap for the repair

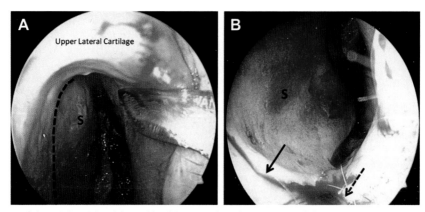

Fig. 5. (*A*) Initial incision (*dotted line*) is started at the junction of the upper lateral cartilage and the septum (*S*). (*B*) The lower incision (*solid arrow*) is carried all the way to the floor of the nose with a #15-blade scalpel (*dotted arrow*).

of larger defects.[7] We do not recommend the use of bone or cartilage in the repair as it has not been found to add stability to the skull-base repair. Rather, it adversely affects the seal by pushing the graft away from the dural edges and bony rim of the defect.

The placement of a lumbar drain in CSF leak repair is noted in the literature. However, its use is controversial, especially in the presence of a larger defect. If a lumbar drain is placed after the repair of large defects, it may increase the risk for meningitis, pneumocephalus, and even brain herniation. However, proponents of drainage state that it may decrease protrusion rates and increase adherence rates by lowering intracranial pressure and preventing CSF pressure fluctuations. In the case of meningoencephalocele, brain pulsations may lead to graft protrusion, which theoretically may be diminished with a lumbar drain.[8,9] However, many surgeons today opt not to place a lumbar drain in the case of CSF leak repair or meningoencephalocele repair. Casiano and colleagues[4,10] demonstrated a 97% successful closure rate of skull-base defects in adults without lumbar drainage. It is our preference not to place lumbar drains because the seal was solid and the drain requires specialized nursing care. A leak that occurs after the packing is removed will initially be managed with a lumbar drain. It is important that the patient have a quiet recovery from general anesthetic without coughing or straining on the endotracheal tube. To prevent such coughing or straining, our patients are extubated at a relatively deep level of anesthesia, have the tube replaced by a laryngeal mask, or have the surgery done with a laryngeal mask alone. This choice depends upon the anesthetist's preferences and level of expertise.

CASE TWO: 45-YEAR-OLD MALE WITH BILATERAL NASAL OBSTRUCTION

A 45-year-old male presented with bilateral nasal obstruction, which he said he had been experiencing for several years. He had no facial pain, pressure, anosmia, or rhinorrhea. He occasionally noticed postnasal drip, which was mild in nature. He had no history of sinusitis and denied any seasonal or perineal allergies. He had an active youth and recalled several times when his nose was hit and traumatized during sporting events. He had no significant past medical history and took no medications. His symptoms failed to improve with several courses of rhinocort and regular saline rinses. Physical examination revealed an S-shaped septal deviation starting posterior to the upper lateral cartilages and large bony spur to the right. The inferior turbinates were enlarged and boggy in appearance. Nasal endoscopy was negative for polyps, masses, or signs of chronic sinusitis.

Preoperative Considerations

This patient was a candidate for both a septoplasty and reduction of inferior turbinates with the goal to improve his nasal airway. The option of performing only a septoplasty or only a reduction was rejected because either alone would likely lead to minimal improvement of the patient's symptoms. The maximal airflow through the nasal cavity passes between the middle and inferior turbinate. Thus, enlargement of the inferior turbinate and septal deviation could both significantly compromise the airflow tract. Once the decision was made to proceed with surgery, the surgeon had to decide whether to perform the septoplasty open or endoscopically and to choose a technique for reducing the size of the inferior turbinates. For several reasons, we favored an endoscopic approach to address the deviated septum. First, the endoscopic approach makes it possible to perform the entire dissection under direct visualization. This allows the surgeon to precisely address any areas of deviation while keeping a well-stabilized dorsal-caudal strut. Second, the use of the endoscope makes it easier to see and address superior septal deflections, which are often missed when performed openly. Lastly, the use of the endoscope means that isolated septal pathology and spurs may be accurately identified and dissected free of surrounding mucosa and removed in a less traumatic manner. Success of endoscopic septoplasty relies on the use of the appropriate instrumentation (ie, suction Freer elevator, endoscope lens cleaner) and identifying the correct plane between the septum and mucoperichondrial flap. Cases where there is an extremely anterior septal deviation may be difficult to approach with an endoscope. In such cases, an open approach is preferred for the first part of the dissection.

There are many ways to address the enlarged inferior turbinate, including submucosal turbinoplasty, partial turbinectomy, diathermy, carbon dioxide laser turbinoplasty, and powered turbinoplasty. The rates for short-term efficacy, long-term efficacy, and complications vary for each technique. Our preferred method to address the inferior turbinate is by powered inferior turbinoplasty. Powered inferior turbinoplasty, by removing the soft tissue along the lateral wall and bone, preserves the medial wall of the turbinate while effectively reducing its size. With this technique, the turbinate may be reduced by 50%. This method preserves the nasal airflow receptors along the medial and superior walls of the inferior turbinate and prevents the "empty nose syndrome" commonly encountered after complete turbinectomy. In addition, removal of only the lateral surface and turbinate bone leaves a minimal amount of raw surface, therefore reducing postoperative crusting and limiting postoperative bleeding.

Surgical Technique

Septoplasty

After induction of general anesthesia, the septum was injected submucoperichondrally with lidocaine 2% and 1:80,000 adrenaline and the nose was topicalized with neuropatties soaked in a mixture of 10% cocaine, adrenaline, and lidocaine. Using a 0° endoscope, the nasal cavity and septum were reexamined without the anatomic distortion of the nasal speculum. Next, using a #15-blade scalpel, a Killian's incision was made on the left side of the septum starting high up just posterior to the leading edge of the upper lateral cartilage (see **Fig. 5**A). The incision was carried inferiorly toward the floor of the nose curving slightly posterior (see **Fig. 5**B). Using a suction Freer elevator, the mucosa was elevated off the septum moving posteriorly first before moving inferiorly toward the floor of the nose (**Fig. 6**). Subsequently the mucosa was elevated off the maxillary crest to the floor of the nose. The cartilaginous-bony junction was visualized and disarticulated (**Fig. 7**). The suction Freer elevator was used to elevate the subperichondrial flap on the opposite side in a similar manner. The inferior aspect of the cartilaginous septum was incised horizontally and this incision was carried anteriorly (**Fig. 8**). The cartilage piece was mobilized from the surrounding mucosa and removed atraumatically with a Blakesley forceps (**Fig. 9**). Next, the deviated bony septum was removed under direct visualization. This allowed for visualization of the posterior bony spur along the right maxillary crest. The subperichondrial flap was taken down to the anterior edge of the spur. The flap was next raised over the spur using the suction Freer elevator. This elevation frequently leads to a tear in the mucosal flap because of the pressure on the flap by the spur during dissection of the mucosa off the spur. It is therefore important to keep one septal flap intact to minimize the risk of a postoperative septal perforation. The spur was mobilized and removed with a straight Blakesley forceps. Finally, the anterior bend in the cartilaginous septum was addressed with relaxing incisions. A #15-blade scalpel was used to score the cartilage along its concave side. This weakens the cartilage, allowing it to relax and straighten. At the end of the septoplasty, the endoscope was placed in the nasal cavity to check for patency of the airway. The septal flaps were approximated with a quilting stitch using a 3-0 Vicryl suture on a cutting needle (**Fig. 10**). A knot at one end of the suture was made and the needle was passed from one side of the nose through the septum to the other side. This was repeated, placing the suture 1 cm anterior to its last exit point. This was carried forward to close the mucosal edges of the incision.[11] At the vestibule, the suture was tied on itself through the vestibular skin (**Fig. 11**). No septal splints were placed.

Powered turbinoplasty

First, the anterior end of the inferior turbinate was injected with lidocaine 2% and 1:80,000 (or 1:100,000) adrenaline. The posterior inferior border of the turbinate was injected using a spinal needle and the same infiltration (**Fig. 12**A). The inferior turbinate was fractured medially with a Freer elevator, creating space for instruments to be placed medially to the turbinate. Using a 0° endoscope and a straight microdebrider blade in oscillation mode, the soft tissue over the lateral aspect of the turbinate was removed leaving the bone and tissue over the medial mucosal surface intact

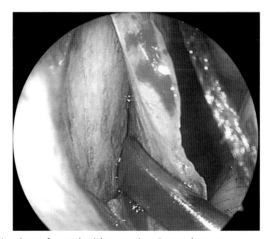

Fig. 6. Flap elevation is performed with a suction Freer elevator.

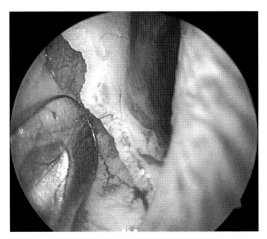

Fig. 7. The bony-cartilaginous junction is incised with a Freer elevator.

(**Figs. 12**B, C). To achieve the greatest reduction in turbinate size without compromising function, the bone of the turbinate was removed, leaving the medial wall intact. A suction Freer or dental elevator was used to mobilize the mucosa and free up the turbinate bone to be removed (**Fig. 12**D). The bone was removed with a straight Blakesley forceps. If there are any remaining small remnants of bone, these can be removed with a pediatric backbiter and small malleable probe. The residual medial mucosa was rolled upon itself covering the raw surfaces (**Fig. 13**). This step promotes optimal healing and minimizes postoperative crusting. A piece of Surgicel was placed lengthwise along the rolled turbinate to keep it in place and prevent the mucosal edges from unfolding (**Fig. 14**). No other packing was used. Postoperatively, the patient was started on saline rinses within a few hours and given a 5-day course of antibiotics. The patient was seen back in the office at 2 weeks. Then, an examination showed that the Surgicel had been absorbed and the turbinate was effectively reduced in size. The septum was midline and the mucosal incision was healing nicely. To date, the patient remains free of symptoms.

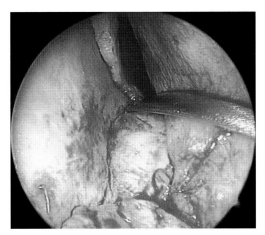

Fig. 8. A horizontal incision is made in the cartilage above the maxillary crest. This is carried anteriorly toward the caudal edge of the septum.

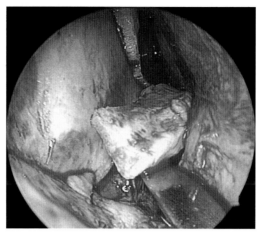

Fig. 9. The excess cartilage found inferiorly along the maxillary crest is removed.

Discussion

Endoscopic septoplasty

The case above is a typical example of a patient with a symptomatic septal deviation who has responded nicely to an endoscopic septoplasty. It is the authors' choice to perform endoscopic septoplasty on most patients presenting with nasal obstruction due to septal pathology. Several studies have shown endoscopic septoplasty to be a viable alternative to the traditional approach with a headlight, citing similar outcomes, complications, and operating room time.[12,13] The endoscope allows for more directed and precise removal of the deviated areas of the septum with improved visualization and magnification. Isolated septal pathology, such as posterior deviations or spurs, may be addressed with minimal disturbance of the remaining septum. When making the initial incision with the endoscope, there is a tendency to start the mucosal flap farther posterior than intended. A good landmark to use to avoid this

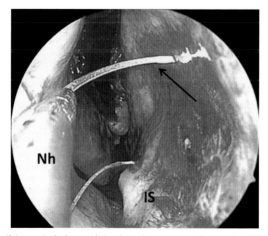

Fig. 10. A septal quilting stitch (*arrow*) is placed to secure the septal flaps. The initial stitch (IS) can be seen more posteriorly behind the needle tip. Nh, needle holder.

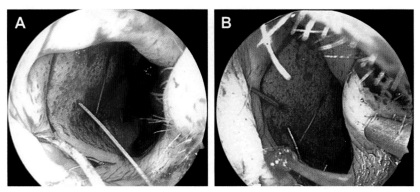

Fig. 11. (*A*) The final quilting stitch approximates and closes the incision. (*B*) The stitch is tied upon itself at the nasal vestibule.

is the curve of the upper lateral cartilage. To make the incision, the back of the scalpel blade is used to pick up the anterior edge of the upper lateral cartilage, allowing the incision to start directly behind its insertion into the septum. This incision is then brought forward almost to the mucocutaneous junction before curving posteriorly toward the maxillary crest. The key to the surgery is identification of the correct plane between the septal cartilage and mucosal flap. The correct plane is identified when

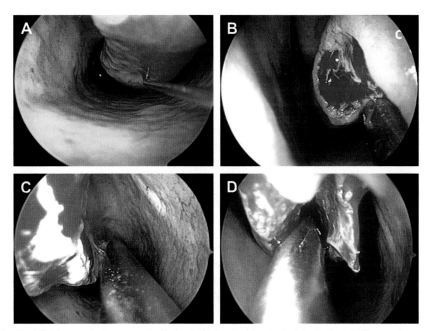

Fig. 12. (*A*) The posterior aspect of the inferior turbinate is injected with lignocaine and adrenaline. (*B*) The anterior aspect of the turbinate is shaved and the shaver blade is placed along the lateral aspect of the turbinate. (*C*) The mucosa over the lateral aspect of the turbinate is removed with a straight microdebrider blade. (*D*) The mucosa (M) over the medial aspect of the turbinate is freed up from the surrounding turbinate bone (*B*), which is removed with a through-cutting instrument.

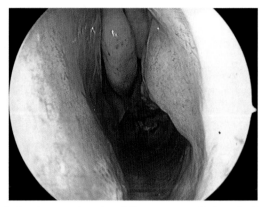

Fig. 13. The turbinate has been reduced and the mucosa rolled against the raw surface.

cartilage glistens white, without any soft tissue covering it. The mucosal flap should elevate quite easily in the correct plane and bleeding should be minimal. A suction Freer is an essential instrument for flap elevation as it allows for the correct plane to be identified and elevated in a bloodless manner. Septal cartilage anterior to the head of the middle turbinate may be removed with a Blakesley forceps in a rocking manner. Removal at this location, anterior to the cribriform plate, poses no risk of causing a CSF leak. More posteriorly, rocking motion of the upper septum should be avoided because it may lead to a fracture in the cribriform plate. The endoscope may be used at the end of the case to visualize the patency of the nasal airway. Palpation of the septum with a Freer elevator can confirm residual septal deviations and the endoscope can be reintroduced between the septal flaps to correct the defect.

Powered turbinoplasty

There are over a dozen reported ways to surgically address the hypertrophic inferior turbinate, each with its own advantages and disadvantages. Powered turbinoplasty has been shown to be successful in reducing the size of the inferior turbinate and improve patient symptoms both short and long term.[14] The authors favor this technique because it has been shown to improve symptoms without compromising

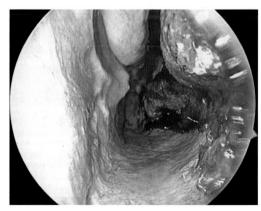

Fig. 14. A small piece of Surgicel is placed lengthwise along the turbinate.

function, has minimal complications, and has proven long-term efficacy. If the dissection is performed only on the lateral side of the turbinate, preserving the medial soft tissue and mucosa (which contains the cavernous sinuses and inferior branches of the sphenopalatine artery), the risk of intraoperative or postoperative bleeding is minimal. Diathermy is rarely needed during the case, minimizing the risk of postoperative crusting. The key to successful surgery is removal of all lateral soft tissue and mucosa and turbinate bone. This is especially important along the anterior aspect of the inferior turbinate where the nasal airway is the narrowest.

REFERENCES

1. Donnenfeld AE, Hughes H, Weiner S. Prenatal diagnosis and perinatal management of frontoethmoidal meningoencephalocele. Am J Perinatol 1988;5:51–3.
2. Smith DE, Murphy MJ, Hitchon PW, et al. Transsphenoidal encephaloceles. Surg Neurol 1983;20:471–80.
3. Wormald PJ, McDonogh M. 'Bath-plug' technique for the endoscopic management of cerebrospinal fluid leaks. J Laryngol Otol 1997;111:1042–6.
4. Senior BA, Jafri K, Benninger M. Safety and efficacy of endoscopic repair of CSF leaks and encephaloceles: a survey of the members of the American Rhinologic Society. Am J Rhinol 2001;15:21–5.
5. Kanowitz SJ, Bernstein JM. Pediatric meningoencephaloceles and nasal obstruction: a case for endoscopic repair. Int J Pediatr Otorhinolaryngol 2006;70: 2087–92.
6. Lanza DC, O'Brien DA, Kennedy DW. Endoscopic repair of cerebrospinal fluid fistulae and encephaloceles. Laryngoscope 1996;106:1119–25.
7. Hadad G, Bassagasteguy L, Carrau RL, et al. A novel reconstructive technique after endoscopic expanded endonasal approaches: vascular pedicle nasoseptal flap. Laryngoscope 2006;116:1882–6.
8. Lee TJ, Huang CC, Chuang CC, et al. Transnasal endoscopic repair of cerebrospinal fluid rhinorrhea and skull base defect: ten-year experience. Laryngoscope 2004;114:1475–81.
9. Alfieri A, Schettino R, Taborelli A, et al. Endoscopic endonasal treatment of a spontaneous temporosphenoidal encephalocele with a detachable silicone balloon. Case report. J Neurosurg 2002;97:1212–6.
10. Casiano RR, Jassir D. Endoscopic cerebrospinal fluid rhinorrhea repair: is a lumbar drain necessary? Otolaryngol Head Neck Surg 1999;121:745–50.
11. Hari C, Marnane C. Wormwald PJ. Quilting sutures for nasal septum: How we do it. J Laryng Otolol 2008;122:422–3.
12. Chung BJ, Batra PS, Citardi MJ, et al. Endoscopic septoplasty: revisitation of the technique, indications, and outcomes. Am J Rhinol 2007;21:307–11.
13. Getz AE, Hwang PH. Endoscopic septoplasty. Curr Opin Otolaryngol Head Neck Surg 2008;16:26–31.
14. Joniau S, Wong I, Rajapaksa S, et al. Long-term comparison between submucosal cauterization and powered reduction of the inferior turbinates. Laryngoscope 2006;116:1612–6.

Index

Note: Page numbers of article titles are in **boldface** type.

A

Acoustic rhinometry, in nasal obstruction, 217–218, 220–221

Airflow, intranasal, influence of functional endoscopic sinus surgery on, 237

    nasal, sensation of, 228

Airway obstruction, nasal. See *Nasal airway obstruction.*

Anosmia, and resection of middle turbinates, 305–306

B

Bony obstruction, residual, following septoplasty, 270, 271, 272–277

C

Cartilage, resection of, in pediatric septoplasty, 293

Child(ren), nasal obstruction in, factors contributing to, 289

        surgical management of, case studies in, **387–398**

    nasal septum of, anatomy of, 289–290, 291

    septoplasty in, **287–294**

    undergoing functional endoscopic sinus surgery, 236–237

Choanal atresia, and choanal stenosis, **339–352**

    bilateral obstruction in, 341

    craniofacial abnormalities in, 342

    diagnosis of, 342, 343

    embryology of, 340

    endoscopic resection in, 345–346

    genetic causes of, 341

    incidence of, 339–340

    molecular models of, 340–341

    nasal obstruction in, 201–203

    presentation of, 341–342

    retinoic acid and, 340–341

    surgery in, computer-assisted, 348

        laser-assisted, 348

        mitomycin C and, 347

        stents and, 347–348

    surgical strategies in, 343–346

    thioamides and, 341

    transnasal puncture in, 343–344

    transpalatal resection in, 344–345

    unilateral obstruction in, 342

Computer-assisted surgery, in choanal atresia, 348

Otolaryngol Clin N Am 42 (2009) 419–425

doi:10.1016/S0030-6665(09)00029-2

0030-6665/09/$ – see front matter © 2009 Elsevier Inc. All rights reserved.

oto.theclinics.com